SETON HALL UNIVERSITY
Y0-BCF-132

It has been known for many years that physical disease or damage, especially of the brain, is associated with an increased risk for psychosocial disorders. However, the understanding of the mechanisms involved in these biological risk processes, and of the marked individual differences in response, is of much more recent origin.

The role of genetic factors, perinatal brain damage, sex hormones, allergy, drugs and language disorder are among the topics reviewed by this book's expert contributors. Topics were selected to illustrate the wide range of mechanisms involved in the development of psychosocial disorders in childhood or later life. Authors were asked to write for a multidisciplinary audience, to adopt a lifespan approach, to focus on the principles involved, and to highlight the outstanding research and clinical issues in each field.

The result is a readable and highly authoritative overview of the factors responsible for a wide range of behavioural and psychological problems. It is a book that will interest practitioners and research workers in many developmental disciplines, particularly child health and paediatrics, neurology, psychology and psychiatry.

Biological risk factors for psychosocial disorders

European Network on Longitudinal Studies on Individual Development (ENLS).

The European Science Foundation (ESF) is an association of 50 research councils and scientific academies in 20 European countries. The member organizations represent all scientific disciplines – in natural sciences, in medical and biosciences, in social sciences and in humanities. One of its main modes of operation is establishing scientific networks.

In this frame the European Network on Longitudinal Studies on Individual Development (ENLS) was established. By organizing a series of workshops on substantive and methodological topics the network has brought together several hundred scientists from very different fields – criminology, developmental biology, epidemiology, pediatrics, psychiatry, psychology, sociology, statistics and others – all actively involved in longitudinal research. By distributing fellowships to young researchers and twinning grants to researchers for planning common projects and by the development and administration of an inventory covering all major longitudinal projects in Europe, longitudinal research has been further supported and stimulated.

Chairman: David Magnusson
Coordination Committee Members: Paul Baltes, Paul Casaer, Alex Kalverboer, Jostein Mykletun, Anik de Ribaupierre, Michael Rutter, Fini Schulsinger, Martti Taklo, and Bertil Törestad.

Already published

1. *Michael Rutter*, ed., Studies of psychosocial risk: The power of longitudinal data
2. *Anik de Ribaupierre*, ed., Transition mechanisms in child development: The longitudinal perspective
3. *David Magnusson and Lars R. Bergman*, eds., Data quality in longitudinal research
4. *Paul B. Baltes and Margret M. Baltes*, eds., Successful aging: Perspectives from the behavioral sciences
5. *David Magnusson, Lars R. Bergmann, Georg Rudinger and Bertil Törestad*, eds., Problems and methods in longitudinal research: Stability and change

Biological risk factors for psychosocial disorders

Edited by

MICHAEL RUTTER

Honorary Director, MRC Child Psychiatry Unit, and Professor of Child Psychiatry, University of London Institute of Psychiatry

PAUL CASAER

Head of the Division of Paediatric Neurology and of the Developmental Neurology Research Unit, Department of Paediatrics, University Hospital Gasthuisberg, Leuven; and Professor of Paediatric Neurology, Katholieke Universiteit, Leuven

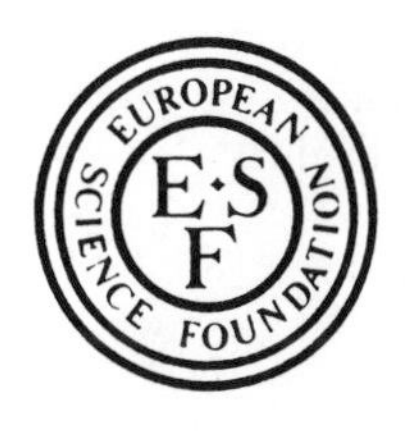

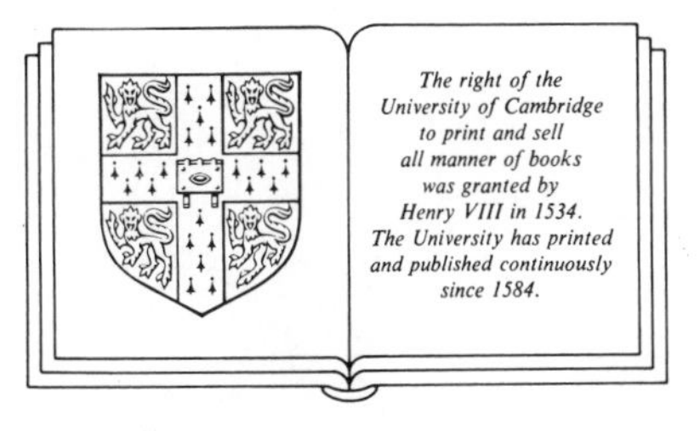

CAMBRIDGE UNIVERSITY PRESS

Cambridge

New York Port Chester Melbourne Sydney

Published by the Press Syndicate of the University of Cambridge
The Pitt Building, Trumpington Street, Cambridge CB2 1RP
40 West 20th Street, New York, NY 10011–4211 USA
10 Stamford Road, Oakleigh, Victoria 3166, Australia

First published 1991

Printed in Great Britain at the University Press, Cambridge

British Library cataloguing in publication data

Biological risk factors for psychosocial disorders.
1. Social psychology
I. Rutter, Michael II. Casaer, Paul
616.89

Library of Congress cataloguing in publication data

Biological risk factors for psychosocial disorders / edited by Michael Rutter and Paul Casaer.
p. cm.
Outgrowth of a workshop organized by the European Science Foundation Network on Longitudinal Studies on Individual Development, held in Como in Oct. 1989.
Includes index.
ISBN 0-521-40103-8 (hardback)
1. Mental illness – Risk factors – Congresses. 2. Mental illness – Etiology – Congresses. I. Rutter, Michael. II. Casaer, Paul Jules Maria. III. European Network on Longitudinal Studies on Individual Development.
[DNLM: 1. Longitudinal Studies. 2. Mental Disorders – epidemiology. 3. Mental Disorders – etiology. 4. Risk Factors.
WM 100 B61487]
RC455.4.R56B56 1991
616.89'071 – dc20 91-11007 CIP

ISBN 0 521 40103 8 hardback

UY

Contents

Principal contributors

Dr J. Bancroft
MRC Reproductive Biology Unit, Centre for Reproductive Biology, Edinburgh, UK

Professor P. Casaer
Division of Pediatric Neurology and Developmental Neurology Research Unit Department of Pediatrics and Neonatal Medicine, University Hospital Gasthuisberg, Leuven, Belgium

Mr P. Fuggle
MRC Register of Children with Congenital Hypothyroidism, Institute of Child Health, London, UK

Dr J.-F. Gadisseux
Service de Neurologie Pédiatrique, Université Catholique de Louvain, Brussels, Belgium

Dr R. Goodman
Department of Child and Adolescent Psychiatry, Institute of Psychiatry, London, UK

Professor P. Graham
Department of Child Psychiatry, Institute of Child Health, London, UK

Professor G. Lyon
Service de Neurologie Pédiatrique, Université Catholique de Louvain, Brussels, Belgium

Dr N. Marlow
Department of Child Health, Royal Hospital for Sick Children, Bristol, UK

Ms L. Mawhood
Department of Child and Adolescent Psychiatry, Institute of Psychiatry, London, UK

Professor M. E. Pembrey
Mothercare Department of Paediatric Genetics, Institute of Child Health, London, UK

Professor R. Plomin
Center for Developmental and Health Genetics, The Pennsylvania State University, USA

Dr C. Rauss-Mason
Department of Child and Adolescent Psychiatry, University of Zurich, Switzerland

Professor M. Rutter
MRC Child Psychiatry Unit, Institute of Psychiatry, London, UK

Professor H.-Ch. Steinhausen
Department of Child and Adolescent Psychiatry, University of Zurich, Switzerland

Professor D. F. Swaab
Netherlands Institute for Brain Research, Amsterdam, The Netherlands

Dr E. Taylor
MRC Child Psychiatry Unit, Institute of Psychiatry, London, UK

Dr L. de Vries
Division of Pediatric Neurology and Developmental Neurology Research Unit, Department of Pediatrics and Neonatal Medicine, University Hospital Gasthuisberg, Leuven, Belgium

Foreword

An individual functions and develops as a totality in a way that can be described as a multidetermined stochastic process. The formulation implies that many factors are involved and operate in a probabilistic, often non-linear way. The functioning of an individual is then characterized by a continuously ongoing, reciprocal interaction among perceptual-cognitive-emotional factors, biological factors in the individual and social and physical factors in the environment. This interactive process is seemingly complex and chaotic but is actually coherent and lawful. It is then a scientific challenge to identify the factors involved and the mechanisms by which they operate.

The view on individual development briefly summarized above has strong theoretical, methodological and research strategical implications. One consequence is that we have to follow the same individuals across time, i.e. to conduct longitudinal research, in order to understand the process of interaction among psychological and biological aspects of individual functioning and social and physical factors in the environment. Another essential consequence is that we have to include biological factors in the models for individual development, in order to understand and explain the total functioning of an individual and how individuals change their way of functioning over the life span as a result of maturation and experience. Without the inclusion of such factors our understanding of individual development will be limited and biased.

From this perspective a natural decision by the Coordination Committee for the European Science Foundation's Network on Longitudinal Studies on Individual Development (ENLS) was to include a workshop on biological risk factors in the series of eight workshops dealing with theoretical, methodological and research strategic issues in longitudinal research. This volume is the outcome of that workshop. The volume presented here covers an important substantive area of central interest for research on individual development.

It is my conviction and that of my colleagues in the Coordination Committee, that by including biological factors in the models for individual functioning we will be better off in understanding and explaining the intricate process of individual development. It is our hope that this volume will contribute to that direction of further research.

David Magnusson
Chairman of the ENLS Coordination Committee

Preface

This volume had its origins in a workshop organized by the European Science Foundation Network on Longitudinal Studies on Individual Development, held in Como in October 1989. The chapters owe much to the discussions during the workshop but they were prepared specifically for the book and the book does not constitute any sort of proceedings of the meeting. Particular thanks are due to the discussants at the workshop: Francesca Brambilla, Giovanni Cavazutti, Thierry Deonna, Joseph Egger, Jaak Jaeken, Josef Parnas, Sandra Scarr, Ake Seiger and Jean-Pierre Fryns. Many of their ideas and suggestions have been incorporated into chapters and, on behalf of all authors, we express our gratitude to them.

It has been appreciated for many years that somatic disease or damage, especially of the brain, is associated with an increased risk for psychosocial disorders. However, an understanding of the mechanisms involved in these biological risk processes, and of the marked individual differences in response is of much more recent origin. Authors were asked to write for a multidisciplinary audience, to adopt a lifespan approach, to focus on the principles involved, to outline the outstanding research and clinical issues and to consider the role of longitudinal studies in furthering knowledge on the psychosocial risks stemming from biological processes. For obvious reasons, there has been no attempt to review all biological risk factors, but those selected for attention were chosen to illustrate the rather diverse range of mechanisms involved. The focus is on the ways in which the psychosocial risks arise and on some of the biological features that determine heterogeneity of outcome. As individual chapters bring out, this is an exciting field in which research advances are causing a rethink on several key matters of theoretical and practical importance. The volume should be of interest to both researchers and practitioners in the fields of paediatrics, neurology, psychiatry, and psychology.

Gilles Lyon and Jean-François Gadisseux set the scene in the first chapter by considering the normal development of the brain and the functional implications of various types of structural abnormalities arising at different points in development. They draw attention to one important feature of brain development; namely, that nerve cells are formed at a considerable distance from their final location and migrate according to an inside-out spatio-temporal pattern. One consequence is that, to a considerable extent, it is possible to determine the timing of an anomaly by its location. It is also probable that, in some instances, the clinical expression of a genetic or prenatally acquired defect may become evident only long after birth at a time when the neurological substrate on which it normally acts arrives at a critical stage of development. For similar reasons Lyon and Gadisseux hypothesize that the structural basis of a cognitive function may shift locus during the course of development.

Robert Goodman takes up the same theme in suggesting that biological factors have a major aetiological role in developmental disorders but that there will often be a lack of concordance between the timing of a brain insult and the timing of its clinical manifestations. He argues that the sequelae of brain damage vary according to whether the damage is incurred during the prenatal period or early infancy, the rest of childhood, or the period after puberty. Attention is drawn to the major reorganization involved in the take-up of functions by normal areas of the brain from damaged parts, and to the negative, as well as positive, consequences, of neuronal reorganization. In interesting, paradoxical fashion, the developing brain is *both* more resilient and more vulnerable than the mature brain.

Dick Swaab points to the extensive evidence on associations between organic brain abnormalities and a wide range of psychopathological conditions in childhood and adult life. He discusses the possible relationships between neurotransmitter development and disturbed brain functioning, drawing attention to a variety of important methodological considerations. The impact of sex hormones on brain organization is also noted.

Marcus Pembrey, in the fourth chapter, provides a lively, up-to-date account of some of the most exciting developments in cytogenetics. In non-technical language, he introduces the very important consequences of the fact that chromosomes are inherited from both parents and, most especially, that it matters which parent provides which chromosome. Thus, it is now known that chromosomes are 'imprinted' during their paternal or maternal transmission; that, probably, there is DNA change during intergenerational transmission; and that one of the two X chromosomes present in each female is inactivated. It might be thought that these matters are of interest only to professional geneticists but that is not so. Thus, for example, it is now known that both Angelman's syndrome (the 'happy puppet' syndrome) and the Prader–Willi syndrome (a disorder associated with pathological over-eating) are due to abnormalities of chromosome 15; the difference is that in the former case the chromosome has a maternal origin and the latter case a paternal one.

Robert Plomin, in a thoughtful wide-ranging review of genetic influences, emphasizes the importance of genetic factors on the *development* of traits, as well as on individual differences in their final manifestation. In that connection, he notes the particular importance of the parent–offspring research design, citing the example of infant IQ. The main focus of this chapter is on the links between the normal and the abnormal and attention is drawn to the potential power of the comparison between group familiality and individual familiality. In illustration, Plomin points to the likely importance of phonological coding as the key genetic element in reading disorder.

In the sixth chapter, Paul Casaer, Linda de Vries and Neil Marlow provide an update on prenatal and perinatal risk factors for psychosocial development. They remind us that severe mental handicap is *not* mainly due to damage during the birth process but rather it derives from genetic and early prenatal causes. Also, they draw attention to the important finding that, while impairments in neonatal care have made little difference to the survival of full-term infants, they have had a big effect on the outcome for very small and very premature babies. Neuroimaging has revolutionized the field in its provision of the means of identifying which babies have brain damage but it has been even more important in showing the particular types of damage. In many ways, the most important feature of this area of research has been the observation of the raised rate of minor motor and behavioural abnormalities, including learning difficulties, in very small babies *without* obvious neurological handicaps. The chain of causal connections is not yet clear but the possibility that periventricular echodensities are associated with early transient dystonia which, in turn, is associated with later minor motor, behavioural and learning difficulties is one possibility that requires testing by systematic prospective longitudinal studies.

Peter Fuggle and Philip Graham, in their insightful discussion of metabolic/endocrine disorders, focus on the contrasts between congenital hypothyroidism (CH), phenylketonuria (PKU), and juvenile onset diabetes. They draw attention to a variety of important issues but perhaps the most crucial question concerns the difference between early and later mechanisms. It is well established that both PKU and CH, if untreated, lead to irreversible brain damage in infancy. However, it now appears that there may be more subtle late effects, operating through different mechanisms, as a result of individual variations in the degree of control over phenylalanine and thyroxine levels.

The media have provided a high level of 'hype' on the possible importance of toxins and allergens on children's behaviour. The consequence has been both an uncritical acceptance by some people of the damage stemming from dietary constituents and, by others, an unthinking dismissal of the suggestion that there are any effects. Eric Taylor acts as knowledgeable pilot in steering a careful course through these troubled waters. While discussing both extremes, and drawing attention to the range of methodological issues, he is forthright in pointing to the real, albeit small, risks that stem from toxins and allergens. Numerous issues remain to be resolved but there are definite effects that require attention.

Michael Rutter and Lynn Mawhood take a somewhat different task in their discussion of the long-term psychosocial sequelae associated with developmental disorders of language. Clinicians and researchers have appreciated for some time that children with delayed language development have an increased rate of socioemotional and behavioural problems. However, usually it has been assumed that the raised rate reflects the difficulties involved in having a language handicap – the reaction, as it were, to an impairment that interferes with normal social life. What is new is the finding that, long after language develops, psychological sequelae persist. Rutter and Mawhood discuss the variety of risk mechanisms that may be involved.

The tenth chapter by John Bancroft tackles the very important topic of the behavioural effects of sex hormones. It is well established that testosterone has effects on behaviour, but it is less widely recognized that the reverse also applies. Winning at tennis raises sex hormone levels but humiliation lowers them! John Bancroft's authoritative review summarizes a wide field of research in a manner that is readily understandable by all. Prenatal hormones have a clear organizing function on brain development in rodents and it is quite possible that something similar applies in humans but the effects are much less certain. In later life, hormonal effects on behaviour are evident but numerous questions remain to be answered. There are well-documented sex differences in psychiatric disorder but are these explicable in terms of hormonal influences? The effects of hormones are not the same in males and females but why is that so and what role do sociocultural factors play?

Hans-Christophe Steinhausen and Carol Rauss-Mason complete the specific review chapters with their careful appraisal of the psychosocial risks associated with epilepsy and treatment by anticonvulsive drugs. As they point out, the associations represent diverse mechanisms. Sometimes epilepsy is genetically determined as a specific abnormality of brain functioning and sometimes it is part of a broader neurodevelopmental disorder. In addition, the psychosocial sequelae need to be considered in terms of the stigmatizing effects of a condition that still remains frightening to the general public. Mystery remains about the possible psychosocial effects of subclinical epilepsy and of possible transient cognitive impairments associated with neurophysiological disturbances that do not give rise to overt fits or seizures. Steinhausen and Rauss-Mason provide informed guidance on these controversial, but clinically important, matters.

In editing this volume, we are acutely aware of our indebtedness to numerous people. First, and foremost, we express our gratitude to the authors, who have delivered their chapters on time and who have responded cheerfully and constructively to the variety of scientific and literary points that we have put to them. It has been a pleasure, as well as a very instructive experience, working with such a responsive and harmonious group of experts. To all of them we express our deep gratitude. Secondly, we would like to express our thanks to David Magnusson whose expert leadership of the Network played such a major role in the success of the series of workshops. Finally, the translation of manuscripts into text is heavily reliant on the skilled clerical work involved in checking references and in reviewing the clarity of expression of ideas and findings. In both tasks we are deeply indebted to Joy Maxwell and Angela Hatton for their help.

M.R.
P.C.

1 Structural abnormalities of the brain in developmental disorders

GILLES LYON AND JEAN-FRANÇOIS GADISSEUX

In this chapter we discuss the existence and nature of prenatal structural abnormalities of the brain that may underlie developmental disorders. If there is a structural basis for such disorders, morphological changes can be appreciated only on the basis of a clear understanding of the normal development of the central nervous system.

PRENATAL DEVELOPMENT OF THE BRAIN AND ITS POSSIBLE DEVIATIONS

Prenatal brain development can conveniently be divided into two periods discussed below (Table 1.1) (Evrard *et al.*, 1984; Lyon *et al.*, 1984).

First phase

The first 20 weeks of fetal life constitute a period of organogenesis, neuronogenesis and neuronal migration. The neural tube closes and the telencephalic vesicles, optic vesicles, olfactory bulbs, corpus callosum and other interhemispheric commissures are formed. Failure to achieve these events leads to some of the most common brain malformations such as a monoventricular brain (holoprosencephaly), arhinencephaly and agenesis of the corpus callosum (see Table 1.2).

A unique feature of the developing central nervous system is that nerve cells are formed at a distance from their final position. Prospective neurons are generated in the ventricular and subventricular proliferative zones and migrate to their definitive site along radial glial fibers (RGF) which extend from the ventricular ependymal lining where their cell body is situated, to the external surface of the cortical plate (Rakic, 1972; Gadisseux & Evrard, 1985; Gadisseux *et al.*, 1990).

Migrating neurons are in close contact with glial guides with which they establish specialized junctions, as *in vitro* studies have demonstrated (see Hatten, 1990). Glial-guided neuronal migration depends on the presence of various 'adhesion molecules" (Edelman, 1984; Lander,

Table 1.1. *Normal and pathological structural events during brain development*

Normal events	Pathology
Cytogenesis – histogenesis 0–20 weeks	
Neuronogenesis	Early developmental microcephalies
Neuronal migration	Disorders of neuronal migration
Regional development	Disorders of telencephalic and commissural development
Growth and maturation 20–40 weeks	
Normal events[a]	Pathology
Neuronal growth, dendritic development, synaptogenesis	Inhibition of neuronal and glial growth & maturation
Gliogenesis, periventricular and local; onset of myelination	→ late developmental microcephaly
Cerebral angiogenesis	Disorders of microvasculature development (type II lissencephaly)
Modulation of neuronal circuitry: axonal elimination, synaptic redistribution, neuronal death, development of neurotransmitters and trophic factors	Disorders of secondary modulation of neuronal circuitry Encephaloclastic brain damage

[a] Events continuing at various degrees after birth.

Table 1.2. *Main structural abnormalities of brain development*

Abnormalities of telencephalic division and formation of cerebral commissures

- *Arhinencephaly–holoprosencephaly*
  Characterized by absence of the interhemispheric commissure, undivided or fused ventricular cavities, absence of olfactory tracts (which may be detected on MRI). Various degrees.
  Frequent, possibly familial (autosomal recessive or dominant) or associated with 13/15 trisomy.
  Except for major lethal forms, moderate or severe mental retardation and evident to mild facial malformations: hypotelorism (on skull x-rays), cleft palate, choanal atresia, fused maxillary central incisors . . . Formes frustes in parents.

- *Agenesis of the corpus callosum*
  Frequent, rarely familial, possibly related to metabolic disorders. No specific clinical syndrome.

Table 1.2. (*cont.*)

Insufficiency in neuronogenesis

- *Early developmental microcephalies*
  Mostly familial, generally autosomal recessive. Usually severe mental retardation.

Disorders of neuronal migration

Rare, frequently familial, autosomal recessive or with chromosomal anomaly. Some are rapidly lethal (type II lissencephaly) or part of a progressive metabolic disorder (Zellweger's disease). Others are constantly associated with severe mental retardation. Type I lissencephaly is associated in 50% of cases with a deletion of chromosome 17.

Disorders involving excessive or insufficient cell death (?) or excessive axonal elimination

Familial hypoplasia of corpus callosum, central white matter and pyramidal tracts.

Disorders of cell growth and maturation

- *Late developmental microcephalies*
  Cause frequently unknown. Mild to moderate mental retardation, various disorders of behavior.
- *Megalencephalies*

Usually familial, various degrees of mental retardation.

Abnormalities of the cerebellar cortex

- *Cerebellar atrophy*
  Practically always associated with mental retardation, although usually no structural abnormality of the telencephalon
  —Acquired: as in fetal alcohol syndrome, hypothyroidism
  —Familial (? autosomal recessive), vermian atrophy with mental retardation and speech disorders. Normal telencephalon at autopsy.
- *Segmental hypoplasia of vermis in autistic children* (?)
- *Complex fusion of molecular layers*: *'cerebellar microgyria'*
- *Heterotopias of fetal granule cells* (*as in* 13/15 *or* 18 *trisomy*) *always with severe mental retardation even if no structural anomaly of the telencephalon.*

Encephaloclastic brain disorders in the second half of pregnancy

Causes: ischemia, hemorrhage, infection

- Polymicrogyria
- Porencephalies and hydranencephalies

? = uncertain

1989). The failure of neurons to contact glial fibers may result in their degeneration. This is, for instance, the fate of granule cells in the cerebellum of the Weaver mouse in which astrotactin, a molecule that mediates neuron–glia binding is missing (Hatten, 1990). RGF are initially grouped in fascicles and are defasciculated by ascending neurons. In the Reeler mouse, defasciculation does not occur, and this could be the cause of the migrational anomaly of this mutant (Gadisseux & Evrard, 1985). Although it has not been convincingly demonstrated, it is conceivable that a genetically controlled defect of the glio-neuronal unit may be at the origin of some human disorders. For instance, it has been suggested that degeneration of the RGF may explain the disorder of migration in Zellweger's disease (Evrard *et al.*, 1978), and a reduction of the number of glio-neuronal units could be at the origin of some extreme developmental microcephalies (see below).

In the cerebral cortex, neuronal migration proceeds according to an inside-out spatio-temporal pattern. The first cells to be formed finally occupy layer I (Cajal–Retzius cells) and layer VII (subplate) which will become the innermost layer of the mature cortex (Marin-Padilla, 1983). Neurons generated later occupy successively more superficial positions in the interval between the two primitive layers (Angevine & Sidman, 1961; Rakic, 1982): those forming layers VI and V are generated first and the last cells to migrate will constitute layer II. The reason for this extraordinary pattern of migration is unknown. One possibility is that it favors cell to cell contacts and the establishment of interneuronal connections. The relatively recent knowledge of this inside-out gradient of neuronal migration has important implications for the interpretation of developmental diseases affecting the cerebral cortex. For instance, an abnormally superficial position of the large pyramidal neurons of layer V indicates that the last neurons to be formed have failed to migrate properly (as for instance in type I lissencephaly). If in any fetal cortical defect there is preservation of a normal layer II (the last to be formed) the anomaly can only have occurred after the end of migration. This is important in establishing the chronology of some disorders as for instance microgyria, a relatively common developmental lesion responsible for mental retardation, which was initially thought to be an early migratory, possibly genetic disease and is now recognized as a late postmigratory condition, because layer II is present.

Whatever their mechanism, defects of neuronogenesis and neuronal migration result either in a marked reduction of the population of neurons (early developmental microcephalies) or in abnormalities in their final position (heterotopias) and in their tangential and radial arrangement (cortical dysplasias) (see Tables 1.1 and 1.2). Such disorders are frequently familial, either inherited as an autosomal recessive trait, or related to a chromosomal aberration (Table 1.2). The importance of the role of acquired pathogenic factors during this period is difficult to assess. It must be remembered that in the telencephalon the entire neuronal population is generated over a limited period of time extending from the fifth to the twentieth week of gestation, i.e. approximately 100 days. Therefore after 20 weeks, neuronogenesis or neuronal migration can in no way be affected by viral infections, intoxications, radiations or ischemia. The assumption that perinatal asphyxia or germinal layer hemorrhage can affect neuronal migration is not warranted.

Theoretically, the germinal matrix and migrating neurons could be the target of various diseases, such as viral infections and intoxications, but this has not been convincingly demonstrated. Concerning viruses, it has often been stated (Naeye, 1967) that brain lesions in fetal cytomegalovirus (CMV) infection are, at least in part, due to a selective involvement of the actively dividing matricial cells, which results in a defect of neuronal migration. However, examination of fetal brains with immunocytochemical methods and careful neuropathological analysis has strongly challenged this view. CMV is only rarely found in the periventricular germinative zone (Gadisseux *et al.*, 1991) and ischemia seems to be the major pathogenic factor of severe brain lesions (Marques Dias *et al.*, 1984). The rubella virus, which is known to produce non-cytopathic mitotic inhibition, could possibly act by this mechanism to restrain the process of neuronogenesis and give rise to microcephaly (Johnson, 1982). The Human Immunodeficiency Virus (HIV) is not known to give anomalies of neuronal migration or a congenital microcephaly.

Fetal alcoholism does not produce a significant abnormality of migration (except for molecular ectopias) or severe microcephaly. However, it could possibly act on the time of origin of neurons and interfere in this way with cortical maturation (Miller, 1987).

To summarize, most disorders affecting the brain in the first 20 weeks of gestation seem to have a genetic origin; neuronogenesis and neuronal migration appear to be relatively immune to the most common external pathogenic factors.

Another feature that could account for the relative stability and resistance to disease of the developmental events during this period is the very early determination of the structural and functional specificity of different classes of neurons. This occurs after their final mitosis and during the early phase of migration (McConnel, 1989; Price, 1989); incoming fibers also show a high degree of specificity in reaching their appropriate cortical target.

It is also important to realize that, while practically no cortical neurons are formed in the telencephalic cortex after 20 weeks of gestation, the external granular cells of the developing cerebellum continue to multiply and migrate into the internal granular layer during the second half of pregnancy and the first 10 to 12 months of life. These cells seem to be more vulnerable to external factors than the germinative cells of the telencephalon. This has, for instance, been shown experimentally in the rat infected with a parvovirus (Lipton & Johnson, 1972). Therefore a disease affecting both the telencephalon and the cerebellum during this period, may have very different morphological consequences (see below).

Second phase

The second half of pregnancy is a period of intense maturation and growth (which will continue well into the first year of life). The brain weight increases considerably and will continue to do so during the first years of life (80 g at 20 weeks gestation, 350 g at 40 weeks and 950 g at one postnatal year). Secondary and tertiary cortical gyri appear, neurons and their dendritic expansions grow considerably, multiple synaptic contacts are established, astrocytes and oligodendrocytes are formed and multiply, and myelination starts in some areas.

The complex adaptation of neuronal networks is modulated by important structural changes: neuronal death (for review see Clarke, 1985), elimination of axonal collaterals (Innocenti *et al.*, 1981), reduction and rearrangement of dendritic expansions and selective synaptic stabilization (see Changeux & Danchin, 1976). Developmental neuronal death, easy to detect in subcortical nuclei, has only recently been shown to exist in all layers of the neocortex in experimental animals by immunocytochemical methods (for reference see Parnavelas & Cavanagh, 1988). Although there is every reason to believe that this phenomenon also occurs in humans, it has not yet been directly demonstrated. The mechanism of neuronal death is still open to discussion, but it is supposed to depend on the availability of 'trophic factors' produced in the target fields. Either these substances are delivered in too limited amounts to profit the whole neuronal population, or they are produced in sufficient quantity, but a number of neurons cannot have access to them because of an insufficient development of their axonal terminals or of synaptic sites on the target cells (Oppenheim, 1989).

During neuronal development in experimental animals, a substantial loss of axons occurs in the corpus callosum, corticospinal tracts, optic nerves and other tracts. In the human corpus callosum, it is thought that axonal loss occurs essentially in the last fetal months and the first three months of life (Clarke *et al.*, 1989).

The elimination or reshaping of neurons and neuronal dendritic and axonal expansions underlines two important biological phenomena of the developing nervous system: an initial cell production far in excess to requirements, and intercellular competition to establish final stable connexions.

Could aberrations of one of these developmental events explain human disorders? There is a theoretical possibility, but absolutely no proof, that excessive developmental neuronal death could explain some of the early developmental microcephalies, and that 'insufficient' neuronal death could play a role in the pathogenesis of dyslexia (Galaburda *et al.*, 1985). It has been argued that an extension of the normal phenomenon of axonal elimination could be at the origin of some familial encephalopathies (Lyon *et al.*, 1990).

Chemical substances also play a role in development. The hypothesis that neuronal survival depends on specific brain-derived neurotrophic factors has still to be convincingly demonstrated (Davies, 1988), although recent experiments provide increasing evidence for a physiological role of nerve growth factors in the central nervous system (Herschman, 1986; Korsching, 1986; Oppenheim, 1989). There is increasing evidence that neurotransmitters are involved in the establishment of neuronal circuits. These substances, used for communication in the mature nervous system, play a role in developmental events such as neurite sprouting, dendritic pruning and possibly cell death (Lipton & Kater, 1989). The establishment of a normally functioning cortex depends in part on the succession of chemical messages – some of them released transitorily – produced at specific times (Chun *et al.*, 1987; Parnavelas & Cavanagh, 1988). It is conceivable that inhibition of a specific trophic factor or the disruption of the chronology of neurotransmitter production could give rise to developmental disorders.

Once established, neuronal circuits in the mammalian brain, far from being rigidly established, display adaptive capacities before and after birth, probably through local synaptic adaptation and sprouting of neuronal processes (Wall, 1988).

It is suggested that during the second half of pregnancy and first weeks of life, a very complex and flexible array of developmental events offers – much more than in the previous period – a multitude of potential targets to acquired or genetically determined disorders. Chromosomal aberrations, intoxications (especially alcohol), inherited metabolic disorders (especially mitochondrial diseases inducing for instance a defect of the corpus callosum (Kolodny, 1989)), viral infections and the deficiency of, as yet unknown, genetic factors may act on developmental events such as cellular growth, synaptogenesis, neuronal death, axonal elimination, and the correct timing of biochemical messages, to give rise to mental retardation and psychological disorders.

If one excepts acquired destructive processes of ischemic, hemorrhagic or infectious origin, structural abnormalities of the developing brain are much less obvious than before 20 weeks of gestation. One of the difficulties in revealing them lies in the limitations of the morphometric, ultrastructural, and immunocytochemical studies on the human brain and in the absence of satisfactory animal models of cerebral developmental disorders (the Reeler mouse does not duplicate a human cerebral malformation). Although it is desirable to construct pathophysiological hypotheses based on present knowledge of normal development, one should draw clearly the line between proof and conjecture in order not to obscure issues and inhibit further research. Advances in this field depend heavily on the development of new techniques, as will be discussed below.

HOW DO STRUCTURAL ABNORMALITIES OF THE BRAIN ACCOUNT FOR DEVELOPMENTAL DISORDERS?

We will address this problem in discussing the significance of some of the morphological anomalies found in developmental disorders and reflect on the frequent absence of any detectable morphological changes with standard neuropathological methods. One important notion will be made clear: in many instances obvious morphological changes do not explain satisfactorily the clinical signs.

Developmental microcephalies

Stunting of head growth (head circumference more than 2 standard deviations (SD) below the mean) may occur in some of the developmental disorders. It is frequently found in severe mental retardation, not uncommon in mild mental retardation, rare in autism and is an element of Rett's syndrome. In such circumstances (except for severe mental retardation), microcephaly is mostly related to non-encephaloclastic developmental defects which may be of genetic or environmental origin, although their exact cause remains frequently unknown.

Theoretically, developmental microcephalies may be the result of one or several of the following mechanisms: reduced production of nerve cells, inhibition of cell growth and enhancement of 'normal' neuronal death. While there is presently no evidence as to the possible occurrence of the latter phenomenon, a reduction in cell numbers (due to a failure of neuronogenesis and/or gliogenesis) or an inhibition of cell growth appear as possible explanations. These mechanisms are, however, difficult to test. Reliable and extensive cell counts have never been done and are probably not feasible in human autopsy material; Golgi impregnation may be used to compare the size of neurons, but the method is not entirely reliable. Two mechanisms have been postulated to explain the early developmental microcephalies: (1) a reduction in the number of radial glio-neuronal units with a normal number of neurons in each radial column, and (2) a numerical reduction of neurons within radial units, which remain in sufficient number (Evrard *et al.*, 1988; Rakic, 1988).

However, these explanations do not account for the fact that in some parts of the central nervous system (especially in the cerebellum and brain stem), neurons do not all migrate along glial fibers, and that glial cells obviously participate in the general reduction of brain volume. If a percentage of glial cells is certainly derived from the radial glia (Schmechel & Rakic, 1979), this is not the sole source of astrocytes and oligodendrocytes (Choi, 1988). The insufficiency of a multipotential germinal cell – which has been shown to exist for instance in the retina (Turner & Cepko, 1987; Wetts & Fraser, 1988), in the avian neural crest (Lumsden, 1989) and in the cerebral cortex of the mouse (Luskin *et al.*, 1988) – could tentatively be postulated.

The occurrence of 'microbrains' (Evrard *et al.*, 1984) provides the demonstration that the mechanisms of neuronogenesis and of neuronal migration may be independent. In this rare, rapidly lethal condition, the brains in neonates born at full term weigh 16 to 50 g i.e. 7 to 20 times less than normal, and the cytoarchitecture of the brain is not significantly modified.

What could then be the relationship between insufficient brain volume and inadequate neuropsychological development? We do not know of any critical level in neuronal number or size below which cognitive functions are affected. There is no linear relationship between the degree of microcephaly and the degree of intellectual impairment. Indeed there is a form of dominant microcephaly (head size 3–5 SD below the normal value) with normal intelligence and behavior (Rossi *et al.*, 1987). It is therefore probable that mechanisms other than insufficient neuronogenesis and cellular growth are at stake, affecting possibly synaptogenesis, neurotransmitter receptors, or a specific protein essential to cortical function.

Delayed morphological and neuropsychological expression of prenatal disorders

In a number of communication disorders (such as Rett's syndrome, moderate mental retardation, and, very occasionally, autism) microcephaly may be detected only several months after birth. When not explained by progressive disorders such as a hereditary metabolic disease or a persistent viral infection (due, for instance, to HIV), it is our opinion, based on our neuropathological experience, that these 'secondary microcephalies' are more often due to an inhibition of brain growth than to actual brain atrophy. They most probably represent the delayed effect of some non-progressive prenatal pathological event. Similarly, non-appearance or apparent loss of neuropsychological abilities (with or without microcephaly) after an early development considered as normal, may be related to prenatal factors. This concept is crucial for further research into the morphological and biological bases of developmental disorders.

It is, in our view, highly probable that in some instances the clinical expression of a genetically determined or prenatally acquired defect of some factor of maturation will become perceptible long after birth, at the time when the neurological substrate on which it normally acts arrives at a critical stage of development and requires the action of this substance for further development. For instance in the Pcd (Purkinje cell degeneration) mouse, the defect of Purkinje cells and the clinical signs appear 3 to 4 weeks after birth.

Such factors of maturation could include neurotransmitters which most probably play a role in neuronal development (Lipton & Kater, 1989) and have been shown to appear for short periods at different times and different levels of the brain (Parnavelas & Cavanagh, 1988). Absence or delayed availability of these transitory biochemical messages might inhibit or delay further maturation. In favour of such a possibility is the finding by Black (1986), on tissue cultures of sympathetic and peripheral nerve cells, that nerve growth factors act at strictly determined periods during development, and that any disruption of their chronology results in important morphological changes.

There are other possible mechanisms to account for the delayed expression of prenatal, non-progressive disorders. As described by Goodman (see Chapter 2, this volume), the structural basis of a cognitive function may shift site during the course of development. One can imagine therefore that in humans, when a fixed prenatal lesion involves a portion of the cortex that will be necessary for a neuropsychological function after a given postnatal time, its clinical expression will be delayed.

Another cause could be an insufficiency of the adaptive capacities of cortical neurons (through synaptic rearrangements, sprouting of neuronal processes or other mechanisms), in response to environmental factors. Wall (1988), for instance, has been able to demonstrate changes in cortical somatosensory maps of rodents, under the influence of prenatal or postnatal changes. Also, in disorders affecting the motor system, congenital hemiplegia provides a clear, if poorly understood, example of the relationship between maturation and clinical expression. After a prenatal or perinatally acquired defect of the motor cortex, paralysis is delayed until the fifth postnatal month, which is the time when voluntary movements of the upper limbs normally appear (Lyon, 1961).

MORPHOLOGICAL CHANGES DESCRIBED IN DEVELOPMENTAL DISORDERS

Apart from destructive lesions due to ischemia, infections or metabolic/degenerative diseases, morphological findings in the central

nervous system in developmental disorders can be said to fall in the following categories:
(a) Major disorders of neuronal migration; (b) minor developmental changes frequently called 'microdysgeneses' or 'microdysplasias' of the cerebral (and also cerebellar) cortex; (c) numerical reduction of specific neuronal populations; (d) regional hypoplasia with changes in relative volumetric development; (e) atrophy of the cerebellum with no detectable morphological changes of the brain; and (f) no detectable change in the central nervous system.

Major disorders of neuronal migration

They are relatively rare, mostly inherited as an autosomal recessive trait or related to a chromosomal aberration (see Table 1.2). Anomalies in neuronal migration constitute a good example of the difficulty in correlating developmental disorders and structural changes. The obvious fact that neurons have not reached their final destination, might not be what is most important in creating cerebral dysfunction: ectopic neurons can make normal connections (Jensen & Killackey, 1984). In the Reeler mouse, in which there is a major change in the cyto-architecture consisting in inversion of the cortical layers, afferent fibers to the cortex nevertheless reach their normal targets (Caviness & Rakic, 1978), and neurotransmitters are normally expressed (Goffinet & Caviness, 1986).

Minor developmental changes of the cerebral (or cerebellar) cortex

A remarkable and intriguing cortical microdysgenesis has been reported by Galaburda *et al.* (1985) in five dyslexic boys and in a child with developmental dysphasia by Cohen *et al.* (1989). There was an excessive number of ectopic clusters of neurons in layer I of the neocortex, and focal minute 'laminar dysplasias'. (A similar anomaly has been found in the New Zealand Black mouse, which has been said to have 'learning disabilities' (Sherman *et al.*, 1987).)

The significance of these minor developmental changes remains to be understood. They are not detected in such quantity in normal brains: they have been found in very small numbers in 26% of controls by Kaufmann & Galaburda (1989). Therefore the anomaly here does not consist in the mere presence of neuronal clusters – as they are found in a quarter of normal individuals – but in their excessive number. This is also true for other types of microdysgenesis. To draw the line between a non-significant morphological peculiarity and a developmental defect one has to rely on quantitative differences, and such criteria are obviously hazardous. On the other hand, it is very difficult to admit that these very mild structural changes have any direct bearing on a language disorder. If unable to explain the disorder, they probably constitute an indicator as to the existence and time of onset (probably the final phase of neuronal migration) of a more widespread 'invisible' developmental defect which underlies the cognitive dysfunction.

There are other examples of minor dysplasias as the only detectable morphological abnormality in children with communication disorders, such as: (a) foci of hypermigration, characterized by strands of neurons crossing vertically the molecular layer into the meninges probably as a result of a localized defect in the external limiting membrane of the brain, are observed in the fetal alcohol syndrome, and in other cases of mental retardation (Robain & Lyon, 1972; Caviness *et al.*, 1978). They have been produced experimentally with 6-hydroxytryptamine (Lidov & Molliver, 1982); (b) periventricular neuronal heterotopias, detectable by magnetic resonance imaging (MRI); (c) isolated heterotopias of fetal granule cells in the dentate nucleus, always associated with mental retardation.

Minor cortical dysgenesis provides another example of the difficulties of morphological interpretation. Some minor limited changes in the usual cortical pattern represent only normal variations; during development it is quite understandable that some neurons do not reach their usual site. However, such normal variations have sometimes been described as developmental abnormalities and considered to be the basis of neurological diseases, for instance primary epilepsy (Meencke & Janz, 1984; 1985). This view has been criticized by Lyon & Gastaut (1985). These authors considered that the minute and rare peculiarities reported by Meencke & Janz were frequently encountered in neurologically normal subjects.

'Hyperinterpretation' of morphological data may lead to undue clinico-structural correlations. One should be aware of the limitations of neuropathological methods in humans. 'Microneuropathology' may lead to 'macro-errors'. The desire to try to establish a morphological basis for developmental disorders is legitimate and certainly very important, but it requires a cautious approach, much experience, the comparison with a sufficient number of controls and the search for new techniques applicable to the human brain. Furthermore, it seems quite possible that in some developmental disorders morphological abnormalities are entirely absent.

Numerical reduction of specific neuronal populations

A reduction in the number of Purkinje cells (Ritvo *et al.*, 1986) and of neurons in the fascia dentata (Bauman & Kemper, 1985) have been reported in autism. However, due to the extreme difficulty of cell counts in the human brain, these observations need confirmation.

The search for the reduction or disappearance of a specific population of neurons is surely an important line of research which has been insufficiently considered up to now. This type of study may prove especially interesting in cases of cognitive disorders without superficial evidence of cortical alteration. In some degenerative disorders, the defect of a specific type of neuron has been shown to occur. For instance, in juvenile lipofuscinosis, Braak & Goebel (1978), using immunocytochemical methods found a selective loss of stellate cells in the cortex. The loss of these local circuit neurons, which contain glutamate acid decarboxylase (the synthetizing enzyme of gamma amino butyric acid (GABA)), could result in a reduction of type II synapses and facilitate paroxysmal and other abnormal activities of the cortex. Selective neuronal degeneration in the striatum is found in Huntington's disease (see Kowall *et al.*, 1987). In the future, the use of immunocytochemical techniques might prove very helpful in tracing defects of certain types of neurons in developmental disorders.

Regional hypoplasia with changes in relative volumetric development

The possible relationship between neuropsychological function and regional hypoplasia of the brain (not atrophy, i.e. shrinkage), as revealed with the MRI or at autopsy, is certainly an important, although still poorly explored, field for research. Underdevelopment of the first temporal gyrus is found in trisomy 21 and insufficient operculation of the sylvian fissure is a feature of the fetal alcohol syndrome (Ferrer & Galofré, 1987). Hypoplasia of lobules VI and VII of the cerebellar vermis has been reported in children with autism by Courchesne *et al.* (1988), but has not been confirmed by others. Short frontal or temporal lobes are sometimes found in children with severe mental deficit on routine neurological examination but no systematic study of these data has been done. Geschwind & Galaburda (1987) have drawn attention to the disappearance of the asymmetry of the planum temporale in dyslexia.

These observations suggest that changes in the relative volumetric development of specific parts of the brain may be characteristic of some neurological disorders. A three-dimensional reconstruction of the brain using computer generated images could be a way to gather more information (Filipek *et al.*, 1988; Caviness *et al.*, 1989), and more attention should be given by neuropathologists to such changes.

Atrophy of the cerebellum with no detectable morphological changes of the brain

The relative frequency of a familial syndrome characterized by the association of usually mild mental handicap with severe language disability, normal brain morphology and cerebellar atrophy (essentially granular) has been shown by systematic MRI screening and in a few neuropathological studies. The cerebellar lesions are usually subclinical.

As discussed by Romano *et al.* (1991), the strongest possibility here is that some pathological event damages simultaneously the cerebellum and the telencephalon and that the morphological differences between these two regions are related to differences in the chronology of their development. The granular layer of the cerebellum (which seems to be selectively affected in this syndrome) is composed of cells which continue to divide and migrate long after postmitotic neurons in the cortex have achieved their migration. Consequently it is understandable that structural changes are more marked in the cerebellum.

This concept is of great potential importance. If one considers that regional differences exist in the chronology of cerebral maturation, one can assume that a disorder affecting the whole brain will produce structural abnormalities (and functional deficits) which will vary according to the degree of maturation of the different parts of the brain at the time of the insult. The relatively immature structures (for instance those in which neuronal migration is not achieved) will be apt to display evident morphological changes which may have no evident clinical expression, whereas more mature regions will show no abnormality. In the latter, there may be subtle changes in neuronal circuitry which, although clinically significant, remain 'invisible' with standard neuropathological methods.

No detectable changes in the central nervous system

In many children with behavioral or cognitive disorders the total absence of morphological changes on neuropathological examination with standard methods comes as a frequent surprise. Shaw (1987) found no significant abnormality at autopsy in 25% of 299 children with severe mental retardation. We have a similar experience, and the proportion of 'normal' brains is most probably higher in mild mental retardation and other communication disorders. A crucial challenge for the neuroscientist in the coming years will be to try to understand the nature of the cerebral disorder in these cases.

The systematic search for a defect or a numerical reduction in synaptic junctions, which comes to mind as one possible explanation, is not easily feasible in humans. The density of synapses measured by Cragg (1975) in cortical biopsies from three mentally handicapped adolescents was found to be normal, but such studies – which should remain quite exceptional if not prohibited – are of limited value because of the very small sample size.

PERSPECTIVES FOR FURTHER RESEARCH

Other possible lines of approach include among others:

- the detection of regional underdevelopment, asymmetries or loss of usual asymmetries, by MRI-based morphometry (Filipek *et al.*, 1988; Caviness *et al.*, 1989) and at autopsy;
- complete cytoarchitectonic studies of the brain after serial sectioning;
- the search for a selective loss of neuronal population by immunocytochemical methods;
- the use of monoclonal antibodies against synaptin (a marker for synapses) in human brains, post-mortem;
- mapping of neurotransmitter receptors in the autopsied brain by way of autoradiography and *in situ* hybridization (Palacios *et al.*, 1986; Young, 1986);
- precise quantification of nerve cells and synapses.

All these methods are extremely promising, but they are time consuming and highly specialized. They can, therefore, be achieved only by way of collaborative studies involving several complementary laboratories. One should also take into account the strong possibility that a primary defect of a specific protein may prevent the normal development of brain function, without giving rise to any structural change.

Finally, no real progress will be made without precise and detailed correlations between clinical, radiological, and neuropathological data.

In ending this chapter, it seems appropriate to cite an opinion expressed by Maxwell Cowan (1981): '. . . perhaps the most serious obstacle in the way of real advance in the study of . . . "higher brain functions" is the absence of theoretical framework . . . If substantial progress is to be made in the understanding of such phenomena as perception, learning, memory and emotion, we shall have to have theories that are cogent and testable . . .'

Theories, however, remain fragile and misleading if not based on solid facts. It is hoped that sufficient progress will be made, with the help of specific neuropathological and neurobiological methodologies and a new awareness of the problems inherent to morphological studies, to allow the elaboration of hypothetical frameworks and models apt to stimulate further research in the field of developmental disorders.

REFERENCES

Angevine, J. B. & Sidman, R. L. (1961) Autoradiographic study of cell migration during histogenesis of cerebral cortex of the mouse. *Nature,* **192,** 766–8.

Bauman, M. & Kemper, T. L. (1985) Histoanatomic observations of the brain in early infantile autism. *Neurology,* **35,** 866–74.

Black, I. B. (1986) Trophic molecules and evolution of the nervous system. *Proceedings of the National Academic of Sciences of the USA,* **83,** 8249–52.

Braak, H. & Goebel, H. H. (1978) Loss of pigment-laden stellate cells: a severe alteration of the isocortex in juvenile neuronal ceroid lipofuscinosis. *Acta Neuropathologica (Berlin),* **42,** 53–7.

Caviness, V. S., Evrard, P. & Lyon, G. (1978) Radial neuronal assemblies, ectopia and necrosis of developing cortex. *Acta Neuropathologica (Berlin),* **41,** 67–72.

Caviness, V. S. & Rakic, P. (1978) Mechanisms of cortical development. A view from mutations in mice. *Annual Review of Neurosciences,* **1,** 297–365.

Caviness, V. S., Filipek, P. A. & Kennedy, D. N. (1989) Magnetic resonance technology in human brain science: blueprint for a program based upon morphometry. *Brain & Development,* **11,** 1–13.

Changeux, J. P. & Danchin, A. (1976) Selective stabilisation of developing synapses as a mechanism for the specification of neuronal networks. *Nature,* **264,** 705–12.

Choi, B. H. (1988) Prenatal gliogenesis in the developing cerebrum of the mouse. *Glia,* **1,** 308–16.

Chun, J. J. M., Makumura, M. J. & Shatz, C. J. (1987) Transient cells of the developing mammalian telencephalon are peptide-immunoreactive neurons. *Nature,* **325,** 617–29.

Clarke, P. H. G. (1985) Neuronal death in the development of the vertebrate nervous system. *Trends in Neurosciences,* **8,** 345–9.

Clarke, S., Kreftsik, R., Van der Loos, H. & Innocenti, G. M. (1989) Forms and measures of adult and developing human corpus callosum: is there sexual dimorphism? *Journal of Comparative Neurology,* **280,** 213–30.

Cohen, M., Campbell, R. & Yagmaai, F. (1989) Neuropathological abnormalities in developmental dysphasia. *Annals of Neurology,* **25,** 567–70.

Courchesne, E., Yeung-Courchesne, R., Press, G. A., Hesselink, J. R. & Jernigan, T. I. (1988) Hypoplasia of cerebellar vermian lobules VI and VII in autism. *New England Journal of Medicine,* **318,** 1349–54.

Cragg, B. C. (1975) The density of synapses and neurons in normal, mentally defective and ageing human brains. *Brain,* **98,** 81–90.

Davies, A. M. (1988) The emerging generality of the neurotrophic hypothesis. *Trends in Neurosciences,* **11,** 243–8.

Edelman, G. M. (1984) Modulations of cell adhesion during induction, histogenesis and perinatal development of the nervous system. *Annual Review of Neurosciences,* **7,** 339–77.

Evrard, P., Caviness, V. S. & Lyon, G. (1978) The mechanism of arrest of neuronal migration in the Zellweger malformation: an hypothesis based upon cytoarchitectonic analysis. *Acta Neuropathologica,* **41,** 109–10.

Evrard, P., Lyon, G. & Gadisseux, J. F. (1984) Les processus destructifs agissant sur le cerveau foetal durant la seconde moitié de la grossesse, durant la période de croissance et de différenciation du tissu nerveux. In *Progrès en néonatologie*, Vol. 4. Bâle: S. Karger, pp. 85–106.

Evrard, P., de Saint-Georges, P., Kadim, H. & Gadisseux, J. F. (1988) Pathology of prenatal encephalopathies. In French, J. H., Hard, S. & Casaer, P. (eds) *Child Neurology and Developmental Disabilities.* Baltimore: Brookes, pp. 153–76.

Ferrer, I. & Galofré, E. (1987) Dendritic spine anomalies in fetal alcohol syndrome. *Neuropediatrics*, **18**, 161.

Filipek, P. A., Kennedy, D. N., Kennedy, S. K. & Caviness, V. S. (1988) Shape analysis of the brain of two siblings based upon magnetic resonance imaging. *Annals of Neurology*, **24**, Abstract, 355–6.

Gadisseux, J. F. & Evrard, P. (1985) Glial-neuronal relationship in the developing central nervous system. *Developmental Neuroscience*, **7**, 12–32.

Gadisseux, J. F., Kadhim, H. J., van den Bosch de Aguilar, P., Caviness, V. S. & Evrard, P. (1990) Neuron migration within the radial glial fiber system of the developing murine cerebrum: an electron microscopic autoradiographic analysis. *Developmental Brain Research*, **52**, 39–56.

Gadisseux, J. F., Van Lierde, M., Lamy, M., Raymond, G. & Lyon, G. (1991) The neuropathology of fetal CMV encephalitis, in preparation.

Galaburda, A. M., Sherman, G. F., Rosen, G. D., Aboitiz, F. & Geschwind, N. (1985) Developmental dyslexia: four consecutive patients with cortical anomalies. *Annals of Neurology*, **18**, 222–33.

Geschwind, N. & Galaburda, A. M. (1987) *Cerebral lateralization.* Cambridge: MIT Press, pp. 1854.

Goffinet, A. M. & Caviness, V. S., Jr, (1986) Autoradiographic localization of beta-adrenoreceptors in the midbrain and forebrain of normal and reeler mutant mice. *Brain Research*, **366**, 193–202.

Goldman-Rakic, P. S., Isseroff, A., Schwartz, M. L. & Bugbee, N. M. (1983) The neurobiology of cognitive development. In Haith, M. M. & Campos, J. J. (eds.) *Mussen's handbook of child psychology*, 4th edn, Vol. II, *Infancy and Developmental Psychobiology*. New York: Wiley, pp. 281–344.

Hatten, M. E. (1990) Riding the glial monorail: a common mechanism for glial guided neuronal migration in different regions of the developing mammalian brain. *Trends in Neurosciences*, **13**, 179–84.

Herschman, H. R. (1986) Polypeptide growth factors and the central nervous system. *Trends in Neurosciences*, **9**, 53–7.

Innocenti, G. M., Fiore, L. & Caminiti, R. (1981) Growth and reshaping of axons in the establishment of visual callosal connections. *Science*, **212**, 824–6.

Jensen, K. F. & Killackey, H. P. (1984) Subcortical projections from ectopic neocortical neurons. *Proceedings of the National Academy of Sciences of the USA*, **81**, 964–8.

Johnson, R. T. (1982) *Viral Infections of the Nervous System.* New York: Raven Press, pp. 207–9.

Kaufmann, W. E. & Galaburda, A. M. (1989) Cerebrocortical microdysgenesis in neurologically normal subjects: a histopathologic study. *Neurology*, **39**, 238–44.

Kolodny, E. H. (1989) Agenesis of the corpus callosum: a marker of inherited metabolic disease? *Neurology*, **39**, 847–8.

Korsching, S. (1986) The role of nerve growth factor in the CNS. *Trends in Neurosciences*, **9**, 570–3.

Kowall, N. W., Ferrante, R. J. & Martin, J. B. (1987) Patterns of cell loss in Huntington's disease. *Trends in Neurosciences*, **10**, 24–9.

Lander, A. D. (1989) Understanding the molecules of neural cell contacts: emerging patterns of structure and function. *Trends in Neurosciences*, **12**, 189–95.

Lidov, H. G. & Molliver, M. E. (1982) The structure of the cerebral cortex in the rat following prenatal administration of the 6-hydroxydopamine. *Developmental Brain Research*, **3**, 81–108.

Lipton, H. L. & Johnson, R. T. (1972) The pathogenesis of rat virus infection in the newborn hamster. *Laboratory Investigations*, **27**, 508–13.

Lipton, S. A. & Kater, S. B. (1989) Neurotransmitter regulation of neuronal outgrowth, plasticity and survival. *Trends in Neurosciences*, **12**, 265–70.

Lumsden, A. (1989) Multipotent cells in the avian neural crest. *Trends in Neurosciences*, **12**, 81–3.

Luskin, M. B., Pearlman, A. L. & Sanes, J. R. (1988) Cell lineage in the cerebral cortex of the mouse studied in vivo and in vitro with a recombinant retrovirus. *Neuron*, **1**, 635–47.

Lyon, G. (1961) First signs and mode of onset of congenital hemiplegia. *Developmental Medicine and Child Neurology. Little Club Clinics*, **4**, 33–8.

Lyon, G., Evrard, P. & Gadisseux, J. F. (1984) Les anomalies du développement du télencéphale humain pendant la période de cytogenèse-histogenèse (1ère moitié de la grossesse). In *Progrès en Néonatologie*, Vol. 4. Bâle: S. Karger, pp. 70–84.

Lyon, G. & Gastaut, H. (1985) Considerations on the significance attributed to unusual cerebral histological findings recently described in eight patients with primary generalized epilepsy. *Epilepsia*, **26**, 365–7.

Lyon, G., Arita, F., Le Galloudec, E., Vallée, L., Misson, J. P. & Ferrière, G. (1990) A disorder of axonal development, necrotizing myopathy, cardiomyopathy, and cataracts: a new familial disease. *Annals of Neurology*, **27**, 193–9.

Marin-Padilla, M. (1983) Structural organization of the human cerebral cortex prior to the appearance of the cortical plate. *Anatomy and Embryology*, **168**, 21–40.

Marques Dias, M. J., Harmany-van Rijckevorsel, G., Landrieu, G. & Lyon, G. (1984) Prenatal cytomegalovirus disease and cerebral microgyria: evidence for perfusion failure, not disturbance of histogenesis, as the major cause of fetal cytomegalovirus encephalopathy. *Neuropediatrics*, **15**, 18–24.

Maxwell Cowan, W. (1981) *The Organization of the Cerebral Cortex*. In Schmitt, F. O., Worden, F. G., Adelman, G. & Dennis, S. G. (eds) Cambridge, Mass: MIT Press, Keynote pp. XI–XXI.

McConnel, S. K. (1989) The determination of neuronal fate in the cerebral cortex. *Trends in Neurosciences*, **12**, 242–349.

Meencke, H. J. & Janz, D. (1984) Neuropathological findings in primary generalized epilepsy: a study of eight cases. *Epilepsia*, **25**, 8–21.

Meencke, H. J. & Janz, D. (1985) The significance of microdysgenesis in primary generalized epilepsy: an answer to the considerations of Lyon and Gastaut. *Epilepsia*, **26**, 368–71.

Miller, M. W. (1987) Effect of prenatal exposure to alcohol on the distribution and time of origin of corticospinal neurons in the rat. *Journal of Comparative Neurology*, **257**, 272–82.

Naeye, R. L. (1967) Cytomegalic inclusion disease: the fetal disorder. *American Journal of Clinical Pathology*, **47**, 738–44.

Oppenheim, R. M. (1989) The neurotrophic theory and naturally occurring motoneuron death. *Trends in Neurosciences*, **12**, 252–5.

Palacios, J. M., Probst, A. & Cortés, R. (1986) Mapping receptors in the human brain. *Trends in Neurosciences*, **9**, 284–9.

Parnavelas, J. G. & Cavanagh, M. E. (1988) Transient expression of neurotransmitters in the developing neocortex. *Trends in Neurosciences*, **11**, 92–3.

Price, J. (1989) When are neurones specified? *Trends in Neurosciences*, **12**, 276–8.

Rakic, P. (1972) Mode of cell migration to the superficial layers of fetal monkey neocortex. *Journal of Comparative Neurology*, **145**, 61–84.

Rakic, P. (1982) Early developmental events: cell lineage, acquisition of neuronal positions and areal and laminar developments. In Rakic, P. & Goldman-Rakic, P. S. (eds.) *Development and modifiability of the cerebral cortex*. Cambridge, Mass: MIT Press, pp. 437–51.

Rakic, P. (1988). Specification of cerebral cortical areas. *Science*, **241**, 170–6.

Ritvo, E. R., Freeman, B. J., Scheibel, A. B., *et al.* (1986) Purkinje cell counts in the cerebella of four autistic subjects: initial findings of the UCLA-NSAC autopsy research report. *American Journal of Psychiatry*, **143**, 862–6.

Robain, O. & Lyon, G. (1972) Les micrencéphalies familiales par malformation cérébrale. *Acta Neuropathologica (Berlin)*, **20**, 96–109.

Romano, A., Motte, J., Del Guidice, E. & Lyon, G. (1991) Mental retardation and latent cerebellar atrophy. Submitted.

Rossi, L. N., Candini, G. & Scarlatti, G. (1987) Autosomal dominant microcephaly without mental retardation. *American Journal of Diseases of Children*, **141**, 655–9.

Schmechel, D. E. & Rakic, P. (1979) A Golgi study of radial glial cells in developing monkey telencephalon: morphogenesis and transformation into astrocytes. *Anatomy and Embryology*, **156**, 115–52.

Shaw, C. M. (1987) Correlates of mental retardation and structural changes of the brain. *Brain and Development*, **9**, 1–8.

Sherman, G. F., Galaburda, A. M., Behar, P. O. & Rosen, G. D. (1987) Neuroanatomical anomalies in autoimmune mice. *Acta Neuropathologica*, **74**, 239–42.

Turner, D. L. & Cepko, C. L. (1987) A common progenitor for neurons and glia persists in rat retina late in development. *Nature*, **328**, 131–6.

Wall, J. T. (1988) Variable organization in cortical maps of the skin as an indication of the lifelong adaptive capacities of circuits in the mammalian brain. *Trends in Neurosciences*, **11**, 549–57.

Wetts, R. & Fraser, S. E. (1988) Multipotent precursors can give rise to all major cell types of the frog retina. *Science*, **239**, 1142–5.

Young, W. S. (1986) In situ hybridization histochemistry and the study of the nervous system. *Trends in Neurosciences*, **9**, 549–51.

2 Developmental disorders and structural brain development

ROBERT GOODMAN

This chapter explores possible relationships between developmental disorders, in the psychological and psychiatric sense, and disorders of development, in the neurobiological sense. In the first section, developmental disorders are defined, and several lines of evidence are presented to suggest that these disorders are rooted, at least in part, in abnormalities in brain development. Can the nature of the underlying neuropathology be inferred from the form of the deficit? The following sections suggest that the answer is 'not necessarily'. Psychological delay does not necessarily reflect neurological delay, nor does psychological deviance necessarily reflect neurological deviance. Similarly, the age of onset or resolution of a psychological disorder does not necessarily reflect the time when the underlying neurological disorder began or ended.

The focus of the chapter then shifts towards developmental neurobiology, summarizing the main phases of brain development. The recent emphasis on the central role of subtractive processes in normal and abnormal development is evident in the subsequent sections on sex differences, sensitive periods, and recovery from early brain damage. Since recovery from early damage to just one hemisphere can be remarkably good, the next section considers whether developmental disorders can reasonably be attributed to lateralized brain abnormalities. On a related theme, the penultimate section examines possible links between developmental disorders and atypical patterns of cerebral lateralization.

There are many plausible neurological explanations for the developmental disorders, and advances in developmental neurobiology continually increase the scope for informed conjecture. These conjectures are valuable, generating a range of alternative hypotheses to explain the known facts. But conjectures are the beginning rather than the end of the scientific process. What about refutation? For researchers, the pressing challenge is to convert neurobiological hypotheses into precise predictions that can be tested empirically, thereby enabling our current conjectures to be refuted or refined. The final section suggests that, despite the limitations in current investigative techniques, alternative neuropathological models of developmental disorders can potentially be translated into testable and clinically relevant predictions.

DEVELOPMENTAL DISORDERS

In this chapter, the term 'developmental disorder' is used to refer to a group of early-onset disorders in which one or more skills develop abnormally, either in rate or in pattern. The ICD-10 category of developmental disorder (World Health Organization, 1989) includes relatively circumscribed abnormalities in the development of speech, language, co-ordination and scholastic skills, and also the 'pervasive developmental disorders' such as autism (involving simultaneous impairments in the development of social interactions, language and play). The DSM-III-R category of developmental disorder (American Psychiatric Association, 1987) is slightly broader, including all the ICD-10 disorders, plus global developmental delay/mental retardation as well. In this chapter, the term 'developmental disorder' is used in a still broader sense, including hyperactivity too. As an early-onset disorder in which attentional skills and activity regulation develop abnormally, narrowly defined hyperactivity (or hyperkinesis (Taylor, 1986)) appears to meet the ICD-10 criteria for a developmental disorder (World Health Organization, 1989).

As defined in this way, the developmental disorders form a coherent group. Different developmental disorders frequently occur together, either affecting the same individual or clustering within the same family. For example, severe and pervasive hyperactivity is commonly accompanied by delayed language or motor development (Taylor *et al.*, 1986), and language disorders are over-represented among the relatives of autistic individuals (e.g. Rutter, 1991).

Several of the associated features of the developmental disorders suggest a major aetiological role for biological factors. Firstly, many of the developmental disorders are particularly over-represented among children with unequivocal brain abnormalities (e.g. Rutter *et al.*, 1970; Hunt & Dennis, 1987). Secondly, family, twin and adoption studies suggest that genes play an important role in many developmental disorders (e.g. Folstein & Rutter, 1977; Goodman, 1989a). Thirdly, boys are more vulnerable than girls to practically all developmental disorders, with a male : female ratio of 4 : 1 or greater in some instances. This male excess may reflect the greater vulnerability of males to a very wide range of derangements of biological development (Taylor & Ounsted, 1972), though psychosocial factors, such as different expectations of boys and girls, could also be relevant (see Huston, 1983). Fourthly, children with a variety of developmental disorders are more likely than controls to have experienced prenatal and perinatal complications (e.g. Nichols & Chen, 1981; Gillberg & Gillberg, 1983). While a link with obstetric complications is persuasive evidence for a biological origin, provided confounding variables such as social class have been allowed for, it remains controversial how far obstetric complications cause developmental disorders, and how far obstetric complications are harmless markers for pre-existing fetal abnormalities, whether genetic or acquired early in prenatal life (see Goodman, 1990). Finally, high rates of left-handedness also provide presumptive evidence for a biological contribution to some developmental disorders (see below).

Psychosocial factors seem less important than biological factors in the aetiology of many developmental disorders. In autism, for example, there is no evidence that child rearing techniques or socioeconomic factors play any causal role whatsoever (see Rutter, 1985). This is not true for all developmental disorders, however. Hyperactivity, for example, is linked to psychosocial factors, such as socioeconomic disadvantage (Goodman & Stevenson, 1989) or early institutional upbringing (Hodges & Tizard, 1989), as well as to biological factors, such as genetic predisposition (Goodman, 1989a) or acquired brain damage (Ingram, 1955, 1956; Ounsted, 1955). The unimportance or subsidiary importance of psychosocial factors in developmental disorders contrasts with the great importance of family and social factors in childhood conduct disorder (e.g. Patterson, 1982), and with the major role of socio-cultural expectations in anorexia nervosa (e.g. Garner & Garfinkel, 1980).

The characteristic early onset of developmental disorders suggests that the biological origins of these disorders may well lie in abnormalities of brain development. A specifically developmental origin is supported by the rarity with which comparable disorders arise in later childhood or adult life. The onset of autism, for example, is characteristically in the first 30 months of life, and later onset, though well recognized, is decidedly rare (see Rutter, 1985). This contrasts with emotional disorders. Although affective disturbances involving anxiety and sadness are common in childhood, broadly similar affective disorders frequently arise *de novo* in adulthood, making a specifically neurodevelopmental origin for affective disorders less plausible.

DELAY AND DEVIANCE: PARALLEL PROCESSES IN BRAIN AND BEHAVIOUR?

Developmental disorders were defined above in terms of abnormalities in the rate or pattern of development. Many authors draw a distinction between delay and deviance. This distinction is straightforward in principle: the delayed individual is making slow progress down a normal developmental pathway, while the deviant individual is progressing down an abnormal developmental pathway.

Does the distinction between delay and deviance allow us to draw any conclusions about the nature of the underlying neuropathology? Several authors have suggested that developmental delays reflect maturational lags in the brain systems mediating the relevant skills (see, for example, Satz & Sparrow, 1970; Bishop & Edmundson, 1987). Other authors have suggested that developmental disorders characterized by deviance reflect qualitatively abnormal (misconnected) brains (see Goodman, 1989b). Despite their apparent plausibility, we should not accept these inferences too readily.

Firstly, the distinction between developmental delay and developmental deviance is often unsatisfactory. Many developmental disorders appear to involve a mixture of delay and deviance. In addition, reliance on quantitative scales may lead us to misconstrue deviance as delay. The use of strength, size and speed subtests could make a donkey appear to be a developmentally delayed horse. Likewise, a tangerine could be construed as a developmentally delayed orange. It is difficult to be sure that we are not making equally absurd errors in the classification of some developmental disorders. For instance, is 'global developmental delay' leading on to 'mental retardation' really an instance of delay, as the names suggest?

Secondly, even when the distinction between delayed and deviant development is straightforward, clinical features may provide a misleading guide to the nature of the underlying neuropathology. For example, delayed development can result from fixed abnormalities of the brain. This possibility is well illustrated by the effect of orbitomedial lesions on delayed-response learning in monkeys (see Goldman-Rakic *et al.*, 1983). In a typical delayed-response task, the monkey observes food being hidden in one of two food-wells, after which both wells are briefly hidden by a screen. Delayed-response learning is judged by the monkey's subsequent success at retrieving food from the correct well. The orbitomedial portion of the prefrontal cortex plays an important part in delayed-response learning in juvenile but not in adult monkeys. Conversely, the dorsolateral portion of the prefrontal cortex is important for delayed-response learning in adult but not in juvenile monkeys. In effect, the neural substrate of delayed-response learning shifts from the orbitomedial to the dorsolateral cortex as a monkey matures. Consequently, when a monkey's orbitomedial cortex is destroyed early in life, the monkey is poor at delayed-response learning as a juvenile (since the orbitomedial cortex is essential at this stage), but is normal at delayed-response learning as an adult (since the intact dorsolateral cortex has taken over by this stage). Behaviourally, this is an instance of delay and subsequent catch-up. Neurologically, this is an instance of a fixed lesion. It would obviously have been wrong to infer neurological delay from the developmental delay.

Conversely, there may be instances of neurological delay that result in psychological deviance rather than psychological delay. If a skill is normally present from birth onwards, a deficiency in that skill will appear deviant even if it results from neurological delay. Visual responsiveness is one instance of a skill that is already relatively well developed in newborn babies (e.g. Antell & Caron, 1985; Bushnell *et al.*, 1989). Consequently, a blind infant is developmentally deviant, since a lack of visual responsiveness is abnormal at any postnatal age. In a developmental disorder known as 'delayed visual maturation', otherwise normal children are slow to see, appearing blind in early infancy but subsequently acquiring normal visual responsiveness, usually before 6 months (see Fielder *et al.*, 1985). The disorder has generally been attributed to delayed maturation of the visual system. If this is so (and Tresidder *et al.* (1990) have recently questioned this), the existence of neurological delay results in transiently deviant visual behaviour.

Some studies suggest that social responsiveness, like visual responsiveness, is surprisingly well developed in the normal human neonate (e.g. Condon & Sander, 1974; Brazelton, 1982; Field *et al.*, 1982). Consequently, if the brain systems mediating early social responsiveness were delayed in their development, the resultant lack of social responsiveness would be deviant, i.e. abnormal for any postnatal age. In his original description of infantile autism, Kanner (1943) speculated that autistic individuals had an 'innate inability to form the usual, biologically provided affective contact with people' (p. 250). This hypothesis is supported by several recent studies, e.g. Hobson (1986), Yirmiya *et al.* (1989). Consequently, neuronal delay in the relevant brain systems might present as a relatively transient autistic disorder. This conjecture receives some support from preliminary evidence that delayed visual maturation and autism can occur together, with the autistic features resolving surprisingly well as the child ages (Goodman & Ashby, 1990). Although the suggestion that neurological delay could underlie some instances of autistic deviance is highly speculative, this possibility is a reminder that the form of a developmental disorder – deviance or delay – does not necessarily mirror the form of the underlying neuropathology. The notion that delay and deviance represent parallel processes in brain and behaviour is a plausible hypothesis to be investigated rather than a corollary that can be taken for granted.

ONSET AND RESOLUTION: DOES PSYCHOPATHOLOGY MIRROR NEUROPATHOLOGY?

It is tempting to suppose that the age of onset or resolution of a developmental disorder provides a useful guide to the age at which the underlying neurodevelopmental abnormalities began or ended. This may be so in some instances, but animal studies suggest that there may well be exceptions. As described above, delayed-response learning in monkeys depends on different portions of the prefrontal lobes at different developmental stages (Goldman-Rakic *et al.*, 1983). In juveniles, the orbitomedial but not the dorsolateral portion is essential, whereas the reverse is true in adults. Consequently, if the dorsolateral portion is damaged in infancy, no deficit is evident initially because the dorsolateral cortex seems to play little or no role at this stage in life, but a permanent deficit in delayed-response learning becomes apparent once the monkey reaches adulthood. The time of onset of the psychological deficit does not reflect the time of onset of the underlying neurological deficit. Conversely, as previously described, if the orbitomedial cortex is damaged in infancy, the monkey is poor at delayed-response learning as a juvenile but 'grows out' of this psychological deficit on reaching adulthood. The time of resolution of the psychological deficit does not reflect the time of resolution of the underlying neurological deficit.

These considerations are potentially relevant to developmental disorders. For example, a minority of autistic children develop relatively normally as infants but undergo a dramatic change in their second year, with the loss of previously acquired skills in social interaction, communication and play. Although it is entirely plausible that this regression reflects brain abnormalities that begin or worsen during the second year, it is also possible that the regression reflects a shift in neural substrate. Imagine, for example, that social interest and awareness depend primarily on one neural system (which we can label S1) in infancy, and primarily on a different neural system (which we can label S2) thereafter. If so, a congenital fault in S2 will have little or no impact during infancy, but will result in loss of social interest and awareness during the transitional phase in the second year when S1 fades out and S2 should take over. According to this model, congenital abnormalities in both S1 and S2 would lead to marked abnormalities in social awareness and interest from early infancy onwards, as seen in most autistic children.

The resolution of developmental disorders could also reflect a shift in neural substrate. Thus although language delay with subsequent catch up plausibly arises from delayed neuronal maturation (cf. Bishop &

Edmundson, 1987), it could potentially reflect a permanent fault in a neuronal system that is essential for language in the early toddler years but not thereafter.

PHASES OF BRAIN DEVELOPMENT

When faced with a malfunctioning 'black box' – a device whose inner workings are unknown to us – we will find it difficult, perhaps impossible, to guess what has gone wrong within the box just from the nature of the malfunction. There are too many possible explanations, and we have no constraints to guide our speculation. The more we know about the components and connections within the box, the easier it is to guess the cause of the malfunction. When the black box is a human brain, and when the malfunction is a developmental disorder, we cannot simply lift the lid and identify the faulty component or connection. Nevertheless, we can use what is known about mammalian brain development in general, and human brain development in particular, to guide our speculations and investigations. Consequently, this section provides a brief outline of one particularly interesting aspect of normal brain development – the succession of additive and subtractive phases.

Additive processes in development can be likened to the production of a car on an assembly line, with a series of parts being added, each in the right place, until the finished product is complete. By contrast, subtractive processes in development resemble the sculpting of a statue from a block of stone, with bits of stone being chipped away until the finished statue remains. Although embryologists have traditionally emphasized additive processes, subtractive processes are involved in the development of practically all biological systems (Glucksman, 1951). During brain development, additive processes determine the broad outline of neuronal organization, with subtractive processes playing a key role in subsequent fine-tuning (Cowan *et al.*, 1984).

For the sake of simplicity, brain development can be divided into a number of overlapping phases (see Sidman & Rakic, 1973; Ebels, 1980). In the human embryo, the initial formation of the neural tube and its derivatives is largely completed by the fifth postconceptual week. Subsequently, cellular proliferation within germinal zones generates neuronal and glial precursors. For example, the cells of the cerebral cortex arise from the subependymal germinal layer surrounding the lateral ventricles. After the completion of the proliferative phase, neuronal losses cannot be made good by additional proliferation. In man, the proliferative phase that gives rise to the cerebral cortex is complete long before birth, while the corresponding proliferative phase in the cerebellum continues well into infancy. Soon after their creation, neuronal precursors migrate away from the germinal zone, lose their motility, and differentiate into specific types of neurones. This phase overlaps with the phase of cellular proliferation, with neurones that were produced early in the proliferative phase having completed their migration long before the proliferative phase comes to an end. Further elaboration of axons and dendrites leads to a progressive growth in the number of synapses. In humans, much of this further elaboration occurs after birth. In the prefrontal cortex, for example, the pyramidal cells may increase their dendritic length tenfold or more in the first six postnatal months (Schade & van Groenigen, 1961).

Subtractive processes lag behind additive processes. In many neuronal systems, roughly half of the original neurones die off during a well-defined period that is characteristic of each neuronal population (see Cowan *et al.*, 1984). In addition, many of the axonal collaterals (branches) of surviving neurones are eliminated during the course of development (see Cowan *et al.*, 1984). Selective neuronal and axonal death is mediated, in part, by competition for essential trophic factors that are in short supply. Selective cell death may eliminate neurones that have formed erroneous connections, as well as helping to match the size of each neuronal population to the size of its target field. Selective elimination of some of the axonal collaterals of an individual neurone can increase the specificity of that neurone's connections (see Cowan *et al.*, 1984). Fine tuning by subtractive processes probably continues throughout childhood. In the human visual cortex, for example, synaptic density reaches a peak in the first year of life and then progressively declines until early adolescence, presumably as a result of subtractive processes (Huttenlocher *et al.*, 1982). In the human prefrontal cortex, peak synaptic density is not achieved until the second year of life, with the subsequent decline in synaptic density continuing until late adolescence (Huttenlocher, 1979). In addition to the synapses that physically disappear, other synapses remain in place but become functionally disconnected – the so-called 'latent synapses' (Wall, 1977). Since these fine-tuning processes continue after birth, they can potentially adjust brain organization in accordance with the individual's postnatal experiences (as discussed in more detail below).

Although this simple outline of successive and overlapping phases of brain development applies to all parts of the brain, different neuronal systems progress through the sequence at different rates. The cerebellar cortex, for example, passes through the phases of proliferation and migration more slowly than the cerebral cortex (Sidman & Rakic, 1973). It is also likely that different regions of the cerebral cortex mature at different rates (though Rakic *et al.* (1986) have presented some contrary evidence). As described above, for example, synaptic density peaks and then declines substantially earlier in the human visual cortex than in the human prefrontal cortex. Similarly, dendritic growth occurs much earlier in the human visual cortex (Takashima *et al.*, 1980) than in the human prefrontal cortex (Schade & van Groenigen, 1961). These differences in rates of histological maturation seem to mirror differences in rates of functional maturation, with human infants acquiring considerable visual competence long before they master tasks that depend, at least in other primates, on the prefrontal cortex (Banks & Salapatek, 1983; Diamond, 1989).

SEX DIFFERENCES

Boys are more vulnerable than girls to practically all developmental disorders. The only possible exception is mild mental handicap, where a male excess has been found in some series (e.g. Hagberg *et al.*, 1981) but not in others (e.g. Broman *et al.*, 1987). It is likely that several biological factors contribute to male vulnerability. Some of the male excess in severe mental handicap can be attributed to sex-linked recessive disorders such as the Lesch–Nyhan syndrome. In other instances, male vulnerability may reflect the slower tempo of male development (Taylor & Ounsted, 1972). Since each phase of development takes longer, boys are vulnerable for longer to any factors that disrupt that phase of development. This longer vulnerable period puts boys at greater overall risk than girls. In addition, sex hormones affect the pattern of brain development in some experimental animals (e.g. Raisman & Field, 1973; Diamond, 1987; Gorski, 1988), and possibly in humans too (e.g. Swaab & Hofman, 1988). Geschwind & Galaburda (1985) have suggested that the male excess of developmental disorders affecting speech, language and reading can be attributed to prenatal testosterone interfering with the proliferative processes that generate the language-related areas of the left cerebral hemisphere. Whereas this theory emphasizes possible effects of testosterone on additive processes in brain development, a recent modification of the theory focuses instead on possible effects of testosterone on subtractive processes in brain development. In the light of a reanalysis of earlier data, Galaburda *et al.* (1987) have suggested that the main action of testosterone is to reduce neuronal and axonal death. Whereas the original theory invoked left-sided proliferative failure to explain instances when language-related areas of cortex were not larger on the left than on the right side of the brain, the new theory explains the same phenomenon in terms of an abnormal lack of selective cell death in the right hemisphere.

SENSITIVE PERIODS AND THE EARLY ENVIRONMENT

In the age of the computer, it is very tempting to use computer analogies when discussing the brain and behaviour. Neuronal organization can be likened to the 'hardware' of silicon chips and magnetic disks, while learned behaviours can be likened to the 'software' of computer programs. Although such analogies may be helpful, they can sometimes be misleading. For example, whereas the hardware of a contemporary computer is not altered by the information it processes, the hardware of a brain can be. In some instances, an individual's early experiences have lasting consequences for neuronal organization.

The relationship between brain development and environmental experience has been extensively studied in experimental animals. The effect of monocular deprivation on the development of a rhesus monkey's primary visual cortex provides one of the clearest instances of the way that brain development can be affected by postnatal experience (see Wiesel, 1982). In the primary visual cortex of a normal juvenile or adult monkey, the number of neurones driven mainly or exclusively by the left eye roughly equals the number of neurones driven mainly or exclusively by the right eye. If just one eye is kept closed for a long period during adulthood (by suturing the eyelids shut on that side), this monocular deprivation does not result in long-term changes in the pattern of ocular preference of the neurones in the visual cortex. By contrast, if a monkey is monocularly deprived as a juvenile, there are marked changes in the pattern of ocular preference in the visual cortex, with the great majority of cells eventually being driven exclusively or mainly by the eye that remained open. Major changes can be induced by relatively brief periods of monocular deprivation in early infancy. During later infancy, comparable changes can only be induced by more prolonged periods of monocular deprivation. Evidently, there is a period in early life when the pattern of ocular dominance is particularly sensitive to monocular deprivation. This sensitivity declines as development proceeds, being lost altogether by adulthood. The changes in neuronal organization induced by early monocular deprivation are permanent if the eye remains closed throughout the sensitive period, but these changes can be reversed, at least partially, if the eye is opened again before the end of the sensitive period. In cats, cortical plasticity can artificially be restored after the end of the sensitive period by local cortical perfusion with noradrenaline (Kasamatsu *et al.*, 1979).

The neuronal reorganization invoked by early monocular deprivation is primarily mediated by changes in subtractive rather than additive processes (Wiesel, 1982). When one eye is closed in early infancy, the geniculostriate axons that carry information from the closed eye to the cortex are more heavily 'pruned' than normal, while the axons from the open eye are less heavily pruned than normal (and may sprout extra collaterials as well). Ascending noradrenergic and cholinergic systems, arising from the locus coeruleus and basal forebrain respectively, modulate cortical plasticity to monocular deprivation (Bear & Singer, 1986). Experience-dependent modifications in the visual cortex probably occur primarily at excitatory axospinous synapses, where axon terminals releasing glutamic acid (or a closely related excitatory neurotransmitter) meet dendritic spines (Bear *et al.*, 1987). The plasticity of these axospinous synapses may be governed by calcium ion flow into the dendritic spine, regulated by the type of post-synaptic glutamate receptor known as the 'NMDA receptor' (Bear *et al.*, 1987). The modulatory role of noradrenaline may be mediated by cyclic-AMP mediated changes in the phosphorylation of cytoskeletal proteins (Aoki & Siekevitz, 1985).

The term 'sensitive period' (or 'critical period') refers to the developmental stage when brain organization is most easily affected by the nature of an individual's experiences. Different brain systems, and different functions of the same system, have different sensitive periods (Harwerth *et al.*, 1986). There is clinical evidence in humans for a sensitive period during which monocular deprivation is particularly damaging (Vaegan & Taylor, 1979; Birch & Stager, 1988). There is also suggestive evidence for a sensitive period in the development of auditory discrimination (Werker & Tees, 1984). Thus at the age of 6 months, infants from English-speaking families can recognize phonetic distinctions that are important in Hindi but not in English. By the end of their first year, however, these infants are no longer able to recognize phonetic distinctions that are unimportant in their native language. It seems likely that infants are born with the innate neural pathways to make many phonetic discriminations, with those pathways that are little used (because the relevant contrasts are unimportant in the infant's native language) being selectively eliminated by about 12 months.

Given the persuasive circumstantial evidence that humans have sensitive periods for visual and auditory perception, it seems reasonable to wonder whether there are sensitive periods for some human 'higher functions' as well. If there are sensitive periods in early life for language, social skill, intelligence, and other 'higher functions', specific sorts of environmental deprivation or adversity during early life should result in permanent deficits, even if the individual subsequently experiences a satisfactory rearing environment. There is limited evidence both for and against this intriguing possibility. On the negative side, longitudinal studies have demonstrated that early adversity has remarkably few long-term consequences if the individual subsequently experiences a normal environment (see Rutter, 1981, 1987). As discussed below, however, there are exceptions to this rule, and these exceptions could reflect the existence of sensitive periods. The findings of behavioural genetics also suggest that early experiences have a relatively limited influence on personality development – with children who grow up together being hardly more similar, on many measures of personality, than would be predicted on genetic grounds alone, suggesting that 'shared environment' (including shared early deprivation or adversity) has relatively little impact (see Plomin & Daniels, 1987). It is possible, however, that behavioural geneticists have underestimated the true impact of shared environment (see Goodman, 1991).

Studies of late adoption provide a particularly good window on the possible long-term consequences of early experiences. It is noteworthy, for example, that in Hodges & Tizard's (1989) longitudinal study, adopted children developed well in most respects despite having spent their early years in institutional care. Despite this generally satisfactory outcome, there were some indications that early adversity can have lasting sequelae, possibly as a result of sensitive period effects. Thus adoption between the ages of 2 and $4\frac{1}{2}$ years was characteristically followed by a dramatic and sustained rise in IQ, averaging about 20 points, whereas the mean IQ of the children who were adopted after the age of $4\frac{1}{2}$ years hardly rose at all. Hodges & Tizard suggest a variety of psychological explanations for this curious finding, but they do not consider a neurological explanation – that there is a sensitive period for the development of the neural underpinnings of intelligence. According to this neurobiological hypothesis, the sensitive period lasts until roughly the age of 5 years, so that placement in a favourable environment before the end of this period can prevent or reverse at least some of the neuronal changes induced by early deprivation. By contrast, if adoption is delayed until after the end of the sensitive period, the neuronal changes induced by early deprivation are irreversible, however favourable the new environment.

Whereas the Hodges & Tizard (1989) study suggests that a sensitive period for intellectual development, if it exists, probably lasts until the age of 5 years or so, the same study provides some circumstantial evidence for a sensitive period for attentiveness that ends well before the age of 5 years. Goldfarb (1944) described prominent hyperactivity in institutionalized children. In the Hodges & Tizard sample, the psychiatric outcome of the adopted ex-institutional children was generally favourable, but even the children adopted before the age of $4\frac{1}{2}$ years had more problems with restlessness and inattention than a group of matched controls, both at 8 and 16 years of age. This persistent hyperactivity, despite more than a decade in favourable family circumstances, is a striking finding. One possible explanation is that the children's biological parents passed on a genetic predisposition to hyperactivity. Alternatively, the attentional problems of the ex-institutional children could reflect the existence of a sensitive period in the development of attention, with institutional care for the first two years or so resulting in lasting damage to the neuronal underpinnings of attention. Studies of maternal depression demonstrate that early environmental factors can influence contemporary attentional skills. Thus

Breznitz & Friedman (1988) found that depressed mothers were poor at sustaining a shared focus of attention with their children – an effect that was probably partly responsible for the children's impaired attention. Institutional care, like maternal depression, may deprive infants and toddlers of opportunities to practise sustained attention. Hodges & Tizard's data are compatible with the notion that this sort of deprivation during the first two or three years of life permanently impairs the neural systems involved in the control of activity and attention.

Since maternal depression can affect a toddler's concentration, it is noteworthy that in Richman *et al.*'s (1982) longitudinal study of a community sample of children, maternal depression when the child was 3 years was a particularly powerful predictor of specific reading retardation when the child was 8 years, and a somewhat less powerful predictor of psychiatric disorder when the child was 8 years. It is striking that 8-year-old outcome was more closely related to maternal depression when the child was 3 years than to maternal depression when the child was 8 years. These findings could be explained by a sensitive period in the development of attention. By depriving an infant or toddler of opportunities to practise sustained attention, early maternal depression may have permanently impaired the development of the neurological systems involved in attention, thereby rendering the child more vulnerable to subsequent academic and psychiatric problems. According to this line of thought, later maternal depression would not have the same consequences because environmental factors do not affect the development of the neural underpinnings of attention after the end of the sensitive period at around the age of 2 or 3 years.

While these speculations about sensitive periods in the development of intelligence and attention are unproven, they do illustrate an interesting and largely unexplored way of conceptualizing the link between early adversity and subsequent development. Although this section has focused on intellectual and attentional development, the existence of sensitive periods could potentially be relevant to some aspects of social and linguistic development as well (see Goodman, 1987).

RECOVERY FROM EARLY BRAIN DAMAGE

Since developmental disorders are particularly common among children with congenital or early-acquired brain damage (Rutter *et al.*, 1970), it is appropriate to review the effects of early injury on brain development. Although recovery from early brain damage can be remarkably good, the high rate of developmental disorders after early damage demonstrates that functional recovery is often incomplete or delayed. It is relevant, therefore, to consider the neural mechanisms involved in recovery, and the factors that influence the degree of recovery. This section provides a brief overview of these important topics, which are reviewed in greater detail elsewhere (Finger & Stein, 1982; Goodman, 1987).

One of the most important factors influencing the degree of recovery from brain damage is how early the brain damage occurs. For some specific skills and abilities, recovery is much better after early brain damage than after comparable later damage. What does 'early' mean in this context? The answer appears to depend partly on whether the damage is bilateral or unilateral. Judging primarily from animal experiments, good recovery from bilaterally symmetrical damage is unlikely unless the damage is sustained very early in development. In monkeys, for example, prenatal damage to the dorsolateral portion of the prefrontal cortex results in little or no long-term impairment, whereas comparable damage in infancy or adulthood results in marked long-term impairment in delayed-response learning (Goldman-Rakic *et al.*, 1983). In this instance at least, early bilateral damage only has a better outcome if it occurs very early indeed. If similar limitations apply to humans, one implication is that recovery from bilaterally symmetrical brain damage (caused, for example, by severe closed head injury) will be roughly as poor after childhood injury as after adult injury. The persistence of 'frontal lobe' symptoms, such as social disinhibition, after severe closed head injuries in childhood supports this gloomy prediction (Brown *et al.*, 1981).

While recovery from bilateral damage may be as poor in children as in adults, different considerations seem to apply to unilateral damage. In particular, when a skill is normally lateralized to one hemisphere, that skill may develop remarkably normally if just one cerebral hemisphere is damaged in early life – even when the skill is normally mediated to the hemisphere that has been damaged. Language acquisition provides the clearest example (see Goodman, 1987). In most individuals, language skills depend principally on the left hemisphere (see Bradshaw & Nettleton, 1983; Springer & Deutsch, 1985). If the left hemisphere is damaged prenatally or during infancy, the individual with an intact right hemisphere can still acquire language that is normal or nearly normal (Smith & Sugar, 1975; Dennis & Whitaker, 1977; Woods & Carey, 1979; Vargha-Khadem *et al.* 1985). When the left hemisphere is damaged in somewhat older children, persistent language deficits are more likely, though these too may be relatively subtle (Woods & Carey, 1979). After puberty, the capacity for left-to-right transfer is still present in some individuals (see Kinsbourne, 1971), but is generally less dramatic than after early brain-damage. It would seem, then, that as brain development progresses, the right hemisphere generally becomes less able to take over the skills that are normally lateralized to the left hemisphere. Conversely, the left hemisphere becomes progressively less able to take over right-hemisphere functions such as visuospatial reasoning (Woods, 1980).

Bringing together the findings on recovery from bilateral and unilateral damage, it seems helpful to distinguish at least three developmental epochs: prenatal life and early infancy; childhood from late infancy to puberty; and adulthood. The acquisition of specific skills may be remarkably normal after either bilateral or unilateral damage during prenatal life or early infancy. During the rest of childhood, recovery from bilateral damage may be just as poor as in adults, whereas recovery from unilateral damage can be much better than in adults. After puberty both bilateral and unilateral damage are likely to result in lasting deficits in specific skills, though some degree of recovery is probably the rule rather than the exception.

The existence of three main epochs can plausibly be explained in terms of underlying neuronal processes. When a brain region is destroyed bilaterally, the functions of the damaged region may be taken over by other regions of the brain. In cats, for example, the parietal lobes can take over some visual functions when the occipital lobes are damaged (Spear, 1979). For good functional recovery, a shift of this sort is likely to require major reorganization of the undamaged portions of the brain. In animal studies, extensive changes in neuronal organization can be induced only by very early lesions (Schneider, 1979; Spear, 1979; Goldman-Rakic *et al.*, 1983). Although these changes may be mediated, in part, by additive processes such as axonal sprouting or re-routing, the recent literature has particularly emphasized the role of damage-induced modifications in subtractive processes, with the sparing of connections that would ordinarily have been eliminated. During childhood, when the basic pattern of neuronal connections is already well established, there may be relatively little scope for substantial reorganization in response to brain damage. Though this may seriously limit recovery from bilateral damage, different considerations seem to apply to recovery from unilateral damage. Shifting a function from a damaged area of one hemisphere to the corresponding area on the other side (e.g. from damaged left temporal lobe to intact right temporal lobe) may not require major neuronal reorganization. Perhaps the normal direction of asymmetry can be reversed by relatively minor changes in the fine-tuning processes that continue throughout childhood. This would explain why the capacity for left-to-right and right-to-left transfer progressively diminishes throughout childhood as the phase of selective axonal pruning moves towards completion.

Although localized brain damage is less likely to result in specific deficits, such as aphasia, when the damage is sustained early in life, early damage is more likely to result in a general lowering of intellectual and scholastic ability (e.g. Rutter *et al.*, 1984). Intuitively, it is tempting to suppose that this loss of intellectual and scholastic 'power' is due to crowding too many functions into too little remaining brain. This simple view is challenged by well-authenticated instances of excellent intellectual and academic outcome after extensive early brain damage (e.g. Smith & Sugar, 1975). Three alternative explanations deserve consideration. Firstly, early localized damage may commonly be accompanied by diffuse generalized damage as well. Secondly, if brain injury disrupts new learning more than it disrupts the retention of previously acquired skills (Hebb, 1942), this effect will inevitably be more handicapping to the individual whose brain damage occurs early in life, before many learned skills have been acquired. Thirdly, animal studies have demonstrated that the neuronal reorganization induced by very early damage can have disadvantages. In some instances, the new connections induced by early brain damage are misconnections that have maladaptive behavioural consequences (Schneider, 1979). This lends some support to the notion that early brain damage in humans can induce widespread misconnections, resulting in irrelevant information ('noise)' being channelled between neurones that would not normally be connected, and thereby disrupting concentration, problem solving and new learning (Goodman, 1989b).

By comparison with the adult brain, the developing brain is both more resilient and more vulnerable to brain damage. As described above, the outcome for specific skills is sometimes better after early damage, whereas the outcome for general intelligence and academic ability is often worse. The developing brain's mixture of resilience and vulnerability applies to susceptibility to brain insults as well as to outcome after brain injury. For example, the newborn brain is particularly vulnerable to herpes simplex infections, but is relatively resistant to anoxia.

To summarize so far, the degree of recovery from brain damage is influenced by a complex interaction of three factors: the age at which the damage was sustained; whether the damage was unilateral or bilateral; and whether the outcome measures emphasize specific skills or general abilities. Several other factors also need to be considered. Even when the focus is on specific skills, there are important differences between skills. For example, whereas the earlier the lesions the better the long-term outcome for language, the same is not true for motor skills (Passingham *et al.*, 1983), contrary to the earlier claims of Kennard (1942).

The degree of recovery from brain injury is also influenced by whether the injury occurs suddenly or gradually. In general, when brain damage occurs gradually, as a result of a slowly expanding lesion or a succession of small injuries, the degree of recovery is greater than when the same amount of damage has occurred suddenly (see Finger & Stein, 1982). By implication, recovery from damage to one hemisphere due to an open head injury may well be less complete than recovery from comparable brain damage due to a slowly expanding abscess or benign tumour.

Finally, the degree of recovery may be affected by whether a region of the brain is totally or partially destroyed. Intuitively, it seems likely that recovery after brain damage will be greater when the area of cortex subserving some particular function is partly spared rather than completely destroyed. This is true in some cases, but animal studies suggest that recovery from early damage is sometimes better after total rather than partial destruction (Carlson, 1984), perhaps because partial destruction interferes with successful reorganization.

UNILATERAL BRAIN ABNORMALITIES AND DEVELOPMENTAL DISORDERS

Asymmetries at various levels of the nervous system have been documented in all vertebrate groups (see Geschwind & Galaburda, 1985). The human cerebral hemispheres provide a particularly striking instance of asymmetrical specialization (see Bradshaw & Nettleton, 1983; Springer & Deutsch, 1985). Several general principles can usefully be extracted from the extensive literature on cerebral asymmetry in adults (see Goodman, 1987). Firstly, both hemispheres are specialized. In a typical right-handed adult, for example, speech depends primarily on the left hemisphere, while face recognition depends primarily on the right hemisphere. Secondly, a major skill may involve component subskills that are lateralized in opposite directions. In the case of communicative skill, for example, the left hemisphere specializes in the grammatical and semantic aspects of language, while the right hemisphere specializes in non-verbal communication by tone of voice, facial expression and gesture. Thirdly, lateral specialization is more often a matter of degree than an all-or-nothing phenomenon. Thus, although the left hemisphere is more specialized in the grammatical and semantic aspects of language, the right hemisphere does have some linguistic capabilities even in these domains. Finally, the degree of lateralization varies between skills and between people.

Although most studies of lateralization have focused on adults, three lines of evidence suggest that hemispheric asymmetry is present in children too (see Kinsbourne & Hiscock, 1983). Firstly, anatomical studies have demonstrated that hemispheric asymmetry arises very early in development. For example, the planum temporale, which is a language-related region of cerebral cortex, is already generally larger on the left side than the right at 29 weeks of gestation (Wada *et al.*, 1975).

Functional studies of normal infants and children provide a second line of evidence for early asymmetries. For instance, cortical evoked responses suggest that the left hemisphere is differentially sensitive to speech sounds even in premature babies (Molfese & Molfese, 1980). Clinical studies of brain-damaged children provide a third line of evidence. From the time language is first acquired, right-hemisphere lesions seem much less likely to produce aphasia than left-hemisphere lesions (Woods & Teuber, 1978). Given this evidence that hemispheric asymmetry dates back to fetal life, the better long-term outcome for language after early left-sided damage than after comparable later damage must clearly be attributed to the developing brain being better at respecialization after injury – and not to the developing brain being unspecialized prior to injury, as used to be taught.

Since hemispheric asymmetry dates back to prenatal life, it is conceivable that early unilateral damage leads to a failure to acquire side-specific skills, just as unilateral damage later in life leads to a loss of side-specific skills. It has been suggested, for example, that congenital abnormalities of the left hemisphere may result in developmental language or reading disorders in much the same way that later injuries to the left hemisphere may result in acquired language or reading disorders (Geschwind & Galaburda, 1985). Similarly, congenital abnormalities of the right hemisphere might lead to a failure to acquire proficiency in non-verbal communication, just as later injuries to the right hemisphere can result in the loss of non-verbal communication skills (Weintraub & Mesulam, 1983). The most obvious objection to these theories is that most children with congenital lesions of just one hemisphere do remarkably well, even when the damage is extensive. As described in the previous section, for example, most children with congenital damage to their left hemisphere have little or no problem with language acquisition. This is clearly a powerful argument against any theory attributing a developmental disorder to unilateral damage. Nevertheless, there are at least four reasons for not dismissing unilateral theories entirely. Firstly, as discussed above, early unilateral damage leads to the long-term sparing of some skills but not others. Secondly, partial damage or dysfunction may be more disruptive of skill acquisition than extensive destruction. Thirdly, there is marked individual variation in most biological capabilities, and there is no reason to suppose that this does not apply to the capacity for the intact hemisphere to take over after early unilateral damage. Finally, the finding that schizophrenia is much commoner after early lesions of the left rather than the right temporal lobe (Taylor, 1975; Ounsted *et al.*, 1987) demonstrates that the laterality of early-acquired brain abnormalities can have striking developmental consequences.

Putting aside these theoretical issues, the empirical evidence for laterality theories of developmental disorders is weak, being derived from a handful of small studies of selected and arguably unrepresentative samples. Galaburda *et al.* (1985) have reported four consecutive cases of dyslexia who came to autopsy, with detailed neuropathological examination revealing patchy areas of cortical dysplasia in each case, particularly affecting language-related areas of the left hemisphere. Both Weintraub & Mesulam (1983) and Voeller (1986) have published small clinical series supporting the notion of a behavioural syndrome due to developmental disorders of the right hemisphere. In both series, congenital or early-acquired abnormalities of the right hemisphere were inferred from clinical or radiological features, with these features being suggestive rather than conclusive in roughly half the cases. In both series, the cases had a characteristic pattern of psychological deficits: poor visuospatial skills; problems with arithmetic; impaired non-verbal communication; interpersonal difficulties; and, in Voeller's series only, attentional deficits. It is worth noting that, judging from case histories, some of the cases would almost certainly have warranted a diagnosis of Asperger's syndrome – a developmental disorder akin to autism (Wing, 1981). Finally, in one small clinical series of children with temporal lobe epilepsy (Stores, 1977), boys with a left-sided focus were more hyperactive than boys with a right-sided focus – findings that were not replicated in girls. Although these various findings are interesting and suggestive, the case for a link between developmental disorders and unilateral abnormalities is far from proven. Consider hyperactivity, for example. A link with right-sided abnormalities was present in Voeller's (1986) series but not in Weintraub & Mesulam's (1983), while a link with left-sided abnormalities was present in Stores' (1977) series, but only for boys. To add to this confusion, the rate of hyperactivity was not apparently influenced by the laterality of damage in several large studies of brain-damaged children (Ingram, 1955, 1956; Ounsted, 1955; Rutter *et al.*, 1970, 1984). The zeitgeist is favourable to laterality explanations, but the supporting evidence is weak.

ATYPICAL CEREBRAL LATERALIZATION AND DEVELOPMENTAL DISORDERS

The two hemispheres are reciprocally specialized. In most individuals, the left hemisphere is particularly specialized in language functions and hand control, while the right hemisphere is particularly specialized in visuospatial functions. In these circumstances, the left hemisphere is sometimes described as the 'dominant hemisphere', though this terminology does little justice to the fact that the right hemisphere predominates in some domains. A substantial minority of the general population have an 'atypical' pattern of cerebral lateralization. In left-handed individuals, for example, language and hand-control commonly lateralize to opposite hemispheres, while language and visuospatial functions may lateralize to the same hemisphere (see Geschwind & Galaburda, 1985). For over half a century, clinicians and researchers have speculated that developmental disorders can be due to incomplete or atypical patterns of cerebral lateralization (e.g. Orton, 1937; Geschwind & Galaburda, 1985). As the most obvious marker for atypical lateralization, left-handedness has attracted particular attention. Left-handedness is over-represented in severe mental handicap, mild mental handicap and autism (Tsai & Stewart, 1982; Soper *et al.*, 1986; Broman *et al.*, 1987). In other instances, a link with left-handedness is more controversial. For example, Geschwind & Behan (1984) reported a striking association between left-handness and developmental reading problems, while no such link emerged from the Isle of Wight study (Rutter & Yule, 1970).

Left-handedness is common, being found in roughly 10% of the general population in a variety of cultures (Oldfield, 1971; Teng *et al.*, 1977; Silverberg *et al.*, 1979). In order to make sense of links between left-handedness and developmental disorders, it is helpful to distinguish between pathological left-handedness, which is relatively rare, and ordinary left-handedness, which is common. Pathological left-handedness arises when damage to the left hemisphere converts someone who would otherwise have developed into a right-hander into a left-hander instead (Satz, 1972). For example, in the extreme case of individuals whose left hemispheres have been extensively and severely damaged before birth, all the individuals become left-handed although about 90% would have become right-handed had they not been brain-damaged. Among individuals with extensive bilateral brain damage, hand control is likely to be poor on both sides, sometimes affecting the left hand worse than the right, but almost equally often affecting the right hand worse than the left. Consequently, the rate of left-handedness is increased by bilateral as well as by left-hemisphere damage. As a result, any developmental disorder that is commonly associated with diffuse or patchy brain abnormalities is almost bound to be associated with an increased rate of pathological left-handedness. A link between left-handedness and a developmental disorder does not prove that atypical lateralization causes the developmental disorder. It is always important to consider the alternative possibility that the developmental disorder and the high rate of left-handedness are independent manifestations of underlying brain abnormalities.

Whereas pathological left-handedness reflects brain damage, ordinary left-handedness reflects genetic predisposition. The familial transmission of left-handedness is well illustrated by the fact that roughly half of the offspring of two left-handed parents are themselves left-handed (Annett,

1983). The most widely accepted genetic model is the 'right shift' theory of Annett (1985). This model postulates a single gene locus with two alleles, that can be represented rs+ and rs−. In the general population, rs+ is commoner than rs−. In the common homozygote (rs++), language and handedness are typically strongly lateralized to the left hemisphere. In the rarer homozygote (rs−−), the degree of lateralization is weaker, both for handedness and for language functions, and the direction of lateralization is equally likely to be to the left or to the right hemisphere. In the heterozygote (rs+−), handedness and language are typically, but not invariably, moderately strongly lateralized to the left hemisphere. The existence of a balanced polymorphism for right- and left-handedness in a variety of populations suggests a heterozygote advantage (as in the case of the sickle-cell polymorphism). If so, individuals who are moderately right-handed (typically due to a rs+− genotype) should be at an advantage compared with individuals who are either left-handed (typically due to a rs−− genotype) or strongly right-handed (typically due to a rs++ genotype). There is now some preliminary evidence that this is so. For example, in a clinic sample of children with developmental reading disorders, there was an over-representation of individuals who were either left-handed or strongly right-handed (Annett & Kilshaw, 1984). An excess of poor readers among both left-handers and strong right-handers has also been found in a recent community survey of schoolchildren aged between 6 and 12 years (Annett & Manning, 1990). It is worth noting, however, that moderate or weak lateralization will not invariably be beneficial. In particular, individuals who have weak or ambiguous handedness due to bilateral brain abnormalities are likely to be at a particularly high risk of developmental disorders. Whereas the link between pathological left-handedness (or pathological mixed-handedness) and developmental disorders probably reflects a shared origin in widespread brain damage, the studies of Annett and her colleagues suggest that the link between ordinary left-handedness (or strong right-handedness) and developmental disorders may be causal, with the degree and direction of cerebral lateralization influencing the rate and pattern of psychological development.

NEUROPATHOLOGICAL MODELS OF DEVELOPMENTAL DISORDERS

In the light of our current knowledge of brain development, it is possible to construct a wide variety of alternative neuropathological models for the developmental disorders. Unfortunately, our capacity for conjecture far outstrips our capacity for refutation. If developmental disorders arise from relatively subtle abnormalities in neuronal organization, these abnormalities will be hard to detect with our current investigative techniques. Few children with well-documented developmental disorders come to autopsy, and existing neuro-imaging techniques can only detect relatively gross abnormalities of structure or function. Neuropsychological and neurophysiological techniques may be more sensitive to subtle changes in neuronal organization, but the interpretation of abnormal test results can be problematic. Abnormalities may simply reflect the developmental disorder without providing any additional clues to the putative neurological underpinnings. For example, if the late components of the visual evoked response (VER) were abnormal in hyperactive children, would this point to neuronal abnormalities in the visual system, or would it simply reflect the children's lack of attention to visual stimuli? Similarly, if an individual with a developmental language disorder obtains an uneven profile on a neuropsychological test battery, does this reflect localized brain damage, or does it simply mean that scores on language-related items are, not surprisingly, more impaired than scores on items unrelated to language?

If neuropathological models are to be useful, they should be testable and clinically relevant. With the techniques currently at our disposal, it is only possible to devise tests for crude and relatively implausible models. To illustrate the potential value of neuropathological models, it is worth considering two simple (and simplistic) models that attribute mental handicap to failures in additive and subtractive processes respectively.

The first model assumes that a widespread failure in the proliferative phase results in a substantially reduced number of neurones in all parts of the brain. Assuming all other phases of neuronal development progress normally, the result will be a scaled-down brain. By comparison with a normal individual of the same age, an individual with a scaled-down brain would probably be less skilled at a wide range of cognitive tasks (in much the same way that, other things being equal, small computers are less powerful than large computers). Although the reasoning skill of the child with a scaled-down brain would be lower than average, the skill would nevertheless be increasing with age because of progressive fine-tuning of the brain by normal subtractive processes.

An alternative model assumes that additive processes and selective cell loss proceed normally, and that the only abnormality in brain development is a slow and incomplete process of axonal and synaptic 'pruning', resulting in a brain that is over-connected by comparison with a normal brain of the same age. This failure in fine tuning, with an accompanying impairment in signal-to-noise ratio, could plausibly impair computational power. Although the problem-solving ability of the child with an over-connected brain is likely to be below average, that ability would nevertheless increase with age as fine tuning progressed (albeit slowly and incompletely).

The over-connected brain is anatomically and physiologically immature, with a degree of subtractive fine-tuning that corresponds to that of a younger normal child. By contrast, the scaled-down brain is of normal anatomical and physiological maturity, with an age-appropriate degree of subtractive fine-tuning. These differences may be reflected in neurophysiological measures. For example, the early components of the flash-evoked VER may have immature wave-forms in individuals with over-connected brains, but age-appropriate wave-forms in individuals with scaled-down brains.

Differences between the two models could potentially explain some of the heterogeneity in the psychiatric accompaniments of mental handicap. For example, in an individual with an over-connected brain, the poor signal-to-noise ratio may result in attentional deficits and hyperactivity. One prediction, then, is that the prevalence of hyperactivity will be higher in a group of children with over-connected brains (as gauged by the VER) than in an IQ-matched group of children with scaled-down brains. Since flash-evoked VERs do not require an individual's active co-operation or attention (Harden, 1982), the use of VERs to distinguish between individuals with over-connected and scaled-down brains would not be invalidated by different rates of hyperactivity in the two groups.

The two models of mental handicap are undoubtedly simplistic. They have been described to demonstrate that neuropathological models of the developmental disorders can potentially be both testable and clinically relevant. Future advances in the neurosciences should make more sophisticated, and correspondingly more plausible, models testable too. It will be up to us to grasp those opportunities.

REFERENCES

American Psychiatric Association (1987) *Diagnostic and statistical manual of the mental disorders*, 3rd edn, revised. Washington D. C.: APA Press.

Annett, M. (1983) Hand preference and skill in 115 children of two left-handed parents. *British Journal of Psychology*, **74**, 17–32.

Annett, M. (1985) *Left, right, hand and brain: the right shift theory.* London: Lawrence Erlbaum Associates.

Annett, M. & Kilshaw, D. (1984) Lateral preference and skill in dyslexics: implications of the right shift theory. *Journal of Child Psychology and Psychiatry*, **25**, 357–77.

Annett, M. & Manning, M. (1990) Reading and a balanced polymorphism for laterality and ability. *Journal of Child Psychology and Psychiatry*, **31**, 511–29.

Antell, S. E. G. & Caron, A. J. (1985) Neonatal perception of spatial relationships. *Infant Behavior and Development*, **8**, 15–23.

Aoki, C. & Siekevitz, P. (1985) Ontogenetic changes in the cyclic adenosine 3′, 5′-monophosphate-stimulable phosphorylation of cat visual cortex proteins, particularly of microtuble-associated protein 2 (MAP2): effects of normal and dark rearing and of the exposure to light. *Journal of Neuroscience*, **5**, 2465–83.

Banks, M. S. & Salapatek, P. (1983) Infant visual perception. In Haith, M. M. & Campos, J. J. (eds.) *Mussen's handbook of child psychology*, 4th edn, vol. II, *Infancy and developmental psychobiology*. New York: Wiley, pp. 435–571.

Bear, M. F., Cooper, L. N. & Ebner, F. F. (1987) A physiological basis for a theory of synapse modification. *Science*, **237**, 42–8.

Bear, M. F. & Singer, W. (1986) Acetylcholine, noradrenaline and the extrathalamic modulation of visual cortical plasticity. *Nature*, **320**, 172–6.

Birch, E. E. & Stager, D. R. (1988) Prevalence of good visual acutiy following surgery for congenital unilateral cataract. *Archives of Ophthalmology*, **106**, 40–3.

Bishop, D. V. M. & Edmundson, A. (1987) Specific language impairment as a maturational lag: evidence from longitudinal data on language and motor development. *Developmental Medicine and Child Neurology*, **29**, 442–59.

Bradshaw, J. L. & Nettleton, N. C. (1983) *Human cerebral asymmetry*. Englewood Cliffs, N. J.: Prentice–Hall.

Brazelton, T. B. (1982) Joint regulation of neonate–parent behavior. In Tronick, E. Z. (ed.) *Social interchange in infancy: affect, cognition, and communication*. Baltimore: University Park Press, pp. 7–22.

Breznitz, Z. & Friedman, S. L. (1988) Toddlers' concentration: does maternal depression make a difference? *Journal of Child Psychology and Psychiatry*, **29**, 267–79.

Broman, S., Nichols, P. L., Shaughnessy, P. & Kennedy, W. (1987) *Retardation in young children: a developmental study of cognitive deficit*. Hillsdale, N. J.: Lawrence Erlbaum Associates.

Brown, G., Chadwick, O., Schaffer, D., Rutter, M. & Traub, M. (1981) A prospective study of children with head injuries: III. Psychiatric sequelae. *Psychological Medicine*, **11**, 63–78.

Bushnell, I. W. R., Sai, F. & Mullin, J. T. (1989) Neonatal recognition of the mother's face. *British Journal of Developmental Psychology*, **7**, 3–15.

Carlson, M. (1984) Development of tactile discrimination capacity in *Macaca mulatta*. III. Effects of total removal of primary sensory cortex (SmI) in infants and juveniles. *Developmental Brain Research*, **16**, 103–17.

Condon, W. C. & Sander, L. W. (1974) Neonatal movement is synchronized with adult speech: interactional participation and language acquisition. *Science*, **183**, 99–101.

Cowan, W. M., Fawcett, J. W., O'Leary, D. D. M. & Stanfield, B. B. (1984) Regressive events in neurogenesis. *Science*, **225**, 1258–65.

Dennis, M. & Whitaker, H. A. (1977) Hemispheric equipotentiality and language acquisition. In Segalowitz, S. J. & Gruber, F. A. (eds.) *Language development and neurological theory*. New York: Academic Press, pp. 93–106.

Diamond, A. (1989) Differences between adult and infant cognition: Is the crucial variable presence or absence of language? In Weiskrantz, L. (ed.) *Thought without language*. Oxford: Oxford University Press, pp. 337–70.

Diamond, M. C. (1987) Sexual differences in the rat forebrain. *Brain Research Reviews*, **12**, 235–40.

Ebels, E. J. (1980) Maturation of the central nervous system. In Rutter, M. (ed.) *Scientific foundations of developmental psychiatry*. London: Heinemann, pp. 25–39.

Field, T. M., Woodson, R., Greenberg, R. & Cohen, D. (1982) Discrimination and imitation of facial expression by neonates. *Science*, **218**, 179–81.

Fielder, A. R., Russel–Eggitt, I. R., Dodd, K. L. & Mellor, D. H. (1985) Delayed visual maturation. *Transactions of the Opthalmological Societies of the United Kingdom*, **104**, 653–61.

Finger, S. & Stein, D. G. (1982) *Brain damage and recovery: research and clinical perspectives*. New York: Academic Press.

Folstein, S. & Rutter, M. (1977) Infantile autism: a genetic study of 21 twin pairs. *Journal of Child Psychology and Psychiatry*, **18**, 297–321.

Galaburda, A. M., Corsiglia, J., Rosen, G. D. & Sherman, G. F. (1987) Planum temporale asymmetry, reappraisal since Geschwind and Levitsky. *Neuropsychologia*, **25**, 853–68.

Galaburda, A. M., Sherman, G. F., Rosen, G. D., Aboitiz, F. & Geschwind, N. (1985) Developmental dyslexia: four consecutive patients with cortical anomalies. *Annals of Neurology*, **18**, 222–33.

Garner, D. M. & Garfinkel, P. E. (1980) Socio-cultural factors in the development of anorexia nervosa. *Psychological Medicine*, **10**, 647–56.

Geschwind, N. & Behan, P. O. (1984) Laterality, hormones, and immunity. In Geschwind, N. & Galaburda, A. M. (eds.) *Cerebral dominance: the biological foundations*. Cambridge, Mass.: Harvard University Press, pp. 211–24.

Geschwind, N. & Galaburda, A. M. (1985) Cerebral lateralization: biological mechanisms, asssociations, and pathology: I. A hypothesis and a program for research. *Archives of Neurology*, **42**, 428–59.

Gillberg, C. & Gillberg, I. C. (1983) Infantile autism: a total population study of reduced optimality in the pre-, peri-, and neonatal period,. *Journal of Autism and Developmental Disorders*, **13**, 153–66.

Glucksman, A. (1951) Cell death in normal vertebrate ontogeny. *Biological Reviews*, **26**, 59–86.

Goldfarb, W. (1944) The effects of early institutional care on adolescent personality. *Journal of Experimental Education*, **12**, 106–29.

Goldman-Rakic, P. S., Isseroff, A., Schwartz, M. L. & Bugbee, N. M. (1983) The neurobiology of cognitive development. In Haith, M. M. & Campos, J. J. (eds.) *Mussen's handbook of child psychology*, 4th edn. Vol. II, *Infancy and developmental psychobiology*. New York: Wiley, pp. 281–344.

Goodman, R. (1987) The developmental neurobiology of language. In Yule, W. & Rutter, M. (eds.) *Language development and disorders. Clinics in developmental medicine, Nos. 101/102.* London: MacKeith Press/Blackwell, pp. 129–45.

Goodman, R. (1989a) Genetic factors in hyperactivity. *British Medical Journal*, **298**, 1407–8.

Goodman, R. (1989b) Neuronal misconnections and psychiatric disorder: is there a link? *British Journal of Psychiatry*, **154**, 292–9.

Goodman, R. (1990) Technical note: are perinatal complications causes or consequences of autism? *Journal of Child Psychology and Psychiatry*, **31**, 809–12.

Goodman, R. (1991) Growing together and growing apart: the non-genetic forces on children in the same family. In McGuffin, P. and Murray, R. (eds.) *The new genetics of mental illness.* Oxford: Heinemann Medical Books, pp. 212–24.

Goodman, R. & Ashby, L. (1990) Delayed visual maturation and autism. *Developmental Medicine and Child Neurology*, **32**, 814–9.

Goodman, R. & Stevenson, J. (1989) A twin study of hyperactivity: I. An examination of hyperactivity scores and categories derived from Rutter teacher and parent questionnaires. *Journal of Child Psychology and Psychiatry*, **30**, 671–89.

Gorski, R. A. (1988) Sexual differentiation of the brain: mechanisms and implications for neuroscience. In: Easter, S. S., Barald, K. F. & Carlson, B. M. (eds.) *From message to mind: directions in developmental neurobiology.* Sunderland, Mass.: Sinauer Associates, pp. 226–302.

Hagberg, B., Hagberg, G., Lewerth, A. & Linberg, U. (1981) Mild mental retardation in Swedish school children. *Acta Paediatrica Scandinavica*, **70**, 441–4.

Harden, A. (1982) Maturation of the visual evoked potentials. In Chiarenza, G. A. & Papakostopoulos, D. (eds.) *Clinical application of cerebral evoked potentials in pediatric medicine.* Amsterdam: Excerpta Medica, pp. 41–59.

Harwerth, R. S., Smith, E. L., Duncan, G. C., Crawford, M. L. J. & von Noorden, G. K. (1986) Multiple sensitive periods in the development of the primate visual system. *Science*, **232**, 235–8.

Hebb, D. O. (1942) The effect of early and late brain injury upon test scores, and the nature of normal adult intelligence. *Proceedings of the American Philosophical Society*, **85**, 275–92.

Hobson, R. P. (1986) The autistic child's appraisal of expressions of emotion. *Journal of Child Psychology and Psychiatry*, **27**, 321–42.

Hodges, J. & Tizard, B. (1989) IQ and behavioural adjustment of ex-institutional adolescents. *Journal of Child Pscyhology and Psychiatry*, **30**, 53–75.

Hunt, A. & Dennis, J. (1987) Psychiatric disorder among children with tuberous sclerosis. *Developmental Medicine and Child Neurology*, **29**, 190–8.

Huston, A. C. (1983) Sex-typing. In Hetherington, E. M. (ed.) *Mussen's handbook of child psychology*, 4th end. Vol IV, *Socialization, personality, and social development*, New York: John Wiley, pp. 387–467.

Huttenlocher, P. R. (1979) Synaptic density in human frontal cortex – developmental changes and effects of aging. *Brain Research*, **163**, 195–205.

Huttenlocher, P. R., de Courten, C., Garey, L. J. & van der Loos, H. (1982) Synaptogenesis in human visual cortex – evidence for synapse elimination during normal development. *Neuroscience Letters*, **33**, 247–52.

Ingram, T. T. S. (1955) A study of cerebral palsy in the childhood population of Edinburgh. *Archives of Disease in Childhood*, **30**, 85–98.

Ingram, T. T. S. (1956) A characteristic form of overactive behaviour in brain damaged children. *Journal of Mental Science*, **102**, 550–8.

Kanner, L. (1943) Autistic disturbance of affective contact. *Nervous Child*, **2**, 217–50.

Kasamatu, T., Pettigrew, J. D. & Ary, M. (1979) Restoration of visual cortical plasticity by local microperfusion of norepinephirne. *Journal of Comparative Neurology*, **185,** 163–81.

Kennard, M. A. (1942) Cortical reorganization of motor function: studies on series of monkeys of various ages from infancy to maturity. *Archives of Neurology and Psychiatry*, **48,** 227–40.

Kinsbourne, M. (1971) The minor cerebral hemisphere as a source of aphasic speech. *Archives of Neurology*, **25,** 302–6.

Kinsbourne, M. & Hiscock, M. (1983) The normal and deviant development of functional lateralization of the brain. In Haith, M. M. & Campos, J. J. (eds.) *Mussen's handbook of child psychology*, 4th edn. vol. II, *Infancy and developmental psychobiology*. New York: John Wiley, pp. 157–280.

Molfese, D. L. & Molfese, V. J. (1980) Cortical responses of preterm infants to phonetic and nonphonetic speech stimuli. *Developmental Psychology*, **16,** 574–81.

Nichols, P. L. & Chen, T.-C. (1981) *Minimal brain dysfunction: a prospective study*. Hillsdale, New Jersey: Lawrence Erlbaum.

Olfield, R. C. (1971) The assessment and analysis of handedness: the Edinburgh inventory. *Neuropsychologia*, **9,** 97–113.

Orton, S. T. (1937) *Reading, writing and speech problems in children: a presentation of certain types of disorders in the development of the language-faculty*. New York: Norton.

Ounsted, C. (1955) The hyperkinetic syndrome in epileptic children. *Lancet*, **ii,** 303–11.

Ounsted, C., Lindsay, J. & Richards, P. (1987) *Temporal lobe epilepsy 1948–1986: a biographical study. Clinics in developmental medicine, No. 103.* Oxford: Blackwells; Philadelphia: Lippincott.

Passingham, R. E., Perry, V. H. & Wilkinson, F. (1983) The long-term effects of removal of sensorimotor cortex in infant and adult Rhesus monkeys. *Brain*, **106,** 675–705.

Patterson, G. R. (1982) *A social learning approach: 3. Coercive family process.* Eugene, Oreg.: Castalia Publishing.

Plomin, R. & Daniels, D. (1987). Why are children in the same family so different from one another? *Behavioral and Brain Sciences*, **10,** 1–60.

Raisman, G. & Field, P. M. (1973) Sexual dimorphism in the neuropil of the preoptic area of the rat and its dependence on neonatal androgen. *Brain Research*, **54,** 1–29.

Rakic, P., Bourgeois, J.-P., Eckenhoff, F., Zecevic, N. & Goldman-Rakic, P. S. (1986) Concurrent overproduction of synapses in diverse regions of the primate cerebral cortex. *Science*, **232,** 232–5.

Richman, N., Stevenson, J. & Graham, P. J. (1982) *Pre-school to school: a behavioural study*. London: Academic Press.

Rutter, M. (1981) *Maternal deprivation reassessed*, 2nd edn. Harmondsworth: Penguin.

Rutter, M. (1985) Infantile autism and other pervasive developmental disorders. In Rutter, M. & Hersov, L. (eds.) *Child and adolescent psychiatry: modern approaches*. 2nd edn. Oxford: Blackwell Scientific Publications, pp. 545–66.

Rutter, M. (1987) Continuities and discontinuities from infancy. In Osofsky, J.

(ed.), *Handbook of infant development*, 2nd edn. New York: John Wiley, pp. 1256–98.

Rutter, M. (1991) Autism as a genetic disorder. In McGuffin, P. & Murray, R. (ed.) *The new genetics of mental illness.* Oxford: Heinemann Medical Books, pp. 225–44.

Rutter, M., Chadwick, O. & Shaffer, D. (1984) Head injury. In Rutter, M. (ed.) *Developmental neuropsychiatry.* Edinburgh: Churchill Livingstone, pp. 83–111.

Rutter, M., Graham, P. & Yule, W. (1970) *A neuropsychiatric study in childhood. Clinics in developmental medicine, Nos. 35/36.* London: S.I.M.P./Heinemann.

Rutter, M. & Yule, W. (1970) Neurological aspects of intellectual retardation and specific reading retardation. In Rutter, M., Tizard, J. & Whitmore, K. (eds.) *Education, health and behaviour.* London: Longman, pp. 54–74.

Satz, P. (1972) Pathological left-handedness: an explanatory model. *Cortex,* **8,** 121–35.

Satz, P. & Sparrow, S. S. (1970) Specific developmental dyslexia: a theoretical formulation. In Bakker, D. J. & Satz, P. (ed.) *Specific reading disability: advances in theory and method.* The Netherlands: Rotterdam Universiy Press, pp. 17–40.

Schade, J. P. & van Groenigen, W. B. (1961) Structural organization of the human cerebral cortex. I. Maturation of the middle frontal gyrus. *Acta Anatomica,* **47,** 74–111.

Schneider, G. E. (1979) It it really better to have your brain lesion early? A revision of the 'Kennard principle'. *Neuropsychologia,* **17,** 557–83.

Sidman, R. L. & Rakic, P. (1973) Neuronal migration with special reference to developing human brains: a review. *Brain Research,* **62,** 1–35.

Silverberg, R., Obler, L. K. & Gordon, H. W. (1979) Handedness in Israel. *Neuropyschologia,* **17,** 83–7.

Smith, A. & Sugar, O. (1975) Development of above normal language and intelligence 21 years after left hemispherectomy. *Neurology,* **25,** 813–8.

Soper, H. V., Satz, P., Orsini, D. L., Henry, R. R., Zvi, J. C. & Schulman, M. (1986) Handedness patterns in autism suggest subtypes. *Journal of Autism and Developmental Disorders,* **16,** 155–66.

Spear, P. D. (1979) Behavioural and neurophysiological consequences of visual cortex damage: mechanisms of recovery. In Sprague, J. M. & Epstein, A. N. (eds.) *Progress in Psychobiology and Physiological Psychology,* Vol. 8. New York: Academic Press, pp 45–90.

Springer, S. P. & Deutsch, G. (1985) *Left brain, right brain.* Revised edition. San Francisco: Freeman.

Stores, G. (1977) Behavior disturbance and type of epilepsy in children attending ordinary school. In Pentry, J. K. (ed.) *Epilepsy: the eighth international symposium.* New York: Raven Press, pp. 245–9.

Swaab, D. F. & Hofman, M. A. (1988) Sexual diffrentiation of the human hypothalamus: ontogeny of the sexually dimorphic nucleus of the preoptic area. *Developmental Brain Research,* **44,** 314–8.

Takashima, S., Chan, F., Becker, L. E. & Armstrong, D. L. (1980) Morphology of the developing visual cortex of the human infant: a quantitative and qualitative Golgi study. *Journal of Neuropathology and Experimental Neurology*, **39**, 487–501.

Taylor, D. C. (1975) Factors influencing the occurrence of schizophrenia-like psychosis in patients with temporal lobe epilepsy. *Psychological Medicine*, **5**, 249–54.

Taylor, D. C. & Ounsted, C. (1972) The nature of gender differences explored through ontogenetic analyses of sex ratios in disease. In Ounsted, C. & Taylor, D. C. (eds.) *Gender differences: their ontogeny and significance*. Edinburgh: Churchill Livingstone, pp. 241–62.

Taylor, E. (1986) *The overactive child. Clinics in developmental medicine, No. 97*. Oxford: Blackwells; Philadelphia: Lippincott.

Taylor, E., Everitt, B., Thorley, G., Schachar, R., Rutter, M. & Wieselberg, M. (1986) Conduct disorder and hyperactivity: II. A cluster analytic approach to the identification of a behavioural syndrome. *British Journal of Psychiatry*, **149**, 768–77.

Teng, E. L., Lee, P., Yang, K. & Chang, P. C. (1977) Handedness in a Chinese population: biological, social, and pathological factors. *Science*, **193**, 1148–50.

Tresidder, J., Fielder, A. and Nicholson, J. (1990) Delayed visual maturation: ophthalmic and neurodevelopmental aspects. *Developmental Medicine and Child Newology*, **32**, 872–81.

Tsai, L. Y. & Stewart, M. A. (1982) Handedness and EEG correlation in autistic children. *Psychiatric Annals*, **17**, 595–8.

Vaegan & Taylor, D. (1979) Critical period for deprivation amblyopia in children. *Transactions of the Ophthalmological Societies of the United Kingdom*, **99**, 432–9.

Vargha-Khadem, F., O'Gorman, A. M. & Watters, G. V. (1985) Aphasia and handedness in relation to hemispheric side, age at injury and severity of cerebral lesion during childhood. *Brain*, **108**, 677–96.

Voeller, K. K. S. (1986) Right-hemisphere deficit syndrome in children. *American Journal of Psychiatry*, **143**, 1004–9.

Wada, J. A., Clarke, R. & Hamm, A. (1975) Cerebral hemispheric asymmetry in humans: cortical speech zones in 100 adult and 100 infant brains. *Archives of Neurology*, **32**, 239–46.

Wall, P. D. (1977) The presence of ineffective synapses and the circumstances which unmask them. *Philosophical Transactions of the Royal Society of London (Series B)*, **278**, 361–72.

Weintraub, S. & Mesulam, M.-M. (1983) Developmental learning disabilities of the right hemisphere: emotional, interpersonal and cognitive components. *Archives of Neurology*, **40**, 463–8.

Werker, J. F. & Tees, R. C. (1984) Cross-language speech perception: evidence for perceptual reorganization during the first year of life. *Infant Behavior and Development*, **7**, 49–63.

Wiesel, T. N. (1982) Postnatal development of the visual cortex and the influence of environment. *Science*, **299**, 583–91.

Wing, L. (1981). Asperger's syndrome: a clinical account. *Psychological Medicine*, **11**, 115–29.

Woods, B. T. (1980) The restricted effects of right-hemisphere lesions after age one: Wechsler test data. *Neuropsychologia*, **18**, 65–70.

Woods, B. T. & Carey, S. (1979) Language deficits after apparent clinical recovery from childhood aphasia. *Annals of Neurology*, **6**, 405–9.
Woods, B. T. & Teuber, H.-L. (1978) Changing patterns of childhood aphasia. *Annals of Neurology*, **3**, 273–80.
World Health Organization (1989) *ICD-10, 1989 draft of chapter V: categories F00–F99, mental and behavioural disorders (including disorders of psychological development). Clinical descriptions and diagnostic guidelines.* Geneva: World Health Organization.
Yirmiya, N., Kasari, C., Sigman, M. & Mundy, P. (1989) Facial expressions of affect in autistic, mentally retarded and normal children. *Journal of Child Psychology and Psychiatry*, **30**, 725–35.

3 Relation between maturation of neurotransmitter systems in the human brain and psychosocial disorders

D. F. SWAAB

INTRODUCTION

Developmental hypotheses and psychosocial disorders

An increasing number of psychosocial disorders have been associated with developmental risk factors. This includes: mental retardation and behavioral abnormalities stemming from hypoxic perinatal brain damage (Benveniste *et al.*, 1984; Bosley *et al.*, 1983), dyslexia (Kemper, 1984), disturbed language development, sleep disorders, schizophrenia, autism, sudden-infant death syndrome (SIDS), hyperkinetic syndrome, depression and anxiety (for references, see Swaab *et al.*, 1988). Left handedness, gender identity and sexual preference are also thought to be determined during early development although they are expressed much later (Dörner, 1979, 1986; Gladue *et al.*, 1984; Ellis *et al.*, 1988). It is important to note that developmental sequelae are often multifactorial and that the same outcomes may have different origins. Sexual differentiation, for instance, may be influenced not only by hormones and other neuroactive compounds (Dörner, 1979; Swaab & Mirmiran, 1986; Rudeen *et al.*, 1986; Zimmerberg & Reuter, 1989), but also by stress (Anderson *et al.*, 1985; Ellis *et al.*, 1988; Dörner, 1979, 1986). This makes the distinction between biological and environmental explanations of developmental disorders obsolete (e.g. Swaab & Hofman, 1988). It is also the case that similar situations or compounds may lead to different developmental sequelae. Maternal stress may lead to differences in sexual orientation of the offspring (Ellis *et al.*, 1988), but also to neurological dysfunction, developmental delays and behavior disturbances (Stott, 1973; Meijer, 1985). Diethylstilbestrol (DES) administration to pregnant women may lead to an increased frequency of bisexuality or homosexuality in their daughters (Ehrhardt *et al.*, 1985) and to more frequent depression and anxiety in sons and daughters (Vessey *et al.*, 1983; Meyer-Bahlburg & Ehrhardt, 1987).

Psychosocial disorders, brain structures and transmitters

Some of the developmental disturbances mentioned above are postulated to be related to alterations in particular brain structures or certain transmitter systems during brain development. Thus, some *sleep disturbances* in children have been related to clonidine taken by the mother during pregnancy and affecting the noradrenergic system of the child (Huisjes *et al.*, 1986). In SIDS a dramatic disappearance of luteinizing hormone releasing hormone (LHRH) fibres has been found in the mediobasal periventricular and paraventricular nuclei (Najimi *et al.*, 1989). Smoking during pregnancy may affect the *school performance* of the child (Butler & Goldstein, 1973; Abel, 1980). In brains of *schizophrenic patients*, disorganized hippocampal pyramid cells (Conrad & Scheibel, 1987) and heterotopic displacement of nerve cells in the entorhinal cortex (Jakob & Beckmann, 1986) have been described, suggesting the presence of factors causing around mid-gestation a disturbance of neuronal migration. In addition, schizophrenia has been associated with alterations in the dopaminergic innervation of the prefrontal cortex and other limbic brain areas (Weinberger, 1988).

Autism is a developmental disorder that results in severe deficits in social, communicative and cognitive functioning. In his initial report, Kanner (1943) emphasized the apparent biological origin of this disorder as reflected by its onset during the first two years of postnatal life. Others have considered it to be a psychological disorder resulting from environmental factors (see Sanua, 1986). The study of Courchesne *et al.* (1988), however, showed that this condition involves abnormal neuroanatomical development of the cerebellum. The authors obtained magnetic resonance scans of the cerebella of 18 patients with autism and without other medical disorders. By using planimetry the neo-cerebellar vermal lobules VI and VII were found to be significantly smaller than those of controls. The small size of the cerebella appeared to be the result of developmental hypoplasia rather than shrinkage after full development since there was no sign of sulcal widening. It is not clear whether the cerebellar abnormality directly or indirectly impairs cognitive functions or occurs concomitantly with damage to other neural sites. Since autism has been observed in association with, for example, congenital rubella and with the preconceptional exposure of the parents to chemicals (Coleman, 1979), autism can at present be regarded as a developmental neurobiological disorder which is probably caused by a number of different factors (e.g. chemical, viral, genetic) before birth. The detection of these factors clearly demands a multidisciplinary approach in the following decades.

Hypoxic, *hypoglycaemic* and *ischaemic encephalopathy* leading to cerebral palsy, mental retardation or epilepsy is presently thought to be mediated by an increased release and extracellular concentration of excitatory amino acids, such as glutamate (Benveniste *et al.*, 1984; Bosley *et al.*, 1983). One should note, however, that brain injuries related to birth are generally overdiagnosed. Many of them may, in fact, rather be due to prenatal brain damage. Prenatal brain damage often predisposes to difficult birth, which leads to the false impression that the birth itself is responsible for disorders such as mental retardation (Chaney *et al.*, 1986). This can be understood since the fetal brain is playing an active role in the process of labour, e.g. by accelerating its course (Swaab *et al.*, 1977).

Gilles de la Tourette's syndrome is thought to be due to abnormal dopamine function as indicated by the therapeutic effect of haloperidol, to abnormal noradrenaline metabolism by the effect of clonidine, and to serotonin on the basis of reduced levels of cerebrospinal fluid (CSF) metabolites. In addition, alterations in encephalin, dynorphim and substance-P have been reported in this condition (Haber *et al.*, 1986). The biochemistry of this disease is, however, far from clear (Messiha, 1988) and obviously needs systematic investigation of postmortem brain tissue of these patients by modern neurobiological techniques.

All these observations certainly need to be replicated and followed up further by studying in a systematic way other brain systems and structures in patients with these conditions. Although the data obtained to date suggest that certain neurotransmitter systems and brain structures are affected during human brain development, it is certainly not yet clear how particular psychosocial disorders may result from the reported alterations.

Syndrome specificity and the functional implications of the structural changes still have to be shown. However, for the time being, the reported structural changes, e.g. in schizophrenia and autism, can be considered as an important index for the period in which the disorder arose, even if the lesions do not at present explain the psychosocial disorders.

Neurotransmitters

Neurotransmitters (i.e. acetylcholine, amines, amino acids and peptides) play a key role in the investigation of the development of psychosocial disorders. Thus, firstly, they may constitute the substrate of such disorders (see above). Secondly, they may mediate risk factors and brain damage. Clonidine causes sleep disturbances, probably by acting on the noradrenergic system. Perinatal hypoxia causes brain damage by stimulating the release of excitatory amino acids. Thirdly, they may mediate therapeutic effects. As examples, the effect of haloperidol or clonidine on Gilles de la Tourette's syndrome may be mentioned, as well as the attempts to prevent perinatal brain damage due to hypoxia by NMDA blockers.

For research in brain ontogeny and the development of brain disorders, neurotransmitters are, moreover, important as markers for the developmental stage of brain structures or systems, and as markers for the delineation of brain structures or systems that are otherwise not visible. As an example, one may mention the human suprachiasmatic nucleus that is not visible in conventionally stained sections, but that can clearly be delineated following staining of one of its main peptide neurotransmitters, i.e. vasopressin (Swaab *et al.*, 1985).

DEVELOPMENT OF TRANSMITTER SYSTEMS IN THE HUMAN BRAIN

There are various major neurotransmitter systems such as cholinergic, aminergic, amino acid containing and peptidergic systems. From all four systems, examples can be given that show their early presence during development in the human fetal brain.

Cholinergic systems

Kostovic (1986), using acetylcholinesterase (AChE) activity as a histochemical marker for the developing human cholinergic system, observed activity in the nucleus basalis complex anlage as early as 9 weeks of gestation. Basal forebrain fibres are sent from there to the anlage of the neocortex and the limbic cortex by the end of the second trimester. Biochemical measurements (Brooksbank *et al.*, 1978) revealed the presence of AChE in the earliest fetuses studied (i.e. 18 weeks of gestation) and an increase in AChE activity in the cerebral cortex with neonatal development to a level higher than that found in the adult. The cerebellum was much richer in AChE than the cerebral cortex and there was a modest developmental increase, the highest concentrations being found in the adult cerebellum. In addition, an increase was found in choline-acetyltransferase (CAT) activity from 18 weeks of gestation towards term, in both the cerebral cortex and the forebrain. The activity had not reached adult levels at birth (Brooksbank *et al.*, 1978). Muscarinic binding sites were present in the brainstem and midbrain of the human fetus at 12 weeks of gestation (Schlumpf & Lichtensteiger, 1987). Muscarinic receptor development (i.e. quinuclidinyl benzilate (QNB) binding sites concentration) appears in the corpus striatum at 16 weeks of gestation (Ravikumar & Sastry, 1985) and reached adult levels at term. In contrast, cerebellar maximal CAT activity was attained at 26–42 weeks of gestation and the highest concentration of QNB binding was reached at 18–22 weeks of gestation (Brooksbank *et al.*, 1978). The sequence observed in the development of QNB and CAT, viz. postsynaptic receptor development preceding the neurotransmitter enzyme or synapse formation, is a phenomenon that has been reported in other systems (in the GABAergic system: see below, for other examples see Brooksbank *et al.*, 1978). This phenomenon also implies that brain areas might be affected during development by exogenous neurotransmitter-like substances well before such a structure is innervated by the endogenous neurotransmitter.

Aminergic systems

The distribution of structures containing catecholamine (CA) and indolamine (IA) in human fetuses has been described by means of the Falck–Hillarp method from 7 weeks of gestation onwards (Nobin & Björklund, 1973; Olson *et al.*, 1973). At 3–4 months of gestation, four CA- and three IA-containing cell groups were present and major axonal pathways were already visible. CA-containing varicose fibres occurred in the hypothalamus, basal ganglia, septum and olfactory regions. By means of tyrosine hydroxylase immunoreactivity, also the locus coeruleus and substantia nigra showed reactivity by 9–10 weeks of gestation (Pearson *et al.*, 1980). Varicose IA fibres were observed only in the rostral pons. The cerebral and cerebellar cortices had no or only very few CA-containing fibres. The overall stage of development of the monoamine neuron systems in these 3–4 months old human fetuses seemed to be comparable with that of the rat during the first or second week after birth. The concentrations of dopamine noradrenaline and serotonin in the human fetal brain are rather low with the exception of a high hypothalamic dopamine level (Hyyppä, 1972). The CA in the lower brain stem of the human infant has also been described by immunocytochemical techniques (Robert *et al.*, 1984).

Amino acid containing systems

The development of the γ-aminobutyric acid (GABA) system has been studied biochemically in the human cerebral cortex and cerebellum by estimating glutamate decarboxylase (GAD) and binding for muscimol. GAD activity in the cerebral cortex at term was only 20% of the adult value that was reached after 60 weeks gestational age. The concentration of muscimol binding sites rose more rapidly than GAD activity. In the cerebellum, however, GADspecific activity reached approximately 40% of its adult level at term and muscimol binding only 10%, and was still increasing at 60 weeks gestational age (Brooksbank *et al.*, 1981). Benzodiazepine binding sites have already been observed in the brainstem and midbrain of the human fetus at 12 weeks of gestation (Schlumpf & Lichtensteiger, 1987), whereas glutamate, NMDA and quisqualate binding sites were found in the hippocampus at mid-gestation (Represa *et al.*, 1989). The concentration of taurine in the human fetal brain is higher than in the adult brain, and decreases with the course of gestation between 7 and 25 cm crown/rump length (Sturman & Gaull, 1975).

Peptidergic systems

Neuropeptides are also present in different brain structures during early human development. Fetal hypothalamic and cortical tissue contained LHRH at $4\frac{1}{2}$–6 weeks of pregnancy (Aksel & Tyrey, 1977; Siler-Khodr & Khodr, 1978; Winters *et al.*, 1974) and LHRH-producing cells were stained at 9–10 weeks of gestation (Bugnon *et al.*, 1977a, Paulin *et al.*, 1977). Thyroid releasing hormone (TRH) was also assayed in the fetal brain as early as 4–5 weeks of pregnancy (Winters *et al.*, 1974) and in the fetal hypothalamus and cortex from 8 weeks of gestation (Aubert, 1979). The presence of TRH in the cerebellum of an anencephalic child (Winters *et al.*, 1974) suggests extrahypothalamic production sites for this material. Somatostatin has been determined in the fetal hypothalamus and in the fetal cerebral cortex at mid-gestation (Paulin *et al.*, 1976; Bugnon *et al.*, 1977b), while α-endorphin staining appeared in the infundibular region from the 11th week of development onwards (Bloch *et al.*, 1978). Substance-P is present at 8 weeks of gestation in the spinal cord and hypothalamus (Paulin *et al.*, 1986). Already in 1953, Dicker & Tyler showed, by means of bio-assays, the occurrence of vasopressin and oxytocin in the human fetal neurohypophysis from 70 days of gestation onwards. Others (Burford & Robinson, 1982; Paulin *et al.*, 1978; Fellman *et al.*, 1979; Visser & Swaab, 1979; Schubert *et al.*, 1981; Khan-Dawood & Dawood, 1984) showed the presence of the same peptides from 11–14 weeks of gestation in the pituitary and hypothalamus, and their exponential increase in the neurohypophysis towards birth. Neurophysins were found from 12–13 weeks onwards. In addition, we observed extrahypothalamic fibres containing neurohypophysial hormones in human fetuses from 17 weeks of gestation (Swaab & Ter Borg, 1981).

THE RELATIONSHIP BETWEEN NEUROTRANSMITTER DEVELOPMENT AND DISTURBED BRAIN DEVELOPMENT

Animal experiments have shown that perturbations of the development of each of the major neurotransmitter classes, i.e. acetylcholine, amines, amino acids or peptides, may result in subtle alterations in brain and behavior. This led to the development of a relatively new field of research, 'behavior' or 'functional teratology' (for review, see Swaab *et al.*, 1988). The developing brain is, in this respect, certainly not only affected by neurotransmitter-like substances. In fact, all those chemical compounds that are capable of influencing the adult brain may also affect brain development (Swaab, 1980). This has been established now, e.g. for sex hormones, corticosteroids, thyroid hormones, neurotransmitters, stimulating compounds (alcohol, nicotine, caffeine, marihuana), anaesthetics and metals.

Since neurotransmitter systems may be the substrate of psychosocial disorders, and may mediate effects of factors influencing brain development and of therapeutic effects, information on their pattern of development may be useful. Excitatory amino acids, for instance, are thought to be involved in hypoxic/ischaemic encephalopathy (Benveniste *et al.*, 1984; Bosley *et al.*, 1983). It will be useful, therefore, to obtain more information on their regional developmental pattern in the human brain. The currently available information on neurotransmitter development in the human brain is, however, only of limited value in this connection, due to a number of factors:

(1) Neuronal systems themselves may already be affected during development before neurotransmitters are expressed, i.e. by factors influencing cell acquisition, cell death, migration, the formation of neurites and synapses or receptor setting. These processes might be disturbed by either alcohol (Swaab *et al.*, 1988) or benzodiazepines (Laegreid *et al.*, 1989).

(2) There has been considerable emphasis on researching when a neurotransmitter can be detected for the first time. It is questionable, however, whether such a line of investigation is very meaningful. Firstly, neurotransmitters are found earlier in development as techniques become more sensitive. Neurotransmitters can even be detected in fertilized egg cells and in the initial phases of neural tube formation (Buznikov *et al.*, 1972; Ignarro & Shideman, 1968). Secondly, such data do not provide the necessary information for estimating when in development a particular system is sensitive to a particular (disturbing) developmental factor, since brain areas may express receptors well before they are innervated by neurotransmitter systems (see above). Consequently, the period during development that a particular neurotransmitter system appears in a certain structure might differ considerably in time with the sensitive phase of that brain area for neurotransmitter-like substances. Important information may, therefore, come from receptor

studies. The transient increase in density of NMDA binding sites in the fetal human hippocampus around 23–40 weeks of gestation (Represa *et al.*, 1989) may well indicate a sensitive period for excitatory amino acids and thus for hypoxia. Also the concentration of muscarinic receptors in fetuses is higher than in adults (Ravikumar & Sastry, 1985). One should, in addition, note that the tissue content of neurotransmitters during development does not hold any information on their release or turnover.

(3) Overall biochemical data on neurotransmitter systems do not reveal information on the marked regional differences in rate of development. The hypothalamic magnocellular vasopressin neurons of the supraoptic and paraventricular nucleus (SON and PVN) have been visualized already at 11 weeks of gestation (Fellman *et al.*, 1979) whereas the majority of the neurons of the nearby suprachiasmatic nucleus (SCN) express vasopressin only after birth (Swaab *et al.*, 1990). 'Molecular anatomical' techniques, such as immunocytochemistry and *in situ* hybridization, are thus preferable.

(4) There are various problems that counteract studies relating developmental sequelae to the causative factors. In the first place, the interval between the time when such factors act on the developing brain and the occurrence of symptoms might be long, extending over years up to decades. In addition, the symptoms might not be specific to the causal factors, or the factors might contribute to multicausal disease entities (Swaab *et al.*, 1988). Longitudinal studies are difficult but essential in the field of functional teratology.

(5) One additional major point of concern for all the data on human brain development is whether or not the measurements are indeed representative for *normal* development, and not influenced by the disease from which the subject died, the administered medicines, the agonal state, or postmortem interval (Swaab & Uylings, 1988). Stable markers of the neurotransmitter systems that show only limited change during a reasonable postmortem interval should be chosen preferentially to follow the development, whereas the clinical state of the subject and the general neuropathology should be extensively documented by a well-organized brain bank (Swaab *et al.*, 1989). In this way, valuable correlations may be established between a change in transmitter development and psychosocial disorders. The causality of such correlations, however, has to be established in animal experiments. Such experimental observations, selecting the right stage of development, are often not available at present.

(6) A final point concerns the way neuropathologists generally screen the brain. Studying brain structures by using one or even a few sections per area can give only an impression of cell density, which is a very poor way of studying cell numbers. Even a factor of 2 more or fewer neurons per structure may pass unnoticed (Swaab & Uylings, 1987). Major changes in the human brain might, therefore, have been missed so far.

ESTIMATION OF THE PERIOD THAT DEVELOPMENTAL SEQUELAE MIGHT HAVE TAKEN PLACE

Analogous to the developmental pattern in animals in which the sensitive period has been established experimentally, it might be possible to estimate the period in which developmental sequelae could take place in the human brain. This point has already been mentioned in relation to the lesions found in schizophrenia and autism, and may also be illustrated by our work on the human hypothalamus.

In rats, sexual differentiation of the sexually dimorphic nucleus (SDN) of the preoptic area in the hypothalamus can be affected around the first postnatal week. This is the period in which the rat SDN becomes sexually dimorphic (Gorski, 1984). In the human brain, sexual differentation of the SDN was found to take place only after 2–4 years postnatally (Figure 3.1). By analogy with the raw data this may be the period in which the SDN is sensitive to factors, either chemical or psychological in nature such as stress, (Swaab & Hofman, 1988) which influence sexual differentiation. Whether such alterations really take place in the human brain has to be studied in subjects who were exposed to factors which possibly could influence sexual differentiation of the human brain in different prenatal and postnatal periods, e.g. Klinefelter, Turner, Prader–Willi and adrenogenital syndromes.

Another example of possible timing of the period of an alteration in development can be given for the suprachiasmatic nucleus, the clock of the hypothalamus. In adulthood, the SCN has some 7000 vasopressin neurons whereas the total cell number of this nucleus is about 46 000. Cell numbers are stable until about 80 years of age (Swaab *et al.*, 1985). Much to our surprise, in two male-to-female transsexuals of 44 and 50 years of age, vasopressin cells and total cell numbers were doubled. This was probably not due to steroid hormone treatment in adulthood, since a patient displaying similar high SCN cell numbers was a 30-year-old woman with Prader–Willi syndrome. This syndrome is characterized by a congenital lack of LHRH and thus a lack of sex hormones (Swaab *et al.*, 1987). Recently, similar high cell numbers have been observed in the SCN of 14 male homosexuals who died of acquired immune deficiency

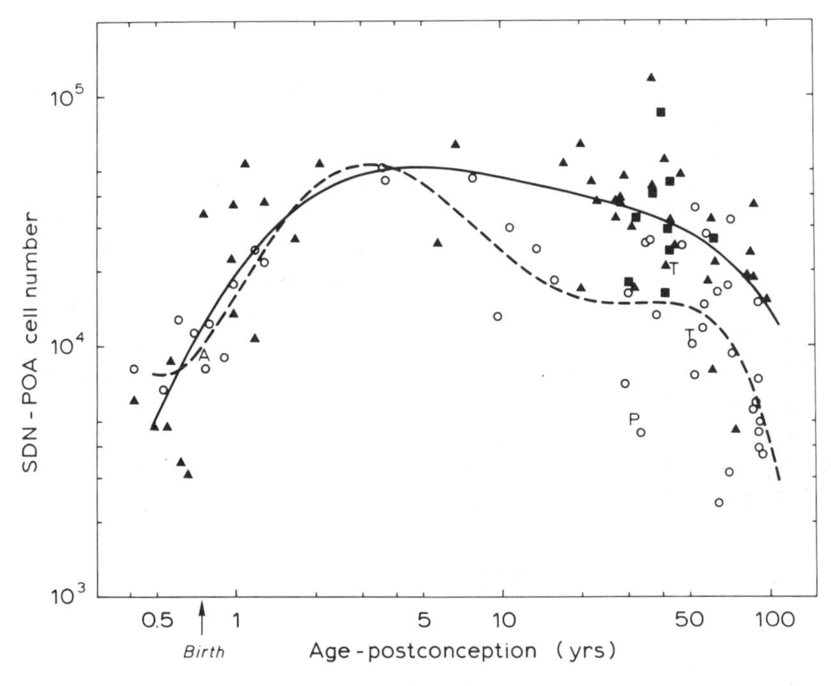

Figure 3.1. Development and sexual differentiation of the human sexually dimorphic nucleus (SDN) of the preoptic area of the hypothalamus. Log-log scale. Note that at the moment of birth the SDN is equally small in boys (▲) and girls (○) and contains only about 22% of the cell number found at 2–4 years of age. The SDN cell number of a female neonate with a pituitary aplasia (A) is fully within the range of other neonates. Cell numbers reach a peak value around 2–4 years postnatally, after which a sexual differentiation occurs in the SDN due to a decrease in cell number in the SDN of women, whereas the cell number in men remains approximately unchanged up to the age of 50. In women cell number decreases for the second time after the age of about 60, after a period of relative stability, dropping to values which are only 10–15% of the cell number found at 2 years postnatally. Note that in men the reduction in cell number in senescence is less dramatic. The largest discrepancy in cell number between men and women is found around 30 years and in people older than 80, whereas the sexual dimorphism in the SDN cell number is at least around the age of 60. The SDN cell number in homosexual men (■) does not differ from that in the male reference group. The cell number of the SDN of two male-to-female transsexuals (T) is within the female range, whereas the SDN of a woman with a Prader–Willi syndrome (P) is small. The curves for quintic polynomial functions fitted to the original data for males (drawn line) and females (dashed line), with $F_s[5, 49] = 10.05$, $P < 0.001$ and $F_s[5, 39] = 7.32$, $P < 0.001$, respectively (from Swaab & Hofman, 1988, with permission).

syndrome (AIDS) (Swaab & Hofman, 1990). The similar large SCN in homosexuals, transsexuals and Prader–Willi syndrome might be related to an alteration in the interaction of sex hormones and brain development. Since it is hard to explain an increased neuron number arising in adulthood, we have studied the developmental pattern of vasopressin cell formation in the SCN (Figure 3.2). It seems that vasopressin expression in the human SCN neurons starts mainly in the neonatal period. Around the first year postnatally, cell numbers are high, i.e. more than twice the number of vasopressin and total cells in the adult (Swaab *et al.*, 1990). These values are comparable to those found in the subject with Prader–Willi syndrome, transsexuals and male homosexuals. After the first postnatal years, cell numbers decrease gradually towards levels seen in adults (Figure 3.2). This developmental study indicates that in these three conditions a factor is preventing the programmed cell death of SCN neurons around the first year of age. Whether or not this factor may be a change in sex hormones should be investigated experimentally. The question whether a large SCN and homosexuality are not directly related but due to a common factor

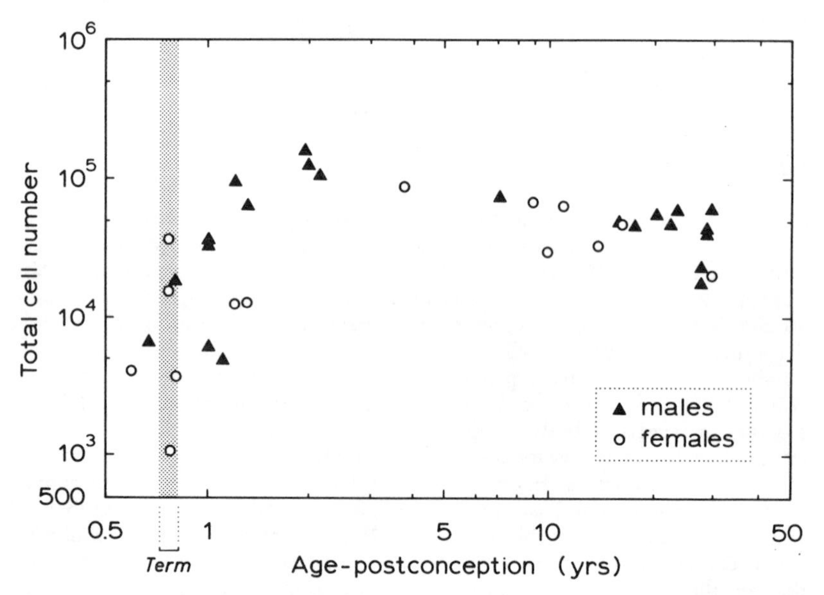

Figure 3.2. Development of the human suprachiasmatic nucleus (SCN) of the hypothalamus. Log-log scale. The period at term (38–42 weeks of gestation) is indicated by the vertical bar. Note that total cell number is low at the moment of birth (21% of the cell number found in adulthood). There is no difference in the developmental course of the SCN in boys and girls. Cell numbers around 1–1½ years postnatally are more than twice the adult cell numbers. After these high levels a decrease to adult total cell number is found. (From Swaab *et al.*, 1990, with permission.)

during brain development or alternatively the SCN is indeed directly involved in partner preference, should also be studied in animal experiments.

Consequently, life-span studies might be useful to pinpoint a particular period in development in which a certain factor might have been active. The ultimate proof that such a relationship is a causal one has to come, however, from animal experiments. This means that studies on human material obtained by a well-organized brain bank on subjects with psychosocial disorders of a possible developmental origin, and on animal experiments should go hand in hand in order to reveal the putative relationship mentioned in the title.

ACKNOWLEDGEMENTS

I want to thank Bert Schillings for his secretarial help and Dr R. Balazs and Dr M. Mirmiran for their critical comments. The human brain from which the data are discussed have been collected by the Netherlands Brain Bank in the Netherlands Institute for Brain Research (coordinator Dr R. Ravid)

REFERENCES

Abel, E. (1980) Smoking during pregnancy: a review of effects on growth and development of offspring. *Human Biology*, **52**, 593–625.

Aksel, S. & Tyrey, L. (1977) Luteinizing hormone-releasing hormone in the hormone in the human fetal brain. *Fertility and Sterility*, **28**, 1067–71.

Anderson, D. K., Rhees, R. W. & Fleming, D. E. (1985) Effects of prenatal stress on differentiation of the sexually dimorphic nucleus of the preoptic area (SDN–POA) of the rat brain. *Brain Research*, **322**, 113–8.

Aubert, M. L. (1979) Ontogènese des fonctions hypothalamiques chez le foetus humain. *Journal de Physiologie* (Paris), **75**, 45–53.

Benveniste, E., Drejer, J., Schousboe, A. & Diemer, N. H. (1984) Elevation of the extracellular concentrations of glutamate and aspartate in rat hippocampus during transient cerebral ischemia monitored by intracerebral microdialysis. *Journal of Neurochemistry*, **43**, 1369–74.

Bloch, B., Bugnon, C., Fellman, D. & Lenys, D. (1978) Immunocytochemical evidence that the same neurons in the human infundibular nucleus are stained with anti-endorphins and other related peptides. *Neuroscience Letters*, **10**, 147–52.

Bosley, T. M., Woodhams, P. L., Gordon, R. D. & Balazs, R. (1983) Effects of anoxia on the stimulated release of amino acid neurotransmitters in the cerebellum in vitro. *Journal of Neurochemistry*, **40**, 189–201.

Brooksbank, B. W. L., Martinez, M., Atkinson, D. J. & Balazs, R. (1978) Biochemical development of the human brain: I. Some parameters of the cholinergic system. *Development in Neuroscience*, **1**, 267–84.

Brooksbank, B. W. L., Atkinson, D. J. & Balazs, R. (1981) Biochemical development of the human brain: II. Some parameters on the GABAergic system. *Development in Neuroscience*, **4**, 188–200.

Bugnon, C., Bloch, B. & Fellman, D. (1977a) Etude immunocytologique des neurones hypothalamiques à LH–RH chez le foetus humain. *Brain Research*, **128**, 249–62.

Bugnon, C., Fellman, D. & Bloch, B. (1977b) Immunocytochemical study of the ontogenesis of the hypothalamic somastostatin-containing neurons in the human fetus. *Cell Tissue Research*, **183**, 319–28.

Burford, G. D. & Robinson, I. C. A. F. (1982) Oxytocin, vasopressin and neurophysines in the hypothalamo-neurohypophysial system of the human fetus. *Journal of Endocrinology*, **95**, 403–408.

Butler, N. R. & Goldstein, H. (1973) Smoking in pregnancy and subsequent child development. *British Medical Journal*, **4**, 573–75.

Buznikov, G. A., Sakkarova, A. V., Manukhin, B. N. & Markova, L. V. (1972) The role of neurohumors in early embryogenesis. IV Fluorometric and histochemical study in cleaving eggs and larvae of sea urchins. *Journal of Embryology and Experimental Morphology*, **27**, 339–51.

Chaney, R. H., Givens, C. A., Watkins, G. P. & Eyman, R. K. (1986) Birth injury as the cause of mental retardation. *Obstetrics and Gynecology*, **67**, 771–5.

Coleman, M. (1979) Studies of the autistic syndromes. In Katzman, R. (ed.) *Congenital and Acquired Cognitive Disorders.* New York: Raven Press, pp. 265–75.

Conrad, A. J. & Scheibel, A. B. (1987) Schizophrenia and the hippocampus: the embryological hypothesis extended. *Schizophrenia Bulletin*, **13**, 577–87.

Courchesne, E., Yeung-Courchesne, B. A., Press, G. A., Hesselink, J. R. & Jernigan, T. L. (1988) Hypoplasia of cerebellar vermal lobules VI and VII in autism. *New England Journal of Medicine*, **318**, 1349–54.

Dicker, S. E. & Tyler, C. (1953) Vasopressor and oxytocic activities of the pituitary glands of rats, guinea-pigs and cats and of human fetuses. *Journal of Physiology*, **121**, 206–14.

Dörner, G. (1979) Psychoneuroendocrine aspects of brain development and reproduction. In Zichella, L. & Pancheri, P. (eds.) *Psychoneuroendocrinology in reproduction, an interdisciplinary approach.* Amsterdam: Elsevier, pp. 43–54.

Dörner, G. (1986) Hormone-dependent brain development and preventive medicine. *Monograph of Neural Sciences*, **12**, 17–27.

Ehrhardt, A. A., Meyer-Bahlberg, H. F. L., Rosen, L. R., Feldman, J. F., Veridiano, N. P., Zimmerman, I. & McEwen, B. S. (1985) Sexual orientation after prenatal exposure to exogenous estrogen. *Archives of Sexual Behaviour*, **14**, 57–75.

Ellis, L., Ames, A. M., Peckham, W. & Burke, D. (1988) Sexual orientation of human offspring may be altered by severe maternal stress during pregnancy. *Journal of Sexual Research*, **25**, 152–7.

Fellman, D., Bloch, B., Bugnon, C. & Lenys, D. (1979) Etude immunocytologique de la maturation des axes neuroglandulaires hypothalamo-neurohypophysaires chez le foetus humain. *Journal de Physiologie* (Paris), **75**, 37–43.

Gladue, B. A., Green, R. & Hellman, R. E. (1984) Neuroendocrine response to estrogen and sexual orientation. *Science*, **225**, 1496–9.

Gorski, R. A. (1984) Critical role for the medial preoptic area in the sexual differentiation of the brain. In de Vries, C. J., de Bruin, J. P. C., Uylings, H. B. M. & Corner, M. A. (eds.) *Sex Differences in the Brain, Progress in Brain Research 61.* Amsterdam: Elsevier, pp. 129–46.

Haber, S. N., Kowall, N. W., Vonsattel, J. P., Bird, E. D. & Richardson, Jr, E. P. (1986) Gilles de la Tourette's Syndrome: a postmortem neuropathological and immunohistochemical study. *Journal of Neurological Sciences*, **75**, 225–41.

Huisjes, H. J., Hadders-Algra, M. & Touwen, B. C. L. (1986) Is clonidine a behavioural teratogen in the human? *Early Human Development*, **13**, 1–6.

Hyyppä, M. (1972) Hypothalamic monoamines in human fetuses. *Neuroendocrinology*, **9**, 257–66.

Ignarro, L. J. & Shideman, F. E. (1968) Appearance and concentrations of catecholamines and their biosynthesis in embryonic and developing chick. *Journal of Pharmacology and Experimental Therapy*, **159**, 38–48.

Jakob, H. & Beckmann, H. (1986) Prenatal development disturbances in the limbic allocortex in schizophrenics. *Journal of Neural Transmission*, **65**, 303–26.

Kanner, L. (1943) Autistic disturbances of affective contact. *Nervous Child*, **2**, 217–50.

Kemper, T. L. (1984) Asymmetrical lesions in dyslexia. In Geschwind, N. & Galaburda, A. M. (eds.) *Cerebral dominance – the biological foundations.* Cambridge, Mass: Harvard University Press, pp. 76–89.

Khan-Dawood, F. S. & Dawood, M. Y. (1984) Oxytocin content of human fetal pituitary glands. *American Journal of Obstetrics and Gynecology*, **148**, 420–3.

Kostovic, I. (1986) Prenatal development of nucleus basalis complex and related fiber systems in man: a histochemical study. *Neuroscience*, **17**, 1047–77.

Laegreid, L., Olegard, R., Walström, J. & Conradi, N. (1989) Teratogenic effects of benzodiazepine use during pregnancy. *Journal of Pediatrics*, **114**, 126–31.

Meijer, A. (1985) Child psychiatric sequelae of maternal war stress. *Acta Psychiatrica Scandinavica*, **72**, 505–11.

Messiha, F. S. (1988) Biochemical Pharmacology of Gilles de la Tourette's Syndrome. *Neuroscience & Biobehavioral Reviews*, **12**, 295–305.

Meyer-Bahlburg, H. F. L. & Ehrhardt, A. A. (1987) A prenatal–hormone hypothesis for depression in adults with a history of fetal DES exposure. In Halbreich, U. (ed.) *Hormones and Depression.* Raven Press, pp. 32–38.

Najimi, M., Chigr, F., Jordan, D., Leduque, P., Bloch, B., Tommasi, M. & Kopp, N. (1989) Anatomical localization of LHRH immunoreactive neurons in the human newborn infant hypothalamus (normal and SIDS). Abstract 38.9, ENA-meeting, Turin, 3–7 September.

Nobin, A. & Björklund, A. (1973) Topography of the monoamine neuron systems in the human brain as revealed in fetuses. *Acta Physiologica Scandinavica*, Supplementum 388, 1–40.

Olson, L., Boréus, L. O. & Seiger, A. (1973) Histochemical demonstration and mapping of 5-hydroxytryptamine- and catecholamine-containing neuron systems in the human fetal brain. *Zeitschrift für die Gesamte Anatomie*, **139**, 259–82.

Paulin, C., Li, J., Bégeot, M. & Dubois, P. M. (1976) La somatostatine et la function somatotrope antéhypophysaire chez le foetus humain. In INSERM, *College de Neuroendocrinologie*, Paris, 129–38.

Paulin, C., Dubois, M. P. & Dubois, P. M. (1977) Immunofluorescence study of LH–RH producing cells in the human fetal hypothalamus. *Cell Tissue Research*, **182**, 341–5.

Paulin, C., Dubois, P. M., Czeenichow, P. & Dubois, M. P. (1978) Immunocytological evidence for oxytocin neurons in the human fetal hypothalamus. *Cell Tissue Research*, **188**, 259–64.

Paulin, C., Charnay, Y., Chayvialle, J. A., Danière, S. & Dubois, P. M. (1986) Ontogeny of substance P in the digestive tract, spinal cord and hypothalamus of the human fetus. *Regulatory Peptides*, **14**, 145–53.

Pearson, J., Brandeis, L. & Goldstein, M. (1980) Appearance of tyrosine hydroxylase immunoreactivity in the human embryo. *Development in Neuroscience*, **3**, 140–50.

Ravikumar, B. V. & Sastry, P. S. (1985) Cholinergic muscarinic receptors in human fetal brain: ontogeny of [^{3}H]quinuclidinyl benzilate binding site in corpus striatum, brainstem, and cerebellum. *Journal of Neurochemistry*, **45**, 1948–50.

Represa, A., Tremblay, E. & Ben-Ari, Y. (1989) Transient increase of NMDA-binding sites in human hippocampus during development. *Neuroscience Letters*, **99**, 61–6.

Robert, O., Miachon, S., Kopp, N., Denoroy, L., Tommasi, M., Rollet, D. & Pujol, J. F. (1984) Immunohistochemical study of the catecholaminergic systems in the lower brain stem of the human infant. *Human Neurobiology*, **3**, 229–34.

Rudeen, P. K., Kappel, C. A. & Lear, K. (1986) Postnatal or in utero ethanol exposure reduction of the volume of the sexually dimorphic nucleus of the preoptic area in male rats. *Drug and Alcohol Dependency*, **18**, 247–52.

Sanua, V. D. (1986) The organic etiology of infantile autism: a critical review of the literature. *International Journal of Neuroscience*, **30**, 195–225.

Schlumpf, M. & Lichtensteiger, W. (1987) Benzodiazepine and muscarinic cholinergic binding sites in striatum and brainstem of the human fetus. *International Journal of Developmental Neuroscience*, **5**, 283–7.

Schubert, F., George, J. M. & Bhaskar Rao, M. (1981) Vasopressin and oxytocin content of human fetal brain at different stages of gestation. *Brain Research*, **213**, 111–7.

Siler-Khodr, T. M. & Khodr, G. S. (1978) Studies in human fetal endocrinology. I. Luteinizing hormone–releasing factor content of the hypothalamus. *American Journal of Obstetrics and Gynecology*, **130**, 795–800.

Stott, D. H. (1973) Follow-up study from birth of the effects of prenatal stresses. *Developmental Medical Child Neurology*, **15**, 770–87.

Sturman, J. A. & Gaull, G. E. (1975) Taurine in the brain and liver of the developing human and monkey. *Journal of Neurochemistry*, **25**, 831–5.

Swaab, D. F., Boer, K. & Honnebier, W. J. (1977) The influence of the fetal hypothalamus and pituitary on the onset and course of parturition. In Ciba

Foundation Symposium 47, *The Fetus and Birth*. Amsterdam: Elsevier, pp. 379–400.

Swaab, D. F. (1980) Neuropeptides and brain development: a working hypothesis. In: Di Benedetta, C., Balazs, R., Gombos, G. & Procellati, P. (eds.) *A Multidisciplinary Approach to Brain Development*. Proceedings of the International Meeting, Selva di Fassano. Amsterdam: Elsevier/North Holland Biomedical Press, pp. 181–96.

Swaab, D. F. & Ter Borg, J. P. (1981) Development of peptidergic systems in the rat brain. In Ciba Foundation Symposium 86, *The Fetus and Independent Life*. London, 271–94.

Swaab, D. F., Fliers, E. & Partiman, T. S. (1985) The suprachiasmatic nucleus of the human brain in relation to sex, age and senile dementia. *Brain Research*, **342**, 37–44.

Swaab, D. F. & Mirmiran, M. (1986) Functional teratogenic effects of chemicals on the developing brain. *Monograph of Neural Science*, **12**, 45–57.

Swaab, D. F., Roozendaal, B., Ravid, R., Velis, D. N., Gooren, L. & Williams, R. S. (1987) Suprachiasmatic nucleus in aging, Alzheimer's disease, transsexuality and Prader–Willi syndrome. In de Kloet, E. R., Wiegant, V. M. & de Wied, D. (eds.) *Neuropeptides and Brain Function*. Progress in Brain Research 72, 301–10.

Swaab, D. F. & Uylings, H. B. M. (1987) Comments on review by Coleman and Flood: "Neuron numbers and dendritic extent in normal aging and Alzheimer's disease". Density measures: parameters to avoid. *Neurobiology of Aging*, **8**, 574–6.

Swaab, D. F., Boer, G. J. & Feenstra, M. G. P. (1988) Concept of functional neuroteratology and the importance of neurochemistry. In Boer, G. J., Feenstra, M. G. P., Mirmiran, M., Swaab, D. F. & van Haaren, F. (eds.) *Biochemical Basis of Functional Neuroteratology*. Progress in Brain Research 73, 3–14.

Swaab, D. F. & Hofman, M. A. (1988) Sexual differentiation of the human hypothalamus: ontogony of the sexually dimorphic nucleus of the preoptic area. *Developmental Brain Research*, **44**, 314–8.

Swaab, D. F. & Uylings, H. B. M. (1988) Potentialities and pitfalls in the use of human brain material in molecular neuroanatomy. In Van Leeuwen, F., Buijs, R., Pool, Chr. & Pach, O. (eds.), *Molecular Neuroanatomy*. Amsterdam: Elsevier, 403–16.

Swaab, D. F., Hauw, J.-J., Reynolds, G. P. & Sorbi, S. (1989) Tissue banking and EURAGE. *Journal of the Neurological Sciences*, **93**, 341–3.

Swaab, D. F. & Hofman, M. A. (1990) An enlarged suprachiasmatic nucleus in homosexual men. *Brain Research*, **537**, 141–8.

Swaab, D. F., Hofman, M. A. & Honnebier, M. B. O. M. (1990) Development of vasopressin neurons in the human suprachiasmatic nucleus in relation to birth. *Developmental Brain Research*, **52**, 289–93.

Vessey, M. P., Fairweather, D. V. I., Norman-Smith, B. & Buckley, J. (1983) A randomized double-blind controlled trial of the value of stilboestrol therapy in pregnancy: long-term follow-up of mothers and their offspring. *British Journal of Obstetrics and Gynaecology*, **90**, 1007–17.

Visser, M. & Swaab, D. F. (1979) Life span changes in the presence of α-melanocyte-stimulating-hormone-containing cells in the human pituitary. *Journal of Developmental Physiology*, **1**, 161–78.

Weinberger, D. R. (1988) Schizophrenia and the frontal lobe. *Trends in Neurosciences*, **11**, 367–70.

Winters, A. J., Eskay, R. L. & Porter, J. C. (1974) Concentration and distribution of TRH and LRH in the human fetal brain. *Journal of Clinical Endocrinological Metabolism*, **39**, 960–3.

Zimmerberg, B. & Reuter, J. M. (1989) Sexually dimorphic behavioral and brain asymmetries in neonatal rats: effects of prenatal alcohol exposure. *Developmental Brain Research*, **46**, 281–90.

4 Chromosomal abnormalities

M. E. PEMBREY

INTRODUCTION

Human chromosomes function in pairs: a legacy of sexual reproduction. This in turn is an evolutionary device for maintaining a winning combination of genes in the face of inevitable mutations at the DNA level, a topic recently reviewed by Kondrashov (1988). There is a huge price to pay for taking this evolutionary route to glory because sexual reproduction itself introduces many new opportunities for disaster! As a central biological phenomenon it is not surprising that it pervades the discussion of psychosocial disorders at all levels from family dynamics to DNA molecules.

Sexual reproduction requires a number of mechanisms to operate effectively at the level of the whole chromosome or at least substantial regions of it. First, homologous chromosomes have to segregate at meiosis during the formation of gametes. For this to be reliable there must first be pairing of homologues and probably also recombination (crossing over to produce visible chiasmata) of chromatids of the homologous chromosomes. Secondly, recombination also has an important role in increasing the assortment of genes in the next generation and to be successful this requires near-perfect alignment of homologous chromosomes in meiosis. Thirdly, sexual reproduction generates sexual dimorphism with sex determination in humans controlled by the inheritance of either an XX or XY complement. It is said that all the Y chromosome does is turn a woman into a man and then sit around feeling pleased with itself. A slight oversimplification perhaps, but there is nevertheless a huge discrepancy in size and active genetic content between the X and Y and this poses a problem of X gene overdose for females. They achieve gene dosage compensation by the mechanism of X-inactivation (Lyon, 1962). Fourthly, since chromosomes and their genes function in pairs, there are the problems of running 'a joint operation'. Dominant or recessive inheritance is, in the final analysis, a question of reliance on one or two active alleles at a gene locus. However, it is also clear that at least in early development there can be a 'division of labour' between some homologous chromosomes, with maternally and paternally derived genes having different effects despite having an identical chromosomal position and DNA sequence. This differential modulation of gene activity, particularly when determined in the germline, is called genomic imprinting (Monk, 1987).

A related area of fundamental importance that has gained enormous momentum during the summer of 1989 is the role of the Hox gene clusters (mammalian homeobox containing genes)* in the segmentation of the early embryonic hindbrain into rhombomeres in the mouse (summarized by Lewis, 1989). In contrast to the mechanisms (as yet less well understood) determining mammalian somite formation, the basic segmentation of the mammalian hindbrain seems to be defined, in part, by a mechanism that is directly comparable to the homoeotic selector gene regulation of whole body segmentation in *Drosophila*. The homeobox encodes a DNA-binding domain on the homeoprotein. Thus it is believed that these genes can orchestrate the activity of whole sets of other genes involved in the next step of development. The homoeotic gene encodes a protein that binds to the controlling region of these other genes acting as a transcription factor. The interest from the chromosomal point of view comes from the fact that the anterior limit of gene expression, of Hox 2.1, 2.6, 2.7 and 2.8 in the mammalian rhombomeres 8, 6, 4 and 2 respectively, corresponds precisely to the sequence of these genes' physical location within the cluster on the chromosome (chromosome 11 in mouse, chromosome 17 in human).

This mirroring of the gene locus order on the chromosome in the segments of expression in the embryo parallels the arrangement in *Drosophila*. If these observations are taken as evidence of a truly ancient homology in embryonic patterning and not some trivial trick of convergent evolution, then we may be able to formulate hypotheses relevant to humans from what we know of *Drosophila* and other insects. Cells of each body region in *Drosophila* become stamped during development with a permanent record of their location along the head-to-tail axis. Experiments suggest that a cell's memory of its anterior–posterior position in the embryo depends on maintenance of the extent of activation along the array of homoeotic selector genes in their clusters on the chromosome. The extent of activation must, to quote Lewis, 'become frozen at the level to which they have been driven by some transient embryonic signal, graded along the body axis'. It

* The term 'box' is used by molecular geneticists to denote DNA motifs that are highly conserved during evolution and therefore regarded as having an important basic function. A network of developmental genes in *Drosophila* has been defined on the basis of homoeotic mutations in which a normally-formed body segment is positioned inappropriately (i.e. legs instead of antennae). All these genes have a conserved DNA sequence of about 180 base pairs – the homeobox.

seems that here we have a molecular mechanism for a cell to memorize a transient event; a form of postzygotic 'imprinting', or learning. Given that the evolutionary process is not one that designs from scratch, but adapts and builds on what already exists for a different purpose, the possibility of some parallel usage of these or similar 'developmental' gene clusters in the learning function of the mature brain may not be so naive as it first appears. There is at least one indication that early embryological development and the learning process in the mature brain may be linked by a key gene activity common to both. The mammalian developmental and transcription factor gene, Krox 20, expresses selectively in the embryonic hindbrain rhombomeres 3 and 5, akin to the process seen with the Hox 2 genes. The activity of a very closely related gene, Krox 24, (Lamaire *et al.*, 1988) was studied by Cole *et al.* (1989) in a well-characterized model of synaptic plasticity in the rat brain – long-term potentiation of the perforant path granule cell (pp-gc) synapse *in vivo.* They found that high frequency stimulation of the pp-gc synapse markedly and selectively increased Krox 24 messenger RNA (mRNA) levels in the ipsilateral granule cell neurons. The stimulus frequency and intensity required to increase Krox 24 mRNA levels were similar to those required to induce long-term potentiation and blocked by the same NMDA-receptor antagonists.

The above is just wild speculation about how disturbances in 'imprinting' of early 'developmental' genes might also disturb mature brain function because the same 'memorized' gene activity is critical to both early embryonic patterning and the learning process. I don't wish to imply that all stored information as a result of learning might be due to combinations of different chemical modifications of various DNA sequences (I have been persuaded that the combination of synaptic connections is central to this), but that the neurobiological substrate for different types of learning and behaviour could be determined in this manner. In particular, the different aptitudes of the infant's two cerebral hemispheres could be predetermined in this way. Indeed one might be so bold as to suggest that because of differential imprinting some critical aspects of brain development and mature function might depend largely on the activity of maternal alleles for one side and paternal alleles for the other side of the brain. It would not surprise me one bit if the so-called higher functions of humans – those that underlie psychosocial development – should prove to be amenable to molecular investigation by a combined experimental animal/clinical approach. It is the structural and functional homology at DNA level that allows the investigator to move relatively freely and reliably between man and other animals.

Much of this chapter focuses on general mechanisms operating at the chromosomal level and how these might moderate the activity of sets of genes or individual genes. It is perhaps important at this stage to clarify the terms used for the functionally significant modifications of DNA during development from parental gametogenesis to physical maturity of the individual. I have already used the terms genomic imprinting (a form of postzygotic 'imprinting') and just 'imprinting'. Any change in the DNA nucleotide sequence is called a mutation. If this arose in an egg or sperm or their precursors, it is a germ-line mutation and will affect all the cells of the offspring. If the mutation occurs during embryological development or subsequently it is a somatic mutation and the individual will be a mosaic. If there is non-mutational modification of the DNA during spermatogenesis and/or oogenesis such that the function of an identical gene differs depending on the sex of the transmitting parent, then the term genomic imprinting is properly used. The widespread modulations of X-inactivation occur in early embryological development so these themselves are not really imprinting, although in some tissues like mouse trophoectoderm there *is* preferential inactivation of the paternal X, so imprinting is involved. It is perhaps permissible to use 'imprinting' when there is some contribution from this differential parental effect.

I believe that it is important to bear these general genetic processes in mind when considering what genetic influences might underlie some psychosocial disorders. However, I would not want this emphasis to detract from the enormous importance of structural chromosomal abnormalities in helping to map and characterize those genes that play a critical role in brain development and function. Defining the role of specific DNA sequence variations in determining the difference between those who cope and those who succumb to adversity is a daunting task. It is, however, one that will become open to systematic study as more and more human genes are characterized as part of the international human genome project (McKusick, 1989).

ERRORS IN MEIOSIS

Chromosomal non-disjunction

The key reduction division in gametogenesis, meiosis, has been the object of study for many years (von Wettstein *et al.*, 1984), but is not easy to observe directly in humans, particularly in the female. Some oogonia become primary oocytes and move into the first meiotic division from about the third month of fetal life but completion of meiosis I will not occur until 15–40 years later, with the second meiotic division coinciding with fertilization. By contrast meiosis I and II in the male are completed by 75 days. Any search for adverse influences must take account of these facts. Chromosomal trisomies and monosomies

Table 4.1. *Estimates of the origin of the non-disjunction in some chromosomal disorders*

Parental origin	Origin of X in Turner's syndrome (45X)	Origin of extra 21 in Down's syndrome		Origin of extra X in Klinefelter's syndrome (47XXY)	
		Meiosis I	Meiosis II	Meiosis I	Meiosis II
Maternal	80%	64%	16%	34%	9%
		80%		43%	
Paternal	20%	12%	8%	53%	—
		20%			
				Postzygotic mitotic error 4%	

Sources: Juberg & Mowrey, 1983; Galt *et al.*, 1989; Jacobs *et al.*, 1988; Hassold *et al.*, 1988.

can arise as errors of either the first (meiosis I) or the second (meiosis II) meiotic division and unambiguous identification of the four parental chromosomes, plus those in the affected child, will usually determine at which meiotic division the error occurred. Some success in classifying trisomies, especially trisomy 21, in this way has been possible using polymorphic variations in the structure and staining properties of chromosomes (Juberg & Mowrey, 1983), but DNA markers in the form of restriction fragment length polymorphisms (RFLPs) should now make this more straightforward in all trisomies (Davies *et al.*, 1984; Jacobs *et al.*, 1988). The same approach allows the parental origin of the extra chromosome in trisomies (or the sole X chromosome in Turner's syndrome) to be determined. Clearly, any attempt to elucidate aetiological factors in aneuploidy will be enhanced by knowledge of the parental origin and meiotic division involved in each particular case. Table 4.1 summarizes some findings on trisomy 21, Klinefelter's syndrome (47XXY) and Turner's syndrome (45X). These are based largely on cytogenetic markers, which are somewhat less reliable than DNA markers with respect to parental origin. The figures may have to be revised as DNA results on unbiased samples are obtained. It already seems that fewer trisomy 21 of paternal origin are being found than indicated in Table 4.1.

Until recently the focus was almost exclusively on attempts to elucidate what might cause the trisomy or monosomy. It was assumed that, as far as the patient was concerned, it didn't matter whether the extra chromosome (or single chromosome in Turner's syndrome) came from mother or father. However, with recognition of the effects of genomic imprinting, it has become important to look for any correlation between the parental origin of the additional or remaining chromosome and the phenotype of the patient.

A great advantage of genetic studies is that they can be done retrospectively and it is going to be interesting to determine the parental origin of the chromosome(s) in those sets of subjects with Turner's syndrome, Klinefelter's syndrome, 47XXX and trisomy 21, in which detailed behavioural and psychometric studies have already been completed to look for phenotypic differences. These comparative data will be difficult to obtain in XXX females since only in 1 of 25 (from the best prospective newborn studies) was the extra X paternal in origin (P. Jacobs, personal communication). In the XXY males of these cohorts, however, about half have the extra X from the father and half the mother.

Mutations due to aberrant recombination

In the 20 years since the discovery of Hb Lepore, a haemoglobin variant in which the non-alpha chain consists of the first part of the normal delta chain fused to the last part of the normal beta chain, there have been a great many examples of mutations generated by unequal crossing over. The price paid for imperfections in chromosome pairing at meiosis is great indeed. Reciprocal exchanges at misaligned homologous chromosomes underlie most of the mutations generating alpha thalassaemia (Nicholls *et al.*, 1987), are the best explanation for several of the mutations causing familial hypercholesterolaemia due to LDL receptor defects (Lehrman *et al.*, 1987) and together with non-reciprocal exchanges – gene conversion events – explain all the mutants so far described at the steroid 21 hydroxylase locus, some of which cause congenital adrenal hyperplasia (T. Strachan, personal communication). These are but common examples. The long list is getting longer by the month. A prerequisite for unequal crossing over is the existence of local repeated homologous or near homologous DNA sequences, for it is in these situations that misalignment due to 'mistaken identity' can occur (much like partnership errors in square dancing with identical twins). The repeated sequences can be duplicated active genes, neighbouring inactive pseudogenes, or dispersed non-coding repeat sequences such as Alu sequences. Chandley (1989) has recently addressed the phenomenon of asymmetrical alignment in the context of discussing the basic underlying mechanism by which eukaryote chromosomes achieve full synapsis at meiotic prophase. She presented data to support her belief that GC-rich repeated sequences in eukaryotes function to initiate pairing between homologous chromosomes at meiosis. The ability of so called G4–DNA to form parallel four-stranded complexes suggests a role for these sequences in meiotic pairing (Sen & Gilbert, 1988). She believed that the highly variable GC-rich tandem repeats or 'minisatellite' DNA of fingerprinting fame in humans are highly variable largely because they suffer repeated unequal crossing over as a result of initial trials at homologous pairing. Meiotic pairing is known to start close to the telomeres of chromosomes and this is where the minisatellite DNA sequences tend to be localized. GC-rich minisatellites elsewhere in the chromosome and Alu-like sequences may also function as initiators of pairing, the latter perhaps providing homology for pairing within gene loci. Asymmetrical alignment during synaptic trial events could, by unequal exchange, generate an infinite variety of mutations from minor allelic changes to structural rearrangements, e.g. deletions, duplications and translocations contributing to genetic disease in man (Chandley, 1989). Thus much of the non-coding so-called 'junk' DNA may function to initiate meiotic pairing and these trials in turn may underlie common mutations such as those for fragile X mental retardation, and the Prader–Willi and Angelman syndrome deletions of the 15q12 region.

There are two further points that may well be relevant to the pathogenesis of brain maldevelopment or dysfunction. (a) Chance mis-pairing and unequal exchanges within GC-repeat sequences can also occur during *mitosis* giving rise to somatic mutations. The extent to which somatic mosaicism established early in development contributes to human genetic disorders is beginning to be explored more fully (Hall, 1988). Again RFLP analysis of different tissues supplements the information gained from traditional chromosome analysis. (b) Repeated illegitimate recombination at either meiosis, or mitotic divisions preceding gamete formation, can lead to amplification of a tandem repeat sequence. This may not directly involve the genes proper, i.e. coding regions, but cause malfunction of genes by altering the chromosomal domain within which they reside. A gene can be transcribed only if RNA polymerase and all the regulatory factors with which it associates have access to the promotor region upstream of the gene. This access could well be a function of the overall configuration of the chromatin in the region. We must at least be prepared to entertain the idea of disorders caused by mutations that indirectly impair the activity of one or more genes by changing the intergenic DNA.

GENOMIC IMPRINTING AND X-INACTIVATION

X-inactivation is a special case of genomic 'imprinting' and one that was recognized long before the general phenomenon because it was so obvious that the second X in females was largely surplus to genetic needs. There is a 'division of labour' between the two Xs. At the first approximation the normal female has functional X monosomy; she is, in fact a mosaic, with one X being active in some cells and the other X being active in the remainder. There are, however, some loci that escape X-inactivation and these could be relevant to the sex chromosome aberrations discussed later. Considering the whole genome it is now clear that although both parental sexes may be contributing equivalent genetic information at most gene loci, this information is not necessarily functionally equivalent. For example, human conceptuses possessing two paternal genomes and no maternal chromosome set form hydatidiform moles (Kajii & Ohama, 1977). This observation could have been attributed to homozygosity for lethal recessive genes, but further study, especially in animals, has shown this not to be the case. Diploid parthenotes possessing two maternal genomes are usually inviable (Markert, 1982) and nuclear transplantation experiments in mice have shown that both parental genomes are necessary for complete embryogenesis. The paternal genome is functionally more important for development of the extra-embryonic tissues, whilst the maternal genome is particularly important for embryonic development (Surani *et al.*, 1987).

Not all of the genome is involved in these parental effects, however, because zygotes with maternal or paternal disomy (i.e. both the chromosomes of the pair being maternal, or paternal in origin respectively) for chromosomes 1, 4, 5, 9, 13, 14 and 15 of the mouse survive normally (Searle *et al.*, 1989). Two striking examples of parental effects in mice were reported by Cattenach & Kirk (1985). Mice disomic for chromosome 11 of maternal origin were smaller than their normal litter-mates and those with paternal disomy 11 larger than normal. Mice with two maternal copies of distal chromosome 2 and no paternal contribution for this region had long flat-sided bodies with arched backs. They became totally inactive within a few hours of birth. The reciprocal type with two paternal copies of the distal chromosome 2 region showed what appeared, at least superficially, to be an opposite phenotype. These mice have short square bodies with broad flat backs and are notably hyperkinetic. They survive several days but do not grow normally and develop abnormal neurological signs.

Studies such as these indicate a modulation of gene activity that is dependent not on changes in DNA sequence but some other modification of the chromosomal DNA. Such modulations would have to be stably maintained through at least the early development of the individual but be erased between generations. The parallel with X-inactivation was obvious. X-inactivation operates in the pre–oogonial cells (Gartler *et al.*, 1975) but both Xs become active in oogonial cells as they move into oogenesis (Gartler *et al.*, 1972). This erasure of all X-inactivation lasts until around the second week after fertilization when one X in each cell becomes inactivated (Gartler & Riggs, 1983). With normal X chromosomes and in most tissues this process is random, but in all descendant progeny cells the same X remains inactive.

The need for some modification of chromatin that could persist stably throughout DNA replication suggested methylation of DNA as a possible mechanism for genomic imprinting. Differential patterns of methylation are stable, heritable (in a somatic sense) and have been implicated in the regulation of gene expression, chromatin configuration and X chromosome expression (Holliday & Pugh, 1975; Monk 1986). The differential effect of parental origin on the pattern of DNA methylation has been reported on at least three occasions in transgenic mice (Reik *et al.*, 1987; Sapienza *et al.*, 1987; Swain *et al.*, 1987). In the latter instance, the transgene was methylated and unexpressed if inherited from the mother, but the same gene tended to be unmethylated and expressed selectively in heart tissue if inherited from the father. DNA methylation may not be the whole story as far as imprinting mechanisms are concerned. It may 'consolidate' inactivation, which arises initially by chromatin configurational changes induced by other means (Monk, 1988).

Genomic imprinting as an influence in human genetic disorders

The role of genomic imprinting in human pathology has so far only been demonstrated in the rather special case of hydatidiform moles (that arise as a result of a duplicated paternal set of chromosomes with loss of the maternal set), in the Prader–Willi syndrome and in the Angelman syndrome.

Myotonic dystrophy and Huntington's disease are both autosomal dominant neurological disorders in which the parental origin of the mutant gene has an influence on disease severity. The severe congenital form of myotonic dystrophy occurs almost exclusively in babies inheriting it from their mothers (Harper, 1979), whilst virtually all those who have the uncommon juvenile onset form of Huntington's disease have inherited it from their fathers (Hayden, 1981). The problem with investigating these examples is that although the mutant loci have been mapped to chromosomes 19 and 4 respectively, the genes themselves have yet to be cloned. Differential methylation may, of course, extend across a whole chromosomal region but evidence from X-linked genes indicates that the differences in methylation between the active and inactive X may be very localized (Vogelstein *et al.*, 1987). It is likely therefore that imprinting and methylation studies will have to await the cloning of the specific genes involved which should not be long in coming.

Two disorders that look increasingly likely as candidates for some form of imprinting effect are the Prader–Willi syndrome (PWS) and Angelman syndrome (AS). Cytogenetic deletions of chromosome 15q11q13, associated with 70% of patients with PWS (Ledbetter *et al.*, 1981, 1982), have recently been reported in AS (Kaplan *et al.*, 1987; Magenis *et al.*, 1987; Pembrey *et al.*, 1988, 1989). Donlon (1988), Knoll *et al.*, (1989) and unpublished results from our own laboratory have shown that the deletions in PWS and AS are *as yet* indistinguishable using several DNA probes from this region. However, clinically the two syndromes are distinct.

AS is associated with moderate to severe mental retardation with absent or near-absent speech, a 'puppet-like' ataxic gait, a happy disposition and seizures (Angelman, 1965; Robb *et al.*, 1989). AS children have characteristic EEG abnormalities which greatly assist the diagnosis in early childhood (Boyd *et al.*, 1988). On the other hand, PWS is characterized by hypotonia and failure to thrive in infancy, variable mental retardation, hypogonadism, short stature, small hands and feet and, later in childhood, hyperphagia leading to obesity (Cassidy, 1984; Niikawa & Ishikiriyama, 1985). The sibling recurrence risk in PWS is very small (<1%) whilst several sets of affected siblings have been reported with Angelman syndrome giving a recurrence risk of 5–10%. We have now been able to study 13 familial cases of AS from 6 families and none show deletions, whilst our original figure of at least 50% of all AS patients showing deletions ((Pembrey *et al.*, 1988) has been substantiated (Williams *et al.*, 1988). Our present data show that 18 out of 24 'sporadic' AS children have deletions. In one AS boy we found what looked like a pericentric inversion 15(inv) 15p11q13 and surprisingly his healthy mother carried the same inversion, a fact that demanded a complex hypothesis to explain the inheritance. We proposed a combination of recessive inheritance and *de novo* cytogenetic deletions involving one or both of duplicated gene loci at 15q11–13 (Pembrey *et al.*, 1989). However, subsequent analysis of the parental origin of the *de novo* 15q11–13 deletions has shifted the focus, and other explanations have to be entertained.

It has been known for some time that the *de novo* deletions causing PWS usually arise in a paternal 15. Deletions in 21 out of 24 PWS patients have been shown either cytologically (Butler *et al.*, 1986) or molecularly (Nicholls *et al.*, 1989a) to be paternal in origin. It should be noted that the use of cytogenetic polymorphisms to determine parental origin may be less reliable than DNA markers, and reassessments are making it more likely that *all* PWS-causing deletions arise on the paternal 15. By contrast the 15q11–13 deletion in AS is maternal in origin. Knoll *et al.* (1989) studied four AS patients molecularly and, adding these to five studied cytogenetically elsewhere, found all 9 deletions were maternal in origin. We have also found all 12 deletions studied so far to be of maternal origin. In a recent abstract (Malcolm *et al.*, 1990) we stated that preliminary cytogenetic evidence suggested that 2 were of paternal origin, but this is now definitely incorrect. Equally striking is our analysis of the affected siblings where our expectation (on the basis of recessive inheritance) was that they would share *both* 15s in common. To date using a combination of cytogenetic and molecular approaches we have shown that they share the maternal 15 in common but may have different paternal 15s making recessive inheritance unlikely. Gonadal mosaicism becomes a distinct possibility, but again the inheritance seems to be selectively from the mother as if the paternal alleles at the AS locus are normally inactive anyway. It should be remembered, however, that genomic imprinting in this chromosomal region, whilst almost certainly playing a part in AS, is not the whole story as far as the curious inheritance pattern is concerned. By contrast very recent work on non-deleted PWS makes it likely that genomic imprinting will explain the genetics of all cases of PWS. Nicholls *et al.* (1989b) studied two cases of PWS without cytogenetic deletions of 15q12 and showed conclusively in one and almost certainly in the second that *both* chromosome 15s in the PWS patient were *maternal* in origin (i.e. there was maternal 15 disomy). These subjects were effectively missing a paternal 15q12 and the two maternal allele(s) were not able to compensate, presumably because they were functionally inactive at the relevant time and place during embryological development. This observation in PWS prompted us to look for *paternal* uniparental disomy in those patients with AS, who did not have any cytogenetic or DNA sequence deletion within 15q11–13. We have very recently demonstrated two such cases of paternal uniparental disomy in typical AS patients with no detectable chromosomal abnormality (S. Malcolm & colleagues, personal communication).

In summary, the data so far indicate that whilst AS and PWS are associated with *as yet* indistinguishable molecular deletions, the parental origin of the deletion seems to be critical for determining which phenotype results. The general importance of clarifying the effect of imprinting in this chromosomal region is illustrated by the fact that Smith *et al.* (1983) have presented evidence that a susceptibility gene for specific reading disability maps to this region of 15, although it should be noted that this linkage has not been confirmed (Fain *et al.*, 1985; Bisgaard *et al.*, 1987).

Experimental approaches to X-inactivation and genomic imprinting

As indicated earlier, X-inactivation is a particular type of genomic 'imprinting', and has been subjected to investigation. The classic late-labelling cytogenetic approach to X-inactivation exploits the fact that inactive X chromosomes replicate their DNA later in the cell cycle than the other chromosomes. Exploiting this fact, these techniques work on the principle of adding DNA precursor substances (e.g. BrdU, tritiated thymidine) late in the cell cycle, and then identifying the precursor cytogenetically. If this late replication is a direct reflection of the chemical modification and altered chromatin configuration associated with inactivation, then detailed analysis of the replication process in the X chromosomes would be one way forward. Reddy *et al.* (1988) have developed such a method for defining the normal replication kinetics of X chromosomes in fibroblasts and lymphocytes. The build-up of band patterns are tissue specific. Although this method is very time consuming, it could be one approach to detecting alterations of X-inactivation at the chromosomal band level if such changes existed. To have higher resolution it is necessary to analyse the DNA direct and here one is dependent on the patterns of methylation of specific CpG dinucleotides in DNA. The active and inactive X have been shown to differ at several gene loci (e.g. HPRT and PGK) with respect to the pattern of DNA methylation (Vogelstein *et al.*, 1987). Fortunately for those studying methylation two isoschizomeric DNA restriction endonucleases respond differently to methylation. MspI cuts the DNA at CCGG sequences whether they are methylated or not; HpaII cuts only the unmethylated sequence.

X gene dosage and X-inactivation in human genetic disorders

The X-inactivation process has to be remarkably reliable. Inappropriate inactivation in a male would be disastrous and failure to maintain inactivation would be equally bad news for a female. X-inactivation erasure between generations must be near perfect. There is evidence in female mice that some genes (e.g. OCT) on the inactive X reactivate in old age (Wareham *et al.*, 1987), but this has not yet been confirmed in humans (Migeon *et al.*, 1988). In thinking about what sort of disease one would get with failure to maintain X-inactivation, I decided (like Riccardi, 1986) that a good candidate would be Rett syndrome (see Rett syndrome Workshop, 1986; Opitz, 1986). Evidence for localization of the Rett locus to the short arm of the X chromosome and a probable role of defective X-inactivation is supported by two recent reports of

X:autosome translocations in girls with Rett syndrome (Journel *et al.*, 1990; Zoghbi *et al.*, 1990). This disorder, very rarely familial, is confined to females and characterized by near-normal early development followed by progressive loss of neurological skills from about 12–18 months. The girls acquire characteristic, sterotypic hand-wringing movements and truncal apraxia/ataxia. Autistic traits in the first year of life are superimposed by severe dementia (Olsson & Rett, 1985) and with pseudoautistic abnormalities (Rolando, 1985). Rett syndrome seems to be a disorder of the central nervous system alone. DNA replication at cell division may be regarded as either an opportunity or a problem for reinforcement of X-inactivation by the enzyme maintenance methylase, so perhaps the central nervous system, with its initial high and eventual low level of cell division, is particularly vulnerable to declining X-inactivation. It was when I was pondering on the above hypothesis that I received the invitation to make a contribution to the workshop on which this book is based and to include a comment on 'possible mechanisms involved in the language (or other neurodevelopmental) delays associated with sex chromosome anomalies'. This is not an area of research with which I am familiar but to me the first hypothesis to exclude for the mechanism underlying learning deficits in those with sex chromosome anomalies would be imbalance in normal X gene dosage. This could come about in two ways: (a) the key genes involved are not normally subjected to X-inactivation, or (b) there is some failure to maintain inactivity of the extra X chromosome(s) or some genes on it.

Dosage effects from genes not normally inactivated

The generally accepted view (as expressed in textbooks) is that the whole of one X chromosome in an XX female is inactivated, except for the tip of the short arm where there is essentially full DNA homology with part of the short arm of the Y chromosome. Obviously genes in this so-called pseudoautosomal region would be candidates to be implicated in some of the developmental abnormalities in the sex chromosome aneuploidies. An additional and unexpected candidate seems to be the ZFY and ZFX genes (that were thought initially to be the putative sex determining gene pair, the gonad determining factor on the Y and its homologue on the X). Another gene on the Y chromosome (SYR – sex determining region of the Y) which has just been cloned now looks to be the definitive maleness-determining gene (Sinclair *et al.*, 1990). The ZFY gene was cloned from a small region of the Y chromosome that had translocated to the X to produce an XX male (Page *et al.*, 1987). The gene is highly conserved in mammals and encodes a zinc finger protein (ZFP). ZFPs can bind DNA and act as transcription factors probably orchestrating the activity of other genes. Interestingly a very similar gene, ZFX, was shown to occur on the X chromosome, and at long last it looked as if sex determination in humans was going to fall into line with many other animals, namely be dependent on the gene dosage of gonad-determining factors. Males would have a double dose from the X and Y, whereas females would have a single dose since one of their two X chromosomes would be inactive. Quite unexpectedly, given its location on the X, the ZFX does not appear to be subjected to X-inactivation (Schneider-Gadicke *et al.*, 1989). The amount of RNA in various tissues, including nervous tissue, is proportional to the number of X chromosomes present. The ZFX and ZFY probes recognize different-sized transcripts on Northern blots, and the predicted proteins are slightly different although they probably bind to the same DNA sequences (i.e. affect the transcriptional activity of the same or similar genes). Thus the effect mediated through an increased dose of ZFP would be somewhat different between XXX, XXY and XYY individuals. Whilst this gene pair alone is now thought not to be the definitive sex-determining mechanism (Ferguson-Smith, 1989; Palmer *et al.*, 1989; Sinclair *et al.*, 1990), it remains an interesting candidate for some of the developmental aberrations in the sex aneuploidies. The challenge is to define the neurodevelopmental deficits characteristic of each sex aneuploidy in such a way that this and other candidate genes can be tested for altered activity in others with the same neurodevelopmental deficits. If some neurophysiological characteristics can be defined, experimental animal work might be a possible means of evaluating candidate genes.

Failure to inactivate additional X chromosomes

The received wisdom is that all additional X chromosomes in the sex aneuploidies are fully inactivated. However, it is known that XXX females have raised levels of coagulant factor VIII even though XX females successfully inactivate one X to produce factor VIII levels no greater than XY males (Mantle *et al.*, 1971). One interpretation is that the XXX female cannot quite cope with maintenance of inactivation of the additional X. This phenomenon might be more widespread, but vary according to both the gene locus and tissue of expression involved. Attempts to maintain inactivation of two X chromosomes during development in XXX females is likely to result in some failure, leading to X gene overdose in a proportion of cells. The problem should be worse in XXXX females with three Xs to keep inactivated. If such a mechanism was operating the neurological deficits should be more marked the more Xs there are. If genes on the Y chromosome have any part to play in X-inactivation, they would presumably act to outlaw inadvertent inactivation of the single X in the male. Thus in XXY males the balance would again be shifted towards failure to maintain X-inactivation in the second X. XYY males on the other hand should not have any neurological deficits by this mechanism, although Y gene overdose will occur.

In crude terms, the above predictions seem to accord with the facts as shown by the pooled data from prospective studies on the sex aneuploidies from birth (see Radcliffe & Paul, 1986). The XYY males have the least intellectual deficit, XXY males next with XXX females having the greatest deficit (Netley, 1986). However, I am not aware that a worsening deficit with time has been demonstrated. Indeed, reduced head circumference at birth would suggest the main problems arise largely before birth, so perhaps replication of extra Xs puts a special burden on DNA methylation. Any neurological deficits in Turner's syndrome, 45X, cannot be due to X gene overdose and therefore would be expected to be qualitatively different from those seen in 'extra X' subjects. 45X females tend to have a verbal IQ that is better than their performance IQ which as a group is shifted downwards, whilst 'extra X' subjects have a verbal IQ that is more reduced than their performance IQ.

It is only possible at this stage to say that the data collected from unbiased prospective studies do not appear to rule out either 'extra X' inactivation failure or the dosage effect of genes like ZFX as a major influence in the cognitive deficits of sex aneuploidies. As regards behavioural characteristics, Netley (1988) has focused his attention on XXY males who are less aggressive, less active and less socially involved than chromosomally normal males. Netley (1988) argues that of the four explanatory options outlined by Bancroft *et al.* (1982), genetically determined abnormalities of a non-hormonal nature are the most likely. The longitudinal studies find evidence against the other three options: (a) familial over-protection induced by parental knowledge of a sex chromosome abnormality; (b) reactions on the part of the 'extra X' male to physical stigmata which may accompany the condition; (c) hormonal abnormalities, in particular androgen deficit, which become evident early in puberty. In support of the view that genetically determined errors of development play a part, Netley & Ravet (1987) and Netley (1988) provide some evidence for left cerebral hemisphere dysfunction in XXY males, and also that activity level and freedom from tendencies towards withdrawal in these subjects are best predicted by the normality of their left hemispheric functioning.

FRAGILE X SYNDROME

Interest in the fragile X syndrome stems from the fact that it is both a common cause of mental retardation and a model for a class of genetic mutations that are as yet ill defined. It represents neither a straightforward chromosomal abnormality nor a single gene defect inherited in a regular Mendelian fashion. In 1981, when an X chromosome specific library of DNA clones first became available, I argued that the fragile X syndrome was a prime candidate for analysis because any chromosomal mutation that is visible by light microscopy must be blatantly obvious at the DNA level. How wrong can one be! 8 years on, the mutant locus has still to be cloned, and clinically useful DNA markers have been developed at a painfully slow rate.

The fragile X syndrome is characterized by mental retardation and the presence of a folate-sensitive fragile site – the appearance of an unstainable gap at Xq27.3. The chromosome at this point looks as though it is broken or about to break. There are many reviews of the fragile X syndrome (Turner & Jacobs, 1983; Sutherland, 1985; Pembrey *et al.*, 1986; Nussbaum & Ledbetter, 1986; Davies, 1989) and the proceedings of each international fragile X workshop are published in the *American Journal of Medical Genetics* (see *Am. J. Med. Genet.* Vol. **17**, January 1984; Vol. **23**, January/February 1986; Vol. **30**, May/June 1988). In this chapter I will focus on selected topics that are currently problematic.

Mental retardation and autism

There is general agreement that mental retardation due to the fragile X syndrome is common. Prevalence rates for people with an intellectual handicap and the fragile X syndrome range from 1 in 2610 males and 1 in 4221 females in an Australian school study (Turner *et al.*, 1986) to 1 in 1000 for both sexes in school children in Coventry, England (Webb *et al.*, 1986). In summarizing all the Coventry based research (Bundey *et al.*, 1985; Webb *et al.*, 1986; Thake *et al.*, 1987; Bundey *et al.*, 1989) which represents some of the most carefully and least biased studies, Dr Bundey recently provided the figures in Table 4.2 for fragile X in *non-specific* mental retardation, i.e. where obvious chromosomal and dysmorphic syndromes had been excluded. These represent some of the highest figures reported and in particular the figure of 1 in 10 for girls with non-specific severe mental retardation (IQ < 50) may be a reflection of small numbers. In commenting on the IQ ranges in special schools in Coventry, Table 4.3, they pointed out that they did not find the verbal IQ to be lower than the performance IQ as previously reported, but the reverse. In a recent review, Hagerman (1989) concluded that language and non-language skills are relatively similar, although isolated areas of language, such as single-word vocabulary, may be significantly higher than isolated non-verbal tasks such as spatial reasoning. This is a reflection of the learning strengths and weaknesses

Table 4.2. *Frequency of fragile X syndrome in Coventry*[a]

Non-specific severe mental retardation	
Boys	1 in 10
Girls	1 in 10[b]
Non-specific mild mental retardation	
Boys	1 in 17
Girls	1 in 10
All school children	
Boys	1 in 1000
Girls	1 in 1000

[a] Fragile X syndrome = Mental retardation *and* fragile X.
[b] This unexpectedly high level may be due to small numbers.

Table 4.3. *IQ ranges in special schools in Coventry*

	Fragile X children		
IQ range	Boys (n = 16)	Girls (n = 13)	Non fragile X children
>70	19%	31%	20%
50–69	50%	46%	43%
35–49	19%	23%	24%
20–34	12%	—	9%
<20	—	—	4%

or cognitive profiles, which are relatively consistent in the fragile X syndrome.

There seems to be a genuine association between the fragile X syndrome and autism, although estimates of the proportion of autistic individuals showing fragile sites at Xq27.3 vary widely from 16% or higher (Blomquist *et al.*, 1985; Brown *et al.*, 1986, Hagerman *et al.*, 1986) to negative reports (Venter *et al.*, 1984). There has been a lot of debate about the relationship of the fragile X syndrome to autism, generating, in my humble view as no expert on autism, more heat than light. An important point to make is that the fragile X syndrome does not seem to account for the few sibling recurrences in Kanner-type autism. Another point is that autism is commoner in those with the fragile X syndrome than in normal males even if one accepts the lower figures such as the 2.4% of 85 autistic males reported by Payton *et al.* (1989). These authors concluded 'the incidence of the fragile X chromosome abnormality in autistic individuals is likely the same as that in the mentally retarded male population and therefore does not increase the risk for autism above that of *mental retardation itself*' (my italics). This latter conclusion seems quite wrong given all the different disorders lumped together under the term 'the mentally retarded male population' some of which may be very rarely associated with autism whilst others may be often associated. A major contribution to such a population of mentally retarded males would be Down's syndrome and whilst autism has been described in association with Down's syndrome it is very rare (Bregman & Volkmar, 1988). It therefore stands to reason that mental retardation *per se* does not cause a standard frequency of autism, and that the fragile X syndrome is one of perhaps many mental retardation syndromes that is positively associated with autism. There may also be a specific neuropsychiatric phenotype in males with the fragile X syndrome (reviewed by Hagerman, 1989). Early work (Brown *et al.*, 1986; Hagerman *et al.*, 1986) focused enthusiastically on autism claiming that a diagnostic evaluation of fragile X male populations indicated that 15–20% meet the DSM–III criteria for infantile autism and nearly 50% may meet criteria for some form of pervasive developmental disorder. However, Dykens *et al.* (1988) found little difference in the rates of autistic symptomatology between males with the fragile X syndrome and males who were retarded for other reasons. In reviewing recent detailed and systematic behavioural assessments, Rutter *et al.* (1990) conclude that although social and language problems are indeed commonly associated with the fragile X syndrome they only occasionally fit the diagnostic criteria for autism.

Varying diagnostic criteria may present problems in these types of studies not only in respect of the phenotype but also the cytogenetic findings. Not only are special cell culture methods necessary to reveal the fragile site in a proportion of lymphocytes, but not all those who can transmit the fragile X mutation show fragile sites. Attempts to enhance the expression of fragile sites in lymphocyte culture in order to reduce 'false negatives' leads to the problems of 'false positives'. The significance of 1–2% fragile sites in an individual who does not come from a clearly established fragile X syndrome family is very difficult to determine, and the difficulties are unlikely to be resolved until the mutational events are characterized at the DNA level. Why I believe this is so becomes clear when considering what is known (or not known) about the genetics of this disorder.

The genetics of the fragile X syndrome

The first point to address is – are we really dealing with an X-linked gene locus? In the early days it was pointed out that the fact that the visible chromosomal change was at Xq27.3 was not proof that the gene defect causing the mental retardation was also located there. Nearly a decade of DNA-based linkage studies has at least resolved this point. If mental retardation alone is used as the disease phenotype, multipoint linkage analysis places the mutant gene responsible right where the fragile site is seen, at least down to the level of high-resolution cytogenetics. Secondly, numerous family studies have demonstrated two key features about this syndrome that are very difficult to explain. A third of female heterozygotes born of mentally normal mothers are intellectually impaired (half the females are affected if the mother is intellectually impaired) and yet in some cases within the same family the grandfather who transmitted the disorder can be intellectually normal. There are only two possible explanations for this with an X-linked mutation. Either there are additional factors, genetic or otherwise, that modify the phenotypic effect of the mutation, or the DNA defect itself is changing.

When I first started fragile X research in 1981, the idea that DNA itself changed within a generation or two in many of the families we saw in clinical practice was heresy. Medical genetics with all the possible gene/gene and gene/environmental interactions at the biochemical and growth and development level was complex enough without the central player, the mutant gene, changing its identity! Nevertheless, family studies have produced data that are extremely difficult to reconcile with autosomal or X-linked modifying genes, cytoplasmic inheritance, modifying mitochondrial genes and even the mother's transplacentral transfer of the normal product of the fragile X locus to protect brain development in her fragile-X-positive male fetus (see Nussbaum & Ledbetter, 1986). To be fair, Israel's (1987) modification of the autosomal modifier hypothesis gets close to a fit with the data, but like all the others does not even attempt to explain the variable 'fragile site' appearance of the X chromosome.

In developing our premutation hypothesis (Pembrey *et al.*, 1985) we drew attention to the fact that the daughters of phenotypically normal transmitting males are virtually never intellectually impaired despite the fact that on the basis of regular X-linked inheritance, they must be all carriers and 30% might be expected to have a cognitive deficit. Sherman *et al.* (1985) confirmed this finding and also emphasized the observation that the mothers of phenotypically normal transmitting males rarely have mentally retarded sons, whilst the daughters of such normal transmitting males often do; an observation that has come to be called the Sherman paradox.

The essence of our premutation hypothesis is that the normal transmitting male has a DNA change (premutation) that does not cause any phenotypic effect *per se* but predisposes to the generation of a full mutation. The fact that this change seems to require transmission through a female suggested to us that the progression from premutation to full mutation was a result of a recombination event between her two X chromosomes, probably unequal crossing over. Nussbaum *et al.* (1986) developed the stepwise progression idea further, arguing that a short repetitive DNA sequence might normally exist at Xq27.3 and was liable to illegitimate, or unequal recombination, thereby amplifying the repetitive DNA sequence. This would represent the 'premutation' stage because, although not enough to disrupt DNA replication and cause a fragile site or interfere with local gene function sufficiently to cause mental retardation, it would nevertheless be highly susceptible to further amplification by illegitimate recombination. Progressive amplification would lead to disruption of local gene function (for example, by too marked a separation of a critical promotor region upstream from the gene itself). It could also delay DNA replication prior to cell division, such that cells will not complete DNA synthesis before chromosome condensation, thereby giving a fragile site.

What is required to explain the Sherman paradox is a biologically relevant factor that can vary between the mother and daughter of a normal transmitting male other than the X chromosome carrying the premutation which by definition (in the premutation hypothesis) is the same in both of them. This variable is their other X chromosome which could differ with respect to its propensity to recombination with the premutation-related sequence. In general terms the premutation hypothesis proposed that the Xq27.3 region contains DNA sequences that act as recombination signals and that this recombination is particularly liable to occur between misaligned X chromosomes; just the sort of phenomenon expected with the initial pairing trials in meiosis at the subtelomeric regions proposed by Chandley (1989). In keeping with this scenario is the increased meiotic recombination observed in general around Xq27.3 (Brown, 1989).

Winter (1987) has calculated the population genetic aspects of a two-stage model (premutation, full mutation) and some of his conclusions are:

(1) 50% of mothers of affected males carry the premutation.
(2) The incidence of carriers for the premutation is 1.35 times the incidence of affected males.
(3) Assuming rates are equal in eggs and sperm, the average mutation rate from normal allele to premutation is approximately 1.67×10^{-4}.

In essence there are large numbers in the population with a DNA change at the fragile X locus that has not yet progressed to the full mutation.

In thinking of phenotypic effects we not only have to accept that we are almost certainly dealing with a progressive change in the DNA defect between generations of the same family, but also have at least to entertain the idea that DNA differences might exist between different tissues in one individual. The particular arrangement of repeat sequences that predispose to unequal crossing over at meiosis may well lead to an equivalent phenomenon occurring between sister chromatids in mitosis (Armour *et al.*, 1989) leading to somatic mosaicism (Hall, 1988). Incidentally, Warren (1988) has proposed that the brain tissue is particularly susceptible to the effects of the Xq telomere being lost as the result of actual breakage at the fragile site. He argues that most other tissues with their high rate of cell turnover are relatively unaffected. Such telomeric deletions may occur commonly (they have been seen in lymphocytes (Fitchett & Seabright, 1984)), but are rapidly selected out during ordinary cell proliferation. To my knowledge this hypothesis has not yet been directly tested, but fresh brain tissue from an affected male should show cellular mosaicism for the absence of the enzyme G6PD (or its mRNA), since G6PD maps to the Xq28 region. The techniques already exist to do this experiment. Returning to the problem of mosaicism, most of us involved in counselling have come across the rare family where there is a discrepancy between the clinical and cytogenetic diagnosis. One such family of ours presented through a young girl with moderate mental retardation who has 16% fragile sites confirmed on repeat samples sent to two laboratories. Her younger brother clearly has learning difficulties, although not so marked as in her, and clinically fits with the picture of the fragile X syndrome (HC > 90 percentile), yet repeated examination of his lymphocytes in two laboratories shows no fragile sites (0/200 cells). Their intellectually normal mother shows no fragile sites (0/200). Perhaps the mother has the premutation which, as far as her son's conception was concerned, was transmitted unchanged in the egg, but the full mutation was generated at mitosis in the early embryo such that the line of cells involving the brain, but not the lymphocyte, was affected. In this situation the way forward (and this illustrates a strategy of general application) is to use the closest linked DNA probes to ask the question – did the two children inherit the same X, or rather the same fragile X locus allele, from their mother? If they did not, then involvement of a fragile X mutation in the boy's learning difficulties would be very unlikely. On the other hand if they received the same X, a fragile X mutation is almost certainly the cause of the boy's learning difficulties whether we are dealing with somatic mosaicism or some other reason for his fragile site negative status. The closest flanking

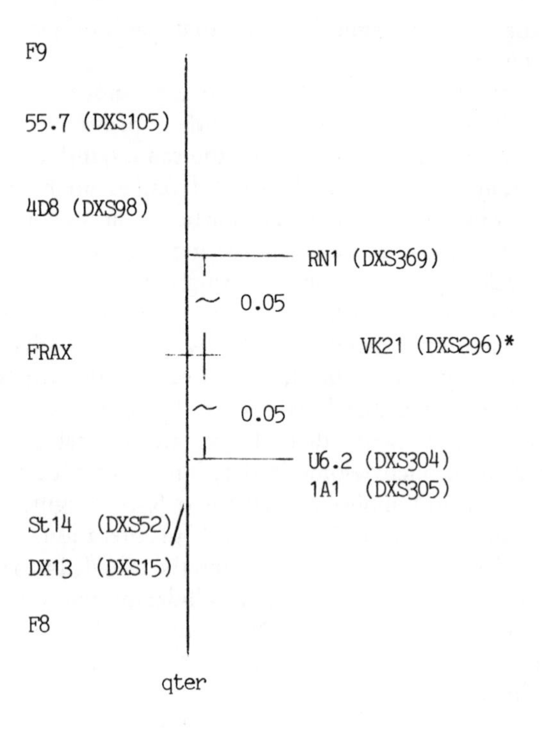

* Limited linkage data, no recombination yet with fragile X (October, 1989), somatic hybrid data indicates it lies between RN1 and U6.2.

Figure 4.1. DNA probes (and their official locus designation) around the fragile X locus (FRAX). Human Gene Mapping Workshop 10, 1989 (Mandel *et al.*, 1989).

DNA markers, as of 1988, showed a recombination between probes (i.e. one DNA result indicated they had inherited the same X from mother whilst the *other* DNA probe predicted that they had inherited the opposite X from each other). However, the new DNA probe RN1 (see Figure 4.1) apparently resolved this point. They both inherited the same X chromosome from their mother. Now that closer probes are coming along, I believe gene tracking within families will be the most powerful way of resolving the influence of DNA variations at the fragile X locus on psychosocial development, particularly where cytogenetic results are negative or difficult to interpret with confidence. Before pursuing this point further, however, it is appropriate to describe one further and significantly different hypothesis concerning the underlying mechanism of the stepwise progression of defective gene function in fragile X families.

Laird's hypothesis (1987) proposed that there is a mutation (in a sense a premutation) on the X chromosome in the region of Xq27.3 that does not cause local gene dysfunction *per se* but results in failure to erase X-inactivation between generations. A normal transmitting male carries this mutation on a fully active X. Any daughter of his will, as an embryo, inactivate one or other X in the usual way. This embryo's pre-oogonial cells will take part in this normal process with approximately 50% having the paternally-derived 'mutant' X inactivated and 50% the normal maternally-derived X inactivated and therefore the 'mutant' X remaining active. However, when these pre-oogonial cells move into oogenesis the normal erasure of inactivation is 'blocked' in the vicinity of the X mutation. Thus the daughter of a normal transmitting male will produce three types of egg from the point of view of X chromosome function: eggs containing the normal X (to give a normal son), eggs containing the mutant X, but derived from a pre-oogonial cell in which it was *not* inactivated (to give a phenotypically normal son), and eggs containing the mutant X derived from a pre-oogonial cell in which it was inactivated so that this X will have genes in the Xq27.3 region permanently inactivated due to failure of erasure (to give an affected son). Laird's hypothesis explains most of the data from family studies but makes one clear prediction that distinguishes it from the premutation/illegitimate recombination hypothesis. Laird's hypothesis predicts that one third of the *phenotypically normal* grandsons of a normal transmitting male will be shown to have inherited the *'mutant' grandpaternal X* by gene tracking with DNA markers. In classical linkage study terms they will appear as 'double recombinants' no matter how genetically close the DNA markers used. The same, however, will not be true of *affected* grandsons – they will be increasingly shown to have inherited the mutant X by gene tracking as closer DNA markers are used.

By contrast, the premutation/illegitimate recombination hypothesis does not predict that 'double recombinants' will be confined to phenotypically normal grandsons. With existing DNA probes they should occur in both phenotypic classes of grandsons, and the proportion of 'double recombinants' will gradually approach zero as closer and closer DNA probes are used.

Figure 4.1 indicates the genetic position of DNA probes around the fragile X locus (FRAX) based on data collated at the Human Gene Mapping Workshop (HGM10) July, 1989 (Mandel *et al.*, 1989).

This brief discussion of the inheritance of the fragile X syndrome serves to indicate how many uncertainties remain, particularly in predicting the influence of DNA variations at the fragile X locus on brain development and function from the cytogenetic findings in lymphocytes.

The significance of fragile sites in lymphocytes

Since the full mutation nearly always produces a significant proportion (>4%) of lymphocytes with fragile sites and mental retardation, could the premutation be a risk factor in some more subtle brain dysfunction and associated with such a low percentage of fragile sites as to be usually scored negative? (e.g. 0/200). If the influence of the premutation (defined as that DNA defect in normal transmitting grandfathers) on psychosocial development and lymphocyte cytogenetic expression of fragile sites is very slight what about intermediate stages of progression of the DNA defect? Could some of these fall short of the full mutation but contribute substantially to psychosocial disorders and be associated with a low expression of fragile sites in the 0.5–2% range? If this were so, the next problem would be – what proportion of those in the general population with the occasional fragile site have a partial progression to the fragile X mutation, and who just have the occasional fragile site as a result of unrelated lymphocyte variations with perhaps very local depletions of nucleotides or other factors necessary for rapid DNA replication of the normal DNA sequence at the fragile X locus? There is some *in vitro* research to support the view that an association exists between the genetic status of an individual (as defined from the pedigree) and the propensity to express fragile sites even below the usual resolution of regular cytogenetic analysis. Ledbetter *et al.* (1986) made rodent/human hybrid cell lines, in which the only human chromosome was the X chromosome, from (a) a mentally-retarded fragile-X-positive (40%) male, (b) a phenotypically normal transmitting grandfather from a proven fragile X family, (c) normal males with no family history of fragile X, (d) a chimpanzee. These cell lines, when subjected to thymidylate (Td) stress and caffeine (which shortens G2 of the cell cycle and therefore the opportunity to complete any DNA synthesis not finished in S phase) revealed fragile sites in the proportions shown in Table 4.4. The fact that there is a progression from 4% in normal males through 12% in the normal transmitting grandfather of an affected boy, to 43% in the affected male, strongly suggests that fragile sites induced under these very artificial and extreme conditions do nevertheless reflect the progressive DNA changes expected when moving from normal males to those with the full manifestations of the fragile X syndrome. Whilst this study supports the view that very low levels of fragile sites might be biologically significant, recent work from the same authors adds yet a further possible complication.

The finding that in the rodent hybrid cell system even chimpanzees showed 2% fragile sites, suggested to the Ledbetters that a common, or constitutive, fragile site (of which there are perhaps 100 or more in the human genome) also exists at Xq27.3. This they confirmed with studies

Table 4.4 *Per cent fragile X expression in parental and hybrid cells from affected males, transmitting males, normal control males and a chimpanzee male*

Cell type treatment	Affected		Transmitting		Normal control		Chimpanzee
	GM4025	DT	MGL66	LC	N1	N2	AG6939A
Parental							
Td stress	29(58/200)	40(60/150)	0(0/200)	0(0/100)	0(0/200)	0(0/200)	—
Hybrids							
Td stress	27(126/468)	23(34/150)	2(22/900)	2(9/400)	2(5/250)	2(3/200)	0.2(1/400)
Caffeine	43(152/350)	30(30/100)	12(62/500)	12(12/100)	4(8/200)	5(9/187)	1.6(4/250)

From Ledbetter *et al.*, 1986.

using aphidicolin (APC) (Ledbetter & Ledbetter, 1988). With relatively high doses of APC, lymphocytes of affected males, normal male controls and chimpanzees had similar levels of fragile sites (6–28%). The tendency for common fragile sites to coincide with the rare folic acid dependent fragile sites on the autosomes, although not reaching statistical significance is suggestive of a biological relationship between the two types. The Ledbetters argue that the common Xq27.3 fragile site may be the initial substrate for the multistep mutation process leading to the full fragile X mutation. In practice the real complication stems from the fact that the ordinary thymidylate stress cultures used to diagnose fragile X may well sometimes induce very low expression (≤1%) of common fragile sites. Thus I am reinforced in my view that until the DNA sequences are cloned (Yu *et al.*, 1991) only extremely rigorous and time-consuming case-control studies will determine the relevance of low levels of fragile X expression to specific psychosocial disorders.

A family study approach to the phenotypic effects of DNA variations at the fragile X locus

As a clinical geneticist it is natural for me to exploit the added information that comes to a complex genotype/phenotype analysis from the fact that the disorder in question is inherited in a simple Mendelian fashion. I know that I have emphasized the irregularity of the inheritance of the fragile X syndrome, but it is still true that it behaves essentially as a monogenic X-linked disorder with no male to male transmission, all daughters of a male who carries the 'mutation' also carrying the mutation, etc.

When we delineate the spectrum and relative frequencies of different abnormalities in an inherited multiple malformation syndrome we start by defining the syndrome by the classic 'full house' of characteristic features; that is we ascertain index cases with a secure diagnosis. We then look at the siblings to find secondary cases and use the following argument. *Given the high prior probability* (in recessive disorders) of 1 in 4 of the siblings inheriting the mutation, we can safely conclude that any sibling with several, but not all the features has inherited the mutation. Even if they only have one feature, or two features very mildly, the relative probabilities are heavily in favour of this being a consequence of this sibling having inherited the mutation rather than having acquired the features for some unrelated reason. This probability can be made a near certainty if linked DNA markers can demonstrate that the secondary case has inherited the same chromosome(s) as the index case. Thus, a systematic study of the secondary cases of fragile X in a family will allow a relatively unbiased assessment of the frequency of certain defined psychosocial disorders in those inheriting the mutation or the range of abnormalities that can be associated with the mutation. Clearly there could be complications in interpreting psychosocial disorders which could arise largely as a result of having a mentally-retarded sibling or a carrier mother who may have a predisposition to certain psychological traits. Here it would be essential to do gene-tracking studies on all the siblings so that those who did not inherit the same X as the index case could be used as a form of control. The error in classification would be as low as the recombination rate between the DNA marker and the disease locus which is now down to 5% or less for fragile X and the 1989 DNA markers.

As the human genome project progresses and loci known to be involved in monogenic disorders of neurodevelopment are mapped and cloned, so the above family study approach will make an important contribution. Less disruptive mutations or DNA variants at these loci can be sought and defined using standard molecular genetic techniques. These can then be tested as genetic influences in the more subtle disorders of behaviour and cognitive functions which on clinical grounds might involve the same neurobiological system. Affected sibling pair analysis is perhaps the best approach when penetrance is still unknown and the pattern of inheritance uncertain. Once the risk is established, the outcome in families of those inheriting the mutation/DNA variant can be assessed, and very precise questions asked of the large population studies, preferably longitudinal, in which many interacting genetic (DNA) variations and environmental variables are being analysed.

ACKNOWLEDGEMENTS

I would like to thank Mrs M. Barham for expert secretarial assistance.

REFERENCES

Angelman, H. (1965) 'Puppet' children: a report on three cases. *Developmental Medicine and Child Neurology*, **7**, 681–3.

Armour, J. A. L., Patel, I., Thein, S. L., Fey, M. F. & Jeffreys, A. J. (1989) Analysis of somatic mutations at human minisatellite loci in tumours and cell lines. *Genomics*, **4**, 328–34.

Bancroft, J., Axworthy, D. I. & Ratcliffe, S. (1982) The personality and psychosexual development of boys with 47, XXY chromosome constitution. *Journal of Child Psychology and Psychiatry*, **23**, 169–80.

Bisgaard, M. L., Eiberg, H., Moller, N., Niebuhr, E. & Mohr, J. (1987) Dyslexia and choromosome 15 heteromorphism: negative lod score in a Danish material. *Clinical Genetics*, **32**, 118–9.

Blomquist, H. K., Bohman, M., Edvinsson, S. O., Gillberg, C., Gustavson, K.-H., Holmgren, G. & Wahlström, J. (1985) Frequency of the fragile X syndrome in infantile autism. A Swedish multicenter study. *Clinical Genetics*, **27**, 113–7.

Boyd, S. G., Harden, A. & Patton, M. A. (1988) The EEG in early diagnosis of Angelman's (happy puppet) syndrome. *European Journal of Pediatrics*, **147**, 508–13.

Bregman, J. D. & Volkmar, F. R. (1988) Autistic social dysfunction and Down's syndrome. *Journal of the American Academy of Child and Adolescent Psychiatry*, **27**, 440–1.

Brown, W. T., Jenkins, E. C., Cohen, I. L., Fisch, G. S., Wolf-Schein, E. G., Gross, A., Waterhouse, L., Fein, D., Mason-Brothers, A., Ritvo, E., Ruttenburg, B. A., Bentley, W. & Castells, S. (1986) Fragile X and autism: a multicenter survey. *American Journal of Medical Genetics*, **23**, 341–53.

Brown, W. T. (1989) DNA studies of the fragile X mutation. In Davies, K. E. (ed.) *The fragile X syndrome*. Oxford: Oxford University Press, pp. 76–101.

Bundey, S., Webb, T. P., Thake, A. & Todd, J. A. (1985) A community study of severe mental retardation in the West Midlands and the importance of the fragile X chromosome in its aetiology. *Journal of Medical Genetics*, **22**, 258–66.

Bundey, S., Thake, A. & Todd, J. (1989) The recurrence risks for mild idiopathic mental retardation. *Journal of Medical Genetics*, **26**, 260–6.

Butler, M. G., Meaney, F. J. & Palmer, C. G. (1986) Clinical and cytogenetic survey of 39 individuals with Prader–Labhart–Willi syndrome. *American Journal of Medical Genetics*, **23**, 793–809.

Cassidy, S. B. (1984) Prader–Willi syndrome. *Current Problems in Pediatrics*, **14**, 1–55.

Cattenach, B. M. & Kirk, M. (1985) Differential activity of maternally and paternally derived chromosome regions in mice. *Nature*, **315**, 496–8.

Chandley, A. C. (1989) Asymmetry in chromosome pairing: a major factor in *de novo* mutation and the production of genetic disease in man. *Journal of Medical Genetics*, **26**, 546–52.

Cole, A. J., Saffen, D. W., Baraban, J. M. & Worley, P. F. (1989) Rapid increase of an immediate early gene messenger RNA in hippocampal neurons by synaptic NMDA receptor activation. *Nature*, **340**, 474–6.

Davies, K. E., Harper, K., Bouthron, D., Krumlauf, R., Polkey, A., Pembrey, M. E. & Williamson, R. (1984) Use of a chromosome 21 cloned DNA probe for the analysis of non-disjunction in Down syndrome. *Human Genetics*, **66**, 54–6.

Davies, K. E. (1989) *The fragile X syndrome*. Oxford: Oxford University Press.

Donlon, T. A. (1988) Similar molecular deletions on chromosome 15q11.2 are encountered in both the Prader–Willi and Angelman syndromes. *Human Genetics*, **80**, 322–8.

Dykens, E., Leckman, J. F., Paul, R. & Watson, M. (1988) Cognitive, behavioural and adaptive functioning in fragile X and non-fragile X retarded men. *Journal of Autism and Developmental Disorders*, **18**, 41–52.

Fain, P. R., Kimberling, W. J., Ing, P. S., Smith, S. D. & Pennington, B. F. (1985) Linkage analysis of reading disability with chromosome 15 (abstract). *Cytogenetics and Cell Genetics*, **40**, 625.

Ferguson-Smith, M. A. (1989) Primary sex determination in the human embryo. *Biology and Society*, **6**, 93–9.

Fitchett, M. & Seabright, M. (1984) Deleted X chromosomes in patients with the fragile X syndrome. *Journal of Medical Genetics*, **21**, 373.

Galt, J., Boyd, E., Connor, J. M. & Ferguson-Smith, M. A. (1989) Isolation of chromosome-21-specific DNA probes and their use in the analysis of nondisjunction in Down syndrome. *Human Genetics*, **81**, 113–9.

Gartler, S. M., Liskay, R. M., Campbell, B. K., Sparkes, R. & Grant, N. (1972) Evidence for two functional X chromosomes in human oocytes. *Cell Differentiation*, **1**, 215–8.

Gartler, S. M., Andina, R. & Grant, N. (1975) Ontogeny of X–chromosome inactivation in the female germ line. *Experimental Cell Research*, **91**, 454–6.

Gartler, S. M. & Riggs, A. D. (1983) Mammalian X-chromosome inactivation. *Annual Review of Genetics*, **17**, 155–90.

Hagerman, R. J., Jackson, A. W., Levitas, A., Rimland, B. & Braden, M. (1986) An analysis of autism in fifty males with the fragile X syndrome. *American Journal of Medical Genetics*, **23**, 359–73.

Hagerman, R. (1989) Behaviour and treatment of the fragile X syndrome. In Davies, K. E. (ed.) *The fragile X syndrome*, Oxford: Oxford University Press, pp. 76–101.

Hall, J. G. (1988) Somatic mosaicism: observations related to clinical genetics. *American Journal of Human Genetics*, **43**, 355–63.

Harper, P. S. (1979) *Myotonic dystrophy*. Philadelphia: W. B. Saunders Company.

Hassold, T., Benham, F. & Leppert, M. (1988) Cytogenetic and molecular analysis of sex-chromosome monosomy. *American Journal of Human Genetics*, **42**, 534–41.

Hayden, M. R. (1981) *Huntington's chorea*. Berlin: Springer-Verlag.

Holliday, R. & Pugh, J. E. (1975) DNA modification mechanisms and gene activity during development. *Science*, **187**, 226–32.

Israel, M. H. (1987) Autosomal suppressor gene for fragile-X: an hypothesis. *American Journal of Medical Genetics*, **26**, 19–31.

Jacobs, P. A., Hassold, T. J., Whittington, E., Butler, G., Collyer, S., Keston, M. & Lee, M. (1988) Klinefelter's syndrome: an analysis of the origin of the additional sex chromosome using molecular probes. *Annals of Human Genetics*, **52**, 93–109.

Journel, H., Melki, J., Turleau, C., Munnich, A. & de Grouchy, J. (1990) Rett phenotype with X/autosome translocation: possible mapping to the short arm of chromosome X. *American Journal of Medical Genetics*, **35**, 142–7.

Juberg, R. C. & Mowrey, P. N. (1983) Origin of nondisjunction in Trisomy 21 syndrome. *American Journal of Medical Genetics*, **16**, 111–6.

Kajii, T. & Ohama, K. (1977) Androgenetic origin of hydatidiform mole. *Nature*, **268**, 633–4.

Kaplan, L. C., Wharton, R., Elias, E., Mandell, F., Donlon, T. & Latt, S. A. (1987) Clinical heterogeneity associated with deletions in the long arm of chromosome 15: report of 3 new cases and their possible genetic significance. *American Journal of Medical Genetics*, **28**, 45–53.

Knoll, J. H. M., Nicholls, R. D., Magenis, R. E., Graham Jr, J. M., Lalande, M. & Latt, S. A. (1989) Angelman and Prader–Willi syndromes share a common chromosome 15 deletion but differ in parental origin of the deletion. *American Journal of Medical Genetics*, **32**, 285–90.

Kondrashov, A. S. (1988) Deleterious mutations and the evolution of sexual reproduction. *Nature,* **336,** 435–40.

Laird, C. D. (1987) Proposed mechanism of inheritance and expression of the human fragile X syndrome of mental retardation. *Genetics,* **117,** 587–99.

Lamaire, P., Revelant, O., Bravo, R. & Charnay, P. (1988) Two mouse genes encoding potential transcription factors with identical DNA-binding domains are activated by growth factors in cultured cells. *Proceedings of the National Academy of Sciences USA,* **85,** 4691–5.

Ledbetter, D. H., Riccardi, V. M., Airhard, S. D., Strobel, R. J., Keenan, B. S. & Crawford, J. D. (1981) Deletions of chromosome 15 as a cause of the Prader–Willi syndrome. *New England Journal of Medicine,* **304,** 325–9.

Ledbetter, D. H., Mascarello, J. T., Riccardi, V. M., Harber, V. D., Airhard, S. D. & Strobel, R. J. (1982) Chromosome 15 abnormalities and the Prader–Willi syndrome: a follow-up report of 40 cases. *American Journal of Human Genetics,* **34,** 278–85.

Ledbetter, D. H., Ledbetter, S. A. & Nussbaum, R. L. (1986) Implications of fragile X expression in normal males for the nature of the mutation. *Nature,* **324,** 161–3.

Ledbetter, S. A. & Ledbetter, D. H. (1988) A common fragile site at Xq27: theoretical and practical implications. *American Journal of Human Genetics,* **42,** 694–702.

Lehrman, M. A., Goldstein, J. L., Russell, D. W. & Brown, M. S. (1987) Duplication of seven exons in LDL receptor gene caused by Alu–Alu recombination in a subject with familial hypercholesterolemia. *Cell,* **48,** 827–35.

Lewis, J. (1989) Genes and segmentation. *Nature,* **341,** 382–3.

Lyon, M. F. (1962) Sex chromatin and gene action in the mammalian X chromosome. *American Journal of Human Genetics,* **14,** 135–48.

Magenis, R. E., Brown, M. G., Lacy, D. A., Budden, S. & LaFranchi, S. (1987) Is Angelman syndrome an alternate result of del(15)(q11q13)? *American Journal of Medical Genetics,* **28,** 829–38.

Malcolm, S., Webb, T., Rutland, P., Middleton-Price, H. R. & Pembrey, M. E. (1990) Molecular genetic studies of Angelman syndrome (abstract). *Journal of Medical Genetics,* **27,** 205–10.

Mandel, J. L., Willard, H. F., Nussbaum, R. L., Romeo, G., Cook, J. M. & Davies, K. E. (1989) HGM10. Report of the committee on the genetic constitution of the X chromosome. *Cytogenetics and Cell Genetics,* **51,** 384–437.

Mantle, D. J., Pye, C., Hardisty, R. M. & Vessey, M. P. (1971) Plasma factor-VIII concentrations in XXX women. *Lancet,* **i,** 58–9.

Markert, C. L. (1982) Parthenogenesis, homozygosity and cloning in mammals. *Journal of Heredity,* **73,** 390–7.

McKusick, V. A. (1989) Mapping and sequencing the human genome. *New England Journal of Medicine,* **320,** 910–5.

Migeon, B. R., Axelman, J. & Beggs, A. H. (1988) Effect of ageing on reactivation of the human X-linked HPRT locus. *Nature,* **335,** 93–6.

Monk, M. (1986) Methylation and the X chromosome. *BioEssays,* **4,** 204–8.

Monk, M. (1987) Genomic imprinting. Memories of mother and father. *Nature,* **328,** 203–4.

Monk, M. (1988) Genomic imprinting. *Genes and Development*, **2,** 921–5.

Netley, C. T. (1986) Summary overview of behavioural development in individuals with neonatally identified X and Y aneuploidy. *Birth Defects: Original Article Series*, **22,** 293–306.

Netley, C. & Ravet, J. (1987) Relations between a dermatoglyphic measure hemispheric specialization and intellectual abilities in 47, XXY males. *Brain and Cognition*, **6,** 153–60.

Netley, C. (1988) Relationships between hemispheric lateralization, sex hormones, quality of parenting and adjustment in 47, XXY males prior to puberty. *Journal of Child Psychology and Psychiatry*, **29,** 281–7.

Nicholls, R. D., Fischel-Ghodsian, N. & Higgs, D. R. (1987) Recombination at the human alpha-globin gene cluster: sequence features and topological constraints. *Cell*, **49,** 369–78.

Nicholls, R. D., Knoll, J. H., Glatt, K., Hersh, J. H., Brewster, T. D., Graham, J. M., Wurster-Hill, D., Wharton, R. & Latt, S. A. (1989a) Restriction fragment length polymorphisms within proximal 15q and their use in molecular cytogenetics and the Prader–Willi syndrome. *American Journal of Medical Genetics*, **33,** 66–77.

Nicholls, R. D., Knoll, J. H. M., Butler, M. G., Karam, S. & Lalande, M. (1989b) Genetic imprinting suggested by maternal heterodisomy in non-deletion Prader–Willi syndrome. *Nature*, **342,** 281–2.

Niikawa, N. & Ishikiriyama, S. (1985) Clinical and cytogenetic studies of the Prader–Willi syndrome: evidence of phenotype–karyotype correlation. *Human Genetics*, **69,** 22–7.

Nussbaum, R. L., Airhard, S. D. & Ledbetter, D. H. (1986) Recombination and amplification of pyrimidine-rich sequences may be responsible for initiation and progression of the Xq27 fragile site: an hypothesis. *American Journal of Medical Genetics*, **23,** 715–22.

Nussbaum, R. L. & Ledbetter, D. H. (1986) Fragile X syndrome: a unique mutation in man. *Annual Review of Genetics*, **20,** 109–45.

Olsson, B. & Rett, A. (1985) Behavioural observations concerning differential diagnosis between Rett syndrome and autism. *Brain and Development*, **7,** 277–89.

Opitz, J. M. (ed.) (1986) The Rett syndrome. *American Journal of Medical Genetics, supplement*, **1,** pp. 1–404.

Page, D. C., Mosher, R., Simpson, E. M., Fisher, E. M. C., Mardon, G., Pollack, J., McGillivray, B., de la Chapelle, A. & Brown, L. G. (1987) The sex-determining region of the human Y chromosome encodes a finger protein. *Cell*, **51,** 1091–104.

Palmer, M. S., Sinclair, A. H., Berts, P., Ellis, N. A., Goodfellow, P. N., Abbas, N. E. & Fellous, M. (1989) Genetic evidence that ZFY is not the testis-determining factor. *Nature*, **342,** 937–9.

Payton, J. B., Steele, M. W., Wenger, S. L. & Minshew, N. J. (1989) The fragile X marker and autism in perspective. *Journal of the American Academy of Child and Adolescent Psychiatry*, **28,** 417–21.

Pembrey, M. E., Winter, R. M. & Davies, K. E. (1985) A premutation that generates a defect at crossing over explains the inheritance of fragile X mental retardation. *American Journal of Medical Genetics*, **21,** 709–17.

Pembrey, M. E., Winter, R. M. and Davies, K. E. (1986). Fragile X mental retardation: current controversies. *Trends in Neurosciences* **9,** 58–62.

Pembrey, M., Fennel, S. J., van den Berghe, J., Fitchett, M., Summers, D., Butler, L., Clarke, C., Griffiths, M., Thompson, E., Super, M. & Buraitser, M. (1988) The association of Angelman syndrome and deletions within 15q11-13 (abstract). *Journal of Medical Genetics,* **25,** 274.

Pembrey, M., Fennell, S. J., van den Berghe, J., Fitchett, M., Summers, D., Butler, L., Clarke, C., Griffiths, M., Thompson, E., Super, M. & Baraitser, M. (1989) The association of Angelman's syndrome with deletions within 15q11-13. *Journal of Medical Genetics,* **26,** 73–7.

Radcliffe, S. G. & Paul, N. (1986) Prospective studies on children with sex chromosome aneuploidy. *Birth defects: original article series,* 2. New York: Alan R. Liss, Inc.

Reddy, K. S., Savage, J. R. K. & Papworth, D. G. (1988) Replication kinetics of X chromosomes in fibroblasts and lyphocytes. *Human Genetics,* **79,** 44–8.

Reik, W., Collick, A., Norris, M. L., Barton, S. C. & Surani, M. A. H. (1987) Genomic imprinting determines methylation of parental alleles in transgenic mice. *Nature,* **328,** 248–51.

(The) Rett syndrome; international workshop on Rett's syndrome (1986) *American Journal of Medical Genetics,* **24,** (Supplement 1).

Riccardi, V. M. (1986) The Rett syndrome: genetics and the future. *American Journal of Medical Genetics,* **24,** 389–402.

Robb, S. A., Pohl, K., Baraitser, M., Wilson, J. & Brett, E. M. (1989) The 'happy puppet' syndrome of Angelman – review of the clinical features. *Archives of Diseases in Childhood,* **64,** 83–6.

Rolando, S. (1985) Rett syndrome: report of eight cases. *Brain and Development,* **7,** 290–6.

Rutter, M., Macdonald, H., Le Couteur, A., Harrington, R., Bolton, P. & Bailey, A. (1990) Genetic factors in child psychiatric disorders II. Empirical findings. *Journal of Child Psychology and Psychiatry,* **31,** 39–83.

Sapienza, C., Peterson, A. C., Rossant, J. & Balling, R. (1987) Degree of methylation of transgenes is dependent on gamete of origin. *Nature,* **328,** 251–4.

Schneider-Gadicke, A., Beer-Romero, P., Brown, L. G., Nussbaum, R. & Page, D. C. (1989) ZFX has a gene structure similar to ZFY, the putative human sex determinant, and escapes X inactivation. *Cell,* **57,** 1247–58.

Searle, A. G., Peters, J., Lyon, M. F., Hall, J. G., Evans, E. P., Edward, J. H. & Buckle, V. J. (1989) Chromosome maps of man and mouse. IV. *Annals of Human Genetics,* **53,** 89–140.

Sen, D. & Gilbert, W. (1988) Formation of parallel four-stranded complexes by guanine-rich motifs in DNA and its implications for meiosis. *Nature,* **334,** 364–6.

Sherman, S. L., Jacobs, P. A., Morton, N. E., Froster-Iskenius, U., Howard-Peebles, P. N., Nielsen, K. B., Partington, M. W., Sutherland, G. R., Turner, G. & Watson, M. (1985) Further segregation analysis of the fragile X syndrome with special reference to transmitting males. *Human Genetics,* **69,** 289–99.

Sinclair, A. H., Berta, P., Palmer, M. S., Ross Hawkins, J., Griffiths, B. L., Smith, M. J., Foster, J. W., Frischauf, A-M., Lovell-Badge, R. & Goodfellow, P. N. (1990) A gene from the human sex-determining region encodes a protein with homology to a conserved DNA-binding motif. *Nature*, **346**, 240–4.

Smith, S. D., Kimberling, W. J., Rennington, B. F. & Lubs, H. A. (1983) Specific reading disability: identification of an inherited form through linkage analysis. *Science*, **219**, 1345–7.

Surani, M. A. H., Barton, S. C. & Norris, M. L. (1987) Influence of parental chromosomes on spatial specificity in androgenetic ↔ parthenogenetic chimaeras in the mouse. *Nature*, **326**, 395–7.

Sutherland, G. R. (1985) The enigma of the fragile X chromosome. *Trends in Genetics*, **1**, 108–12.

Swain, J. L., Stewart, T. A. & Leder, P. (1987) Parental legacy determines methylation and expression of an autosomal transgene: a molecular mechanism for parental imprinting. *Cell*, **50**, 719–27.

Thake, A., Todd, J., Webb, T. & Bundey, S. (1987) Children with the fragile X chromosome at schools for the mildly mentally retarded. *Developmental Medicine and Child Neurology*, **29**, 711–9.

Turner, G. & Jacobs, P. (1983) Marker (X) linked mental retardation. In Harris, H. & Hirschhorn, K. (eds.) *Advances in Human Genetics 13.* New York: Plenum, pp. 83–112.

Turner, G., Robinson, H., Laing, S. & Purvis-Smith, S. (1986) Preventative screening for the fragile X syndrome. *New England Journal of Medicine*, **315**, 607–9.

Venter, P. A., Op't Hof, J., Coetzee, D. J. & van de Welt Retaf, A. E. (1984) No marker X in autistic children. *Human Genetics*, **67**, 107.

Vogelstein, B., Fearon, E. R., Hamilton, S. R. *et al.* (1987) Clonal analysis using recombinant DNA probes from the X chromosome. *Cancer Research*, **47**, 4806–13.

von Wettstein, D., Rasmussen, S. W. & Holm, P. B. (1984) The synaptonemal complex in genetic segregation. *Annual Review in Genetics*, **18**, 331–413.

Wareham, K. A., Lyon, M. F., Glenister, P. H. & Williams, E. D. (1987) Age related reactivation of an X-linked gene. *Nature*, **327**, 725–7.

Warren, S. T. (1988) Fragile X syndrome: a hypothesis regarding the molecular mechanism of the phenotype. *American Journal of Medical Genetics*, **30**, 681–8.

Webb, T., Bundey, S., Thake, J. & Todd, A. (1986) The frequency of the fragile X chromosome among schoolchildren in Coventry. *Journal of Medical Genetics*, **23**, 396–9.

Williams, C. A., Donlon, T. A., Gray, B. A., Stone, J. W., Hendrickson, J. E. & Cantu, E. S. (1988) Incidence of 15q deletions in the Angelman syndrome: a survey of 14 affected persons. *American Journal of Human Genetics*, **43**, supplement A75.

Winter, R. M. (1987) Population genetics implications of the premutation hypothesis for the generation of the fragile X mental retardation gene. *Human Genetics*, **75**, 269–71.

Yu, S., Pritchard M., Kremer, E., Lynch, M., Nancarrow, J., Baker, E., Holman, K., Mulley, J. C., Warren, S. T., Schlessinger, D., Sutherland, G. R. & Richards, R. I. (1991). Fragile X genotype characterized by an unstable region of DNA. *Science,* **252,** 1179–1181.
Zoghbi, H. Y., Ledbetter, D. H., Schultz, R., Percy, A. K. & Glaze, D. G. (1990) A *de novo* X; 3 translocation in Rett syndrome. *American Journal of Medical Genetics,* **35,** 148–51.

5 Genetic risk and psychosocial disorders: links between the normal and abnormal

ROBERT PLOMIN

A crucial category of biological risk factors for psychosocial disorders is genetics. Genetics is likely to be the ultimate cause of many biological risks discussed in this volume, such as structural and neurochemical aspects of neurobiology, as well as endocrine, metabolic, allergic, and cognitive/language risks. The goal of this chapter is to provide a brief overview of current evidence for genetic influence on psychosocial dimensions (variation in the normal range) and on psychosocial disorders in order to address a single specific issue: the extent to which genetic influence on disorders represents the extremes of genetic influence on dimensions.

Much must be excluded in this brief chapter. First, it is not possible to review basic methods of human quantitative genetics such as family, twin, and adoption designs and combinations of them, or more recent advances such as multivariate and model-fitting analyses. Second, techniques derived from the 'new genetics' of recombinant DNA are not described, in part because these techniques have to date been limited to the study of major-gene effects. Few such effects have been found or are likely to be found for psychosocial disorders, as discussed later. Third, although the application of quantitative genetic techniques to the study of environmental influences represents an exciting new direction for such research, this topic must also be ignored. Discussion of these topics can be found in a recent textbook on behavioral genetics (Plomin *et al.*, 1990a).

The longitudinal theme of the ESF network provides an opportunity to discuss the application of quantitative genetic analysis to longitudinal data before turning to the focal issue of this chapter.

GENETICS AND LONGITUDINAL RESEARCH

In 1875, Francis Galton, the progenitor of human behavioral genetics, wrote:

> It must be borne in mind that the divergence of development, when it occurs, need not be ascribed to the effect of different nurtures, but it is quite possible that it may be due to the appearance of qualities inherited at birth, though dormant.

Age-to-age genetic change

The new subdiscipline of developmental behavioral genetics considers change as well as continuity in quantitative genetic parameters during development (Plomin, 1986a). Evidence to date, for example, suggests the counterintuitive notion that when heritability changes during development it increases. The most exciting direction in developmental behavioral genetics is the analysis of longitudinal data in order to explore the etiology of age-to-age genetic change as well as continuity. Genetic continuity and change refers to the genetic correlation, the extent to which genetic deviations that affect a disorder at one age are correlated with genetic deviations that affect the disorder at another age. That is, heritability of a disorder could be high in childhood and in adulthood but different genetic effects might be in operation at the two ages, in which case the genetic correlation is low, which means that genetics contributes to change, not continuity.

Genetic change in developmental behavioral genetics denotes changes in the effects of genes on behavioral differences among individuals, not molecular changes in the transcription of DNA. For example, the same genes need not be transcribed at the two ages even if the genetic correlation is 1.0: the relevant genes at age 2 years might no longer be actively transcribed, but their structural legacy (e.g. differences in neural networks) could produce a genetic correlation between age 1 and age 2 years. Conversely, if a genetic correlation between two ages is zero, actively transcribed genes that affect the trait at age 1 year could continue to be actively transcribed at age 2 years if their gene products no longer have the same effect at that time. In other words, genetic correlation refers to covariance between the genetic deviations that affect two traits rather than to the transcription and translation of the same genes.

Computation of age-to-age genetic correlations and of genetic contributions to phenotypic stability and instability follows from the simple extension of multivariate analysis of covariance to longitudinal data (Plomin, 1986b). Any behavioral genetic design that can estimate genetic and environmental components of the variance of a single trait can also be used to estimate genetic and environmental components of the covariance across time if longitudinal data are available. Genetic change is implicated, for example, when heritabilities exceed phenotypic stability (Plomin & Nesselroade, 1990). In the case of IQ, genetic correlations from childhood to adulthood are surprisingly high (DeFries *et al.*, 1987b), but personality data suggest more genetic change than continuity, especially during childhood (Plomin & Nesselroade, 1990). This suggests that age-to-age genetic change might be important in the development of psychosocial disorders, especially in childhood.

However, not a single longitudinal behavioral genetic study of psychopathology appears to have been reported.

Acknowledging the possibility of genetic change is important in thinking about biological risk factors for psychopathology from a longitudinal perspective. For example, 'high-risk' psychiatric studies tend to assume that genetically-influenced disorders of adulthood will show manifestations early in life. It is quite possible, however, that the genes that affect adult disorders such as schizophrenia show no effects in childhood.

Parent–offspring design as an instant longitudinal study

Longitudinal analyses of year-to-year change require the contemporaneous relationship of twins or the nearly-contemporaneous relationship of siblings. If genetic change is important, the wide age gap between parents and offspring limits the utility of this design for analyses of developmental change. However, parent–offspring data are very useful as a short-cut to approximate a long-term longitudinal analysis (Plomin *et al.*, 1988a). The traditional genetic expectation for the relationship between parents and their offspring is $0.5h^2$, that is, half the heritability. However, this traditional approach assumes that developmental genetic change is unimportant. Heritabilities for parents and offspring are assumed to be the same, and the genetic correlation between adulthood (i.e. parents) and childhood (i.e. offspring) is assumed to be 1.0. The genetic expectation between parents and offspring is better represented as $h_c h_a r_G$ – that is, the product of the square roots of heritabilities in childhood and in adulthood *and* the genetic correlation between childhood and adulthood. In other words, heritability could be substantial in childhood and in adulthood but parent–offspring resemblance will be zero if the genetic correlation between childhood and adulthood is zero.

Thus, genetic resemblance between parents and their offspring requires heritability in childhood, heritability in adulthood and a genetic correlation between childhood and adulthood. In fact, it is difficult to detect parent–offspring resemblance unless all three elements are substantial because they are multiplied to produce the parent–offspring expectation. For example, if a trait is 50% heritable in childhood and in adulthood and the genetic correlation for the trait is 0.50 between childhood and adulthood, the expected parent–offspring correlation is 0.125. In this sense, parent–offspring designs are not powerful for detecting heritability. However, this is a hidden strength of the design: finding significant parent–offspring resemblance (say for biological parents and their adopted-away offspring which sidesteps possible environmental sources of resemblance) implies not only significant heritability in childhood and in adulthood but also significant genetic continuity between childhood and adulthood.

From this genetic perspective, the parent–offspring design can be viewed as an instant longitudinal study from childhood to adulthood. This feature can be exploited to screen biological and behavioral measures in childhood for their ability to predict psychosocial disorders in adulthood. A midparent–midtwin design is especially powerful because it increases the reliability of parent–offspring resemblance (by including both parents and two children per family) and it can disentangle genetic and environmental sources of parent–offspring resemblance. This design is currently being employed to screen infant measures in the first year of life for their ability to predict adult cognitive abilities (DiLalla *et al.*, 1990).

Continuity may be found in change. That is, genetic effects on a behavior at one age might be more highly correlated with genetic effects on a different behavior at a later age. In other words, changing patterns of behavior over time may reflect genetic continuity in underlying traits. Combining multivariate and longitudinal quantitative genetic designs in this way can facilitate the search for such heterotypic continuity in which behavior changes in form but still reflects the same underlying genetic processes. This multivariate perspective is also useful in conceptualizing the longitudinal association between biological risk factors and psychosocial disorders.

EVIDENCE FOR GENETIC INFLUENCE ON PSYCHOSOCIAL DIMENSIONS

One of the most important genetic questions concerning psychosocial disorders is the extent to which genetic factors that affect these disorders represent the quantitative extremes of genetic factors responsible for the normal continua of variability rather than qualitatively different genetic factors. That is, to what extent are psychosocial disorders the result of co-occurrence of many of the same genetic factors that are responsible for dimensional variability in the normal range?

To broach this topic, the chapter begins with an overview of what is known about the genetics of psychosocial dimensions in normal samples and then considers the genetics of psychosocial disorders. This background information is followed by a description of a method and some results that explicitly compare the genetics of the normal and abnormal. The goal of the chapter is to explore the extent to which psychosocial disorders are etiologically part of the normal continua of variability.

Most genetic research on normal behavior can be considered in the two broad categories of cognitive abilities and personality.

Cognitive abilities

IQ scores have been studied more than any other trait, and the evidence from family, twin, and adoption studies converges on a conclusion of substantial genetic influence. Older estimates of as much as 70–80% heritability have given way to estimates closer to 50%. The most recent model-fitting analysis of the IQ literature that takes into account assortative mating and nonadditive genetic variance, suggests a broad heritability estimate of 46% (Chipuer *et al.*, 1990). The magnitude of genetic influence increases during childhood (Fulker *et al.*, 1988). Much less is known about specific cognitive abilities such as verbal, spatial, and memory abilities. Verbal and spatial abilities appear to show as much genetic influence as IQ, but memory is probably less heritable (Plomin, 1988). Recent work has begun to consider information-processing measures of cognitive abilities (McGue & Bouchard, 1990) as well as physiological correlates such as nerve conduction velocity, visual evoked potentials, positron emission tomography, and anatomical abnormalities assessed by magnetic resonance imaging (Reed, 1989).

Personality

More relevant to psychosocial disorders is genetic research on personality. One focus of this research involves two 'super factors', extraversion and neuroticism. Four twin studies in four countries involving over 30 000 pairs of twins yield heritability estimates of about 50% for these two traits (Loehlin, 1989).

Some personality traits, especially extraversion, show evidence for nonadditive genetic variance (Henderson, 1982). Nonadditive effects involve unique combinations of genes that contribute to the similarity of identical twins but not to the resemblance of first-degree relatives. For example, evidence for nonadditive genetic variance was found in a recent large-scale twin study in Australia (Martin & Jardine, 1986) and in two studies of adult twins reared apart (Pedersen *et al.*, 1988; Tellegen *et al.*, 1988). The presence of nonadditive genetic variance may be responsible for the lower estimates of heritability from adoption studies of first-degree relatives (Loehlin *et al.*, 1982, 1985; Scarr *et al.*, 1981), although some of the difference appears to be due to violations of the assumption of equal environments for MZ (monozygotic) and DZ (dizygotic) twins reared together (Plomin *et al.*, 1990c).

Extraversion and neuroticism are global traits that encompass many dimensions of personality. The core of extraversion, however, is sociability, and the key component of neuroticism is emotionality. From infancy to adulthood, emotionality, sociability and activity level have been proposed as the most heritable components of personality, a theory referred to with the acronym EAS (Buss & Plomin, 1984). A review of behavioral genetic data for these three traits in infancy, childhood, adolescence and adulthood lends support to the EAS theory (Plomin, 1986a). The only behavioral genetic study of personality in the last half of the life span also finds evidence for significant heritability of the EAS traits (Plomin *et al.*, 1988b). Although the EAS traits consistently show evidence of substantial genetic influence, it should be noted that many other personality traits also display genetic influence. For this reason it is difficult to prove that the EAS traits are more heritable than others (Loehlin, 1982).

Personality researchers have in recent years shown considerable interest in the so-called 'big five' personality traits (Digman, 1990; McCrae & Costa, 1987; Norman, 1963). Although the names of the factors vary, the 'big two' of the 'big five' are clearly extraversion and neuroticism. The 'other three' are much less well defined but can be referred to as openness to experience, agreeableness and conscientiousness. Only one behavioral genetic study has considered the 'little three' of the 'big five' traits and it suggests that at least one of these traits, agreeableness, shows little genetic influence (Bergeman *et al.*, 1991).

The genetics of personality has not focused on those dimensions of normal personality most likely to be relevant to psychosocial disorders, a problem that looms large in attempts to compare explicitly the genetics of the normal and the abnormal, as discussed below. Although neuroticism involves emotional stability, few studies have considered such traits as depression (sadness), mania, aggressiveness, attention, anxiety, gender identification and attachment. The most relevant personality data come from twin studies of the Minnesota Multiphasic Personality Inventory (MMPI). Table 5.1 lists a summary of twin correlations for the 10 scales of the MMPI averaged over three small studies (a total of 120 MZ and 132 DZ pairs; from Vandenberg, 1967). Table 5.1 also includes results of two recent reports of a sample of twins at Indiana University for composite scales derived from MMPI items (Pogue–Geile & Rose, 1985; Rose, 1988). The six composites in the 1985 report were based on scales developed by Wiggins (1966) and Welsh (1956) and the 1988 report used nine scores derived from factor analyses of MMPI items in normal samples (Costa *et al.*, 1985).

In general, MMPI twin results for normal samples look much like twin results for other personality questionnaires. The median MZ and DZ correlations in Table 5.1 are 0.45 and 0.23, respectively, although the Rose report yields unusual median correlations of 0.56 and 0.41. As in other studies, masculinity–femininity and religiosity show little genetic influence (cf. Waller *et al.*, 1990). In the Rose report, the intellectual interests scale indicates surprisingly little evidence of genetic

Table 5.1. *Twin studies for the Minnesota Multiphasic Personality Inventory*

	Twin correlations					
	Vandenberg		Pogue–Geile		Rose	
Scale	MZ	DZ	MZ	DZ	MZ	DZ
Social introversion	0.45	0.12				
Depression	0.44	0.14	0.43	0.01		
Psychasthenia	0.41	0.11				
Psychopathic deviate	0.48	0.27	0.47	0.15		
Schizophrenia	0.44	0.24	0.50	0.23		
Paranoia	0.27	0.08				
Hysteria	0.37	0.23				
Hypochondriasis	0.41	0.28			0.44	0.23
Hypomania	0.32	0.18				
Masculinity–femininity	0.41	0.35			0.76	0.70
Social maladjustment			0.74	0.28		
Overall adjustment			0.33	0.12		
Religiosity			0.83	0.65	0.71	0.66
Neuroticism					0.41	0.22
Psychoticism					0.70	0.41
Extraversion					0.60	0.42
Inadequacy					0.54	0.22
Cynicism					0.51	0.35
Intellectual interests					0.56	0.48

Note: Vandenberg's (1967) summary pools results for 120 MZ and 132 DZ pairs from two studies by Gottesman (1963, 1965) and one by Reznikoff & Honeyman (1967). The study by Pogue–Geile & Rose (1985) includes 101 MZ and 102 DZ pairs at 20 years of age. The data reported by Rose (1988) are based on 228 MZ and 182 DZ pairs in adolescence and young adulthood.
From Pogue-Geile & Rose, 1985; Rose, 1988; Vandenberg, 1967.

influence; the results for extraversion in this study are also unusual in relation to other studies as discussed above. Twin results for other MMPI scales in these studies consistently suggest genetic influence. It is noteworthy that although depression shows genetic influence, the DZ correlation is less than half the MZ correlation, suggesting the possibility of nonadditive genetic variance or contrast effects (Plomin *et al.*, 1990c). As mentioned above, nonadditive genetic variance might be responsible for lower estimates of genetic influence from adoption studies of first-degree relatives than from twin studies.

Isolated twin studies have considered other relevant traits such as anxiety and depression (Kendler *et al.*, 1986), childhood depression

(Wierzbicki, 1987), obsessions (Clifford *et al.*, 1981), psychosomatic complaints (Wilde, 1964), fears (Rose & Ditto, 1983), childhood behavior problems (O'Connor *et al.*, 1980; Stevenson & Graham, 1988), hyperactivity (Goodman & Stevenson, 1989a,b) and delinquent acts (Rowe, 1983, 1986). As in the case of MMPI data, these studies generally yield results similar to those for other personality questionnaires. One exception may be aggressiveness, which shows less hereditary influence and more evidence of shared environmental influence than other personality dimensions (Plomin *et al.*, 1990b).

The vast majority of research on personality genetics relies on self-report questionnaires and parental rating questionnaires. During the past decade, a few observational studies of twin children have been conducted and these suggest less ubiquitous genetic influence than do questionnaire studies (Plomin, 1986a). These findings should encourage more research on personality using other methods such as observations and interviews despite the greater cost of such studies.

Abnormal behavior

The studies described in the previous section involved normal samples unselected for psychosocial disorder. The focus of such studies is the etiology of inter-individual differences. In contrast, studies of psychosocial disorders focus on the etiology of the difference between diagnosed individuals and the rest of the population.

Mental retardation

Over 100 rare single-gene mutations have been identified that involve mental retardation (McKusick, 1988). Chromosomal abnormalities are also responsible for some retardation, with recent interest focused on the fragile X syndrome (see chapter 4, this volume). None-the-less, most mild retardation appears to be due to multifactorial (polygenic and environmental) factors. Despite the outpouring of genetic research on cognitive abilities, there is surprisingly little genetic research relevant to mental retardation. A few family studies but no twin or adoption studies have been reported.

Reading disability

Reading disability shows considerable familial resemblance (DeFries *et al.*, 1986). One recent twin study found evidence for a genetic basis for this familial resemblance (DeFries *et al.*, 1987a); another twin study found genetic influence on spelling disability but not on other aspects of reading disability (Stevenson *et al.*, 1987). A single-gene effect has been proposed for spelling disability (Smith *et al.*, 1983), but subsequent analyses have not confirmed the linkage (Kimberling *et al.*, 1985; McGuffin, 1987; Smith *et al.*, 1990).

Delinquency and criminality

Although the normal range of variability in delinquent acts shows substantial genetic influence (Rowe, 1983, 1986), six twin studies of juvenile delinquency yielded 87% concordance for MZ twins and 72% concordance for DZ twins, suggesting slight genetic influence and substantial environmental sources of resemblance (Cloninger & Gottesman, 1987; Gottesman *et al.*, 1983). Adoption data also suggest little genetic influence (Cadoret, 1978; Bohman, 1971, 1972), although an adoption study of aggressive conduct disorder found greater evidence for genetic influence (Jary & Stewart, 1985).

In contrast, twin studies of adult criminality yield evidence for substantial genetic influence. On average, MZ and DZ twin concordances are 69% and 33% respectively in one review (Gottesman *et al.*, 1983) and 51% and 22% respectively in another (McGuffin & Gottesman, 1985). Adoption studies are consistent with the hypothesis of some genetic influence on adult criminality, although the evidence is not as strong as in twin studies (Mednick *et al.*, 1984).

Alcoholism

Alcoholism in a first-degree relative is by far the single best predictor of alcoholism (Mednick *et al.*, 1987). About 25% of the male relatives of alcoholics are themselves alcoholics, as compared with fewer than 5% of the males in the general population.

Alcoholism is one area in which acceptance of genetic influence has outpaced the evidence (Searles, 1988). Twin studies of normal drinkers show substantial genetic influence on quantity and frequency of drinking, although the evidence is not clear concerning heavy drinking *per se*. Moreover, no twin studies have focused on diagnosed alcoholism.

Adoption studies suggest genetic influence on alcoholism. One study of 55 adopted-away children of alcoholic biological parents found that 18% were alcoholic as compared to 5% of control adoptees (Goodwin, 1979). Because the two groups did not differ in problem drinking or heavy drinking, the study makes the counterintuitive claim that alcoholism may be genetically distinct from heavy drinking. A Swedish adoption study also provides evidence for genetic influence on alcoholism (Bohman *et al.*, 1987; cf. Peele, 1986). Of 268 adopted sons of biological fathers registered for alcohol abuse in Sweden, 22.8% were diagnosed as alcoholic, in contrast to 14.7% of 571 sons of non-alcoholic parents. In addition, two subtypes of alcoholism, milieu-limited and male-limited, were proposed. The male-limited form, in which biological fathers but not mothers showed early onset of alcoholism, is thought to involve greater genetic risk than the milieu-limited type which is particularly susceptible to postnatal risk such as lower socioeconomic class. About 17% of the male adoptees in the male-limited category were alcoholic.

Schizophrenia

An excellent summary of the extensive behavioral genetics literature on schizophrenia is available (Gottesman & Shields, 1982). In 14 older studies involving over 18 000 first-degree relatives of schizophrenics, the risk for first-degree relatives was about 8%, eight times greater than the population base rate. Recent family studies continue to yield similar results.

Twin and adoption studies suggest that this familial resemblance is due to heredity. Five twin studies since 1966 yield weighted average probandwise concordances of 46% for MZ and 14% for DZ twins (Gottesman & Shields, 1982). The most recent twin study involved all male twins who were US veterans of World War II (Kendler & Robinette, 1983). Twin concordances using ICD-8 criteria were 30.9% for 164 pairs of MZ twins and 6.5% for 268 pairs of DZ twins. The same study indicated that genetic influence on schizophrenia exceeds that for common medical conditions such as diabetes mellitus (18.8% concordance for MZ vs. 7.9% for DZ), ulcers (23.8% vs. 14.8%), chronic obstructive pulmonary disease (11.8% vs. 8.2%), hypertension (25.9% vs. 10.8%), and ischemic heart disease (29.1% vs. 18.3%).

As another example of recent research, a reanalysis of the Danish Adoption Study of Schizophrenia using DMS-III criteria (Kendler & Gruenberg, 1984) confirms earlier reports that schizophrenia occurs more frequently in the biological relatives of schizophrenic adoptees than in biological relatives of control adoptees (Kety, 1987; Kety *et al.*, 1978). The reanalysis also indicated elevated rates of schizotypal personality disorder and paranoid personality disorder (but not delusional disorder, anxiety disorder, or major depressive disorder) in the biological relatives of schizophrenic adoptees, suggesting that these facets of the schizophrenic spectrum are related genetically to schizophrenia.

The goal of much research in psychopathology is to break down the apparent heterogeneity to find etiologically distinct subtypes. Research on heterogeneity of schizophrenia has been less successful than for other disorders, especially the affective disorders. Although schizophrenia is genetically distinct from the affective disorders, the classical subtypes of schizophrenia do not breed true (Farmer *et al.*, 1984), as seen most dramatically in a follow-up of the Genain quadruplets who were concordant for schizophrenia but showed variable symptoms (DeLisi *et al.*, 1984).

Linkage to a dominant gene on chromosome 5 was reported in 1988 for schizophrenia in five Icelandic and two English families with a high incidence of schizophrenia (Sherrington *et al.*, 1988). However, several failures to replicate the linkage have been reported (Detera-Wadleigh *et al.*, 1989; Kennedy *et al.*, 1988; St Clair *et al.*, 1989) and as yet no positive replication has appeared. It can be argued that such conflicting results are due to genetic heterogeneity – different major genes may be responsible for schizophrenia in different families. In this view, polygenic influence is seen at the population level because of the concatenation of different major genes in different families. An opposing view suggested by a quantitative genetic perspective is that, for each individual, many genes make small contributions towards vulnerability to schizophrenia (Plomin, 1990). If correct, this position implies that current linkage strategies, which are able only to detect major-gene effects, will fail. New strategies are needed to detect genes that account for small amounts of behavioral variation.

The best evidence for the multi-gene nature of behavior is selection studies of animal behavior. Response to selection in such studies continues unabated during the course of most selection studies of behavior. If only one or two major genes were responsible for genetic effects on these behaviors, the relevant alleles would be sorted into high and low lines in a few generations. Other animal designs such as the powerful recombinant inbred strain method also suggest that, although any one of many genes can disrupt behavioral development, the normal range of behavioral variation is orchestrated by a system of many genes each with small effect. Recent research on complex characteristics in plants clearly shows that most genes account for less than 1% of the variance of complex traits (e.g. Edwards *et al.*, 1987). It seems unlikely that human behavior is any less complex than such traits in plants.

Affective disorders

Although twin studies of affective disorders indicate even greater genetic influence than for schizophrenia, adoption studies suggest less genetic influence (Loehlin *et al.*, 1988). For example, the largest twin study of affective disorders yields concordances of 67% and 18% for MZ and DZ, respectively (Bertelsen *et al.*, 1977). In contrast, in one recent adoption study, affective disorders were diagnosed in only 5.2% of biological relatives of affectively-ill adoptees, although this risk is greater than the risk of 2.3% found in the biological relatives of control adoptees (Wender *et al.*, 1986). The biological relatives of affected adoptees also showed greater rates of alcoholism (5.4% vs. 2.0%) and attempted or actual suicide (7.3% vs. 1.5%) than controls.

Greater progress has been made in analyzing heterogeneity of affective disorders than of schizophrenia. Unipolar depression appears to be distinct from manic-depressive disorder in that relatives of manic-depressives have higher rates of manic-depressive disorder than do relatives of unipolar depressives (Vandenberg *et al.*, 1986). The most recent study of unipolar depression consisted of 235 probands with major depressive disorder and their 826 first-degree relatives (Reich *et al.*, 1987). Major depression was diagnosed for 13% of the male relatives and for 30% of the female relatives. Several studies indicated that the prevalence of depression is increasing and that the onset of depression is occurring earlier in young cohorts, a change that has occurred too quickly to be accounted for by genetic factors. The familial risk for bipolar illness is lower, 5.8% in eight studies of over 3000 first-degree relatives of bipolar probands as compared with a risk of 1.1% in a control sample (Rice *et al.*, 1987). No gender difference was found for bipolar illness.

A novel finding has emerged from a study of the offspring of identical twins discordant for manic-depressive illness (Gottesman & Bertelsen, 1989). Surprisingly, the risk of affective disorder was similar for the offspring of discordant identical twins regardless of whether the parental twin was affected. This suggests that the identical twin who does not evidence manic-depressive illness none-the-less transmits the illness to his or her offspring to the same extent as does the affected co-twin.

In 1987, linkage to the short arm of chromosome 11 was reported for bipolar depression in one family pedigree of 81 Old Order Amish individuals, 19 of whom were affected (Egeland *et al.*, 1987). As in the case of the claim of linkage for schizophrenia, analyses of other pedigrees excluded the reported linkage (Detera-Wadleigh *et al.*, 1987; Gill *et al.*, 1988; Hodgkinson *et al.*, 1987). The Amish results have now essentially been withdrawn (Kelsoe *et al.*, 1989) because follow-up work on the original Amish pedigree yielded two new diagnoses of manic-depressive illness that reduced the evidence for linkage to nonsignificance, and an extension of the original pedigree has also failed to replicate the original result.

Developmental disorders

Genetic factors in child psychiatric disorders have recently been reviewed (Rutter *et al.*, 1990). In addition to research on reading disability and delinquency mentioned earlier, a recent small twin study has suggested genetic influence for anorexia nervosa (56% MZ and 5% DZ concordance; Holland *et al.*, 1984). Other twin studies have found evidence for genetic influence on specific speech disruptions (Howie, 1981); enuresis (Bakwin, 1973); and sleepwalking (Bakwin, 1970). Although adoption studies using retrospective reports of hyperactivity suggest genetic influence, as does a recent twin study using teacher ratings (Goodman & Stevenson, 1989a, b), no conclusions can as yet be made concerning the role of genetic factors in hyperactivity (Rutter *et al.*, 1990). Several relevant family studies have been reported recently that indicate familial resemblance, although family studies cannot untangle genetic and environmental effects.

Work on autism is particularly interesting. Up to a decade ago there was no evidence of genetic influence for autism (Hanson & Gottesman, 1976). However, studies during the past decade have shown that autism is familial, with a sibling risk of 2.9% (Smalley *et al.*, 1988). Genetic influence has been demonstrated in a twin study that yielded MZ and DZ concordances of 36% and 0%, respectively (Folstein & Rutter, 1977), and a replication study is producing comparable findings (Le Couteur *et al.*, 1989).

None-the-less, quantitative genetic research in developmental psychopathology has just begun and much work needs to be done to answer the most basic question of the extent of genetic involvement for most areas of developmental psychopathology. For example, no twin or adoption studies with reasonable sample sizes have been reported for mental retardation, anxiety disorders, childhood depression, gender identity disorders, or the 'other disorders' of Axis 1 of DSM-III. Thus, for the vast majority of developmental disorders, we cannot yet say whether genetic influence is significant, let alone estimate its effect size.

Other psychopathology

Attention has begun to turn to other disorders. Examples of recent research include family studies of anxiety disorder and panic disorder (Crowe *et al.*, 1983); a twin study that suggests genetic factor agoraphobia and panic disorder but not generalized anxiety disorder (Torgersen, 1983); family and adoption studies of somatization disorder that involves multiple and chronic physical complaints of unknown origin (Bohman *et al.*, 1984; Cloninger *et al.*, 1986; Guze *et al.*, 1986); a family study and a twin study of Tourette's syndrome (Pauls *et al.*, 1981; Price *et al.*, 1985); family studies of the association between Tourette's syndrome and obsessive–compulsive symptoms (Montgomery *et al.*, 1982; Pauls *et al.*, 1986); and an adoption study of drug abuse (Cadoret *et al.*, 1986).

NORMAL AND ABNORMAL BEHAVIOR

The previous reviews of psychosocial dimensions and disorders lead to two general conclusions. First, genetic influence is significant and often substantial for most aspects of behavior, both for disorders (categories) and for the normal range of inter-individual variability (dimensions). In the normal range where estimates of proportions of variance are more straightforward, results indicate that 30–50% of the phenotypic variance can usually be assigned to genetic factors. Only for a few disorders is it as yet possible to estimate the magnitude of heritability – for most disorders, the question is whether genetic effects are significant. Indeed most investigations of psychosocial disorders are even more preliminary in that they attempt to establish familial resemblance via family studies that cannot disentangle genetic and environmental effects. None-the-less, where adequate data are available, it appears that psychosocial disorders, like the multiple facets of personality, show some genetic influence.

A second conclusion from the foregoing overview of behavioral genetic research is that there is little correspondence between the measures used in studies of normal and abnormal behavior. One exception is IQ; mental retardation is assessed using IQ measures relevant to the normal range of variability. However, there are few behavioral genetic studies of mental retardation. Quantitative genetic studies of specific cognitive abilities and information processing have no analogs in studies of mental retardation. Similarly, behavioral genetic studies of personality have little direct bearing on behaviors that are the focus of psychosocial disorders. Exceptions include studies of the MMPI and isolated studies of problem behaviors in normal samples. These studies generally yield results similar to those from studies of normal dimensions of personality.

Closer correspondence between studies of the normal and abnormal will benefit both types of research. For example, the abnormal provides societal significance for the study of the normal range of variability. That is, understanding genetic and environmental contributions to normal variability in drinking alcohol may be important in its own right, but its societal value derives from its possible applicability to alcohol abuse. Why should researchers interested in diagnosed disorders also pay attention to research in the normal range of variability? One answer could be that studying the normal range of variability can elucidate processes involved in the development of a disorder.

There is now a more compelling answer to the question: only by studying the abnormal in the context of the normal is it possible to assess the extent to which disorders represent the extreme of the normal continuum of variability. That is, the mechanisms responsible for abnormal behavior might be only quantitatively, not qualitatively, different from those that cause normal variability. As Rutter (1988) has indicated, there can be no presupposition that normal and abnormal development do, or do not, involve the same mechanisms; rather there must be a concern empirically to test for similarities and dissimilarities.

Quantitative genetics provides an as-yet unexploited approach to the hoary problem of the relationship between the normal and abnormal. If quantitative (dimensional) data are obtained on probands, probands' relatives and the population, it is now possible to assess the extent to which the genetic and environmental etiologies of abnormality differ from the etiologies of normality (DeFries & Fulker, 1985, 1988; DeFries *et al.*, 1987a).

Mental retardation as an example

The origins of the new quantitative genetic approach to this issue can be seen in research on mental retardation by Roberts in 1952. Although the body of data used by Roberts has been criticized for methodological shortcomings (Kamin, 1974), recent work by Nichols (1984) using more adequate data has yielded results similar to those of Roberts.

The key to Roberts' work was to focus on mean IQ differences between retarded individuals and their siblings in order to address the etiology of retardation, that is, the etiology of the average IQ difference between retarded individuals and the rest of the population. Roberts suggested that the etiology of mild and severe retardation differs. Siblings of mildly retarded individuals were below average in IQ, whereas siblings of severely retarded individuals had IQs in the normal range. These findings suggested that mild mental retardation is familial (the siblings on average resemble the mildly retarded probands) and that severe retardation is not familial. The next step is to note that variability of IQ scores in the normal range shows substantial familial resemblance (Bouchard & McGue, 1981). This suggests that mild retardation which is also familial may be etiologically connected with the rest of the IQ distribution. Severe retardation, on the other hand, is etiologically distinct from the rest of the IQ distribution because severe retardation shows no familial resemblance. Thus, mild retardation might merely be the low end of the distribution of genetic and environmental factors that affect the rest of the IQ distribution. Severe retardation, on the other hand, differs etiologically from the rest of the IQ distribution.

Roberts could have ignored the IQ scores of the probands, their siblings, and the population and merely examined concordance for retardation as is usually done in research on disorders. Concordances would have led to similar conclusions about mild and severe retardation because siblings show moderate concordance for mild retardation and they show no concordance for severe retardation. However, as explained later, dichotomizing IQ data into discrete categories of normal and not normal loses important information needed to estimate the magnitude of genetic and environmental influence. Also, it should be noted that Roberts' approach does not address differences between familiality at the low end of the IQ distribution and familiality for the rest of the distribution. Familiality for the low end of the distribution refers to the origins of IQ differences among retarded individuals; rather, Roberts' method addresses the etiology of the average difference between retarded individuals and the rest of the population.

Nichols' data make the same point that mild retardation is familial but severe retardation is not. Siblings of mildly-retarded children (IQs from 50 to 69) showed familial resemblance in that their average IQ was 85. This low average IQ occurred because the distribution was shifted downward, not because a few siblings were retarded. In contrast, siblings of severely retarded children (IQs less than 50) had an average IQ of 103 which indicates an absence of familial resemblance. Similar results, suggesting that mild retardation is familial but severe retardation is not, have been found in parent–offspring analyses (Johnson *et al.*, 1976). No twin or adoption studies have as yet been reported that sort out the genetic and environmental underpinnings of these family studies. Moreover, the argument from these studies is qualitative rather than quantitative. That is, the argument is that severe retardation is not at all familial, that mild retardation is familial and, implicitly, that mild retardation is just as familial as the rest of the IQ distribution.

Few relevant data are available for psychosocial disorders other than mental retardation, primarily because quantitative measures such as the IQ test are rarely available in quantitative genetic studies of psychosocial disorders. Rather, studies of disorders usually employ measures that lead to dichotomously-defined diagnoses in order to compare risk for biological relatives of probands to the risk for control groups or for the general population. For example, genetic influence on diagnosed depression is suggested because the risk of diagnosable depression for biological relatives adopted away from depressed probands exceeds the risk for the general population. This result suggests that the difference between diagnosed depression and normality is to some extent genetic in origin. As we have seen, measures of differences in the amount of depression among individuals in the general population also indicate genetic influence. Thus, one might conclude that, as in the example of mild retardation, diagnosed depression is etiologically connected to individual differences in depression in the normal range. However, this would be a tenuous conclusion for the two reasons mentioned above: (a) the measures are different – the diagnosis of depression is dichotomous whereas the measure of individual differences is continuous; and

(b) only the existence of genetic influence, not its magnitude, has been compared in the abnormal and normal groups.

Individual and group familiality

As discussed later, concordance data for dichotomous diagnoses can be converted to liability correlations that assume an underlying continuous distribution. Although qualitative diagnoses will benefit by being considered in a quantitative framework, we need to measure these dimensions rather than to assess diagnostic dichotomies and then assume that continua underlie the dichotomies. The ability of quantitative genetic analyses to compare the etiologies of the normal and abnormal should provide a fresh impetus to move in this direction because this approach requires the use of quantitative measures of dimensions. In a series of papers by DeFries and colleagues (DeFries & Fulker, 1985, 1988; DeFries *et al.*, 1987a), the approach has been described in relation to the twin method which compares MZ and DZ twins reared together.

The conceptual framework for the approach is illustrated in Figure 5.1 in relation to the more straightforward case of siblings rather than twins of probands. For a quantitative measure relevant to a particular disorder, diagnosed probands will fall towards the extreme of the distribution. The mean of the siblings ($\bar{S}$ in Figure 5.1) of the probands will regress to the unselected population mean (μ) to the extent that familial factors are unimportant in the etiology of the disorder. In

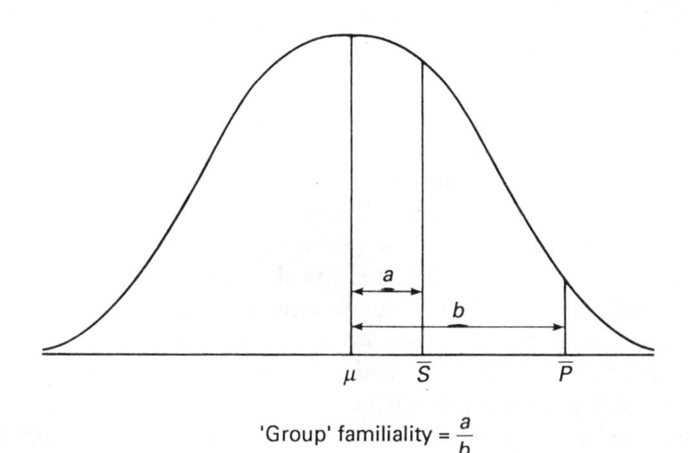

Figure 5.1. Hypothetical distribution of behavioral variation on a quantitative measure showing means of the probands ($\bar{P}$), of the siblings of the probands ($\bar{S}$), and of the population (μ). (Adapted from twin analysis proposed by DeFries, Fulker & LaBuda, 1987.)

contrast, if familial factors are important, the mean of the siblings of the probands will be greater than the population mean.

The use of quantitative measures is important because they permit an estimate of the magnitude of familial resemblance. The extent to which the mean difference between the siblings and the population approaches the mean difference between the probands ($\bar{P}$) and the population provides a quantitative estimate of the extent to which the mean difference between the probands and the population is due to familial factors.

This estimate (a/b in Figure 5.1) is called 'group' familiality to distinguish it from the usual 'individual' familiality which is based on analyses of individual differences in the normal range. The critical point is that group familiality can differ from individual familiality. If group familiality differs from individual familiality, this means that the etiology of deviant scores differs from the etiology of individual differences in the normal distribution. If group familiality is not different from individual familiality, this suggests that differences in the abnormal range may represent the extreme of the normal continuum of variability. This outcome (group familiality equals individual familiality) is not as clearly interpretable as the outcome for severe retardation (group familiality does not equal individual familiality). When group familiality differs from individual familiality as in the case of severe retardation, there seems to be no explanation other than that the disorder is etiologically different from variation for the rest of the distribution. In contrast, finding as in the case of mild retardation that group familiality is similar to individual familiality does not prove that the etiology of the disorder and the distribution are the same. That is, the disorder and the distribution may yield the same magnitude of familiality even though the factors that produce the familiality differ. For example, although group familiality for mild retardation is similar to individual familiality for IQ, some cases of mild retardation may be the result of familial organic disorders that play a negligible role in variation of IQ in the rest of the distribution.

In Roberts' (1952) and Nichols' (1984) reports on mental retardation, group familiality was not calculated and the mean IQ of probands was not reported. None-the-less, a rough estimate of group familiality can be obtained from Nichols' data for mild and severe retardation. For mild retardation, the probands had IQs between 50 and 69. Assuming an average IQ of 65, the mean IQ difference between the probands and the unselected population is −35 (i.e. 65 − 100) and the mean difference between the siblings of these probands and the unselected population is −15 (i.e. 85 − 100). This suggests a group familiality of 0.43 (i.e. the ratio of −15 to −35), as illustrated in Figure 5.2.

In other words, about 40% of the difference between mildly retarded

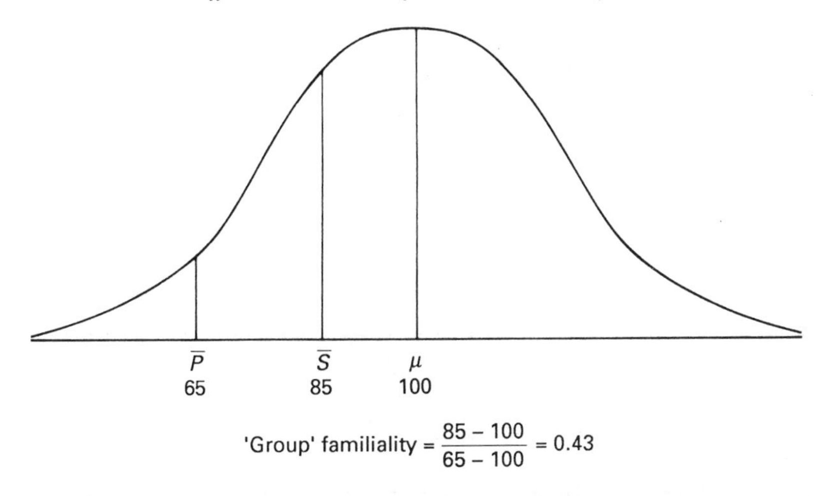

$$\text{'Group' familiality} = \frac{85 - 100}{65 - 100} = 0.43$$

Figure 5.2. Familial retardation: IQ means for mildly-retarded probands, their siblings, and the population. (Data from Nichols, 1984.)

probands and the rest of the distribution is due to familial factors. This group familiality is quite similar to estimates of individual familiality. For example, the average weighted sibling correlation for IQ is 0.45 in 69 studies involving 26 473 sibling pairs (Bouchard & McGue, 1981), which implies that individual familiality is 45% for IQ. Thus, this rough analysis of mild retardation suggests that group familiality is comparable to individual IQ familiality, which is consistent with the hypothesis that mild mental retardation represents the low end of the IQ distribution.

For severe retardation, in contrast, group familiality is negligible because the mean IQ of siblings of severely retarded probands regresses completely to the mean IQ of the population, as shown in Figure 5.3. This implies that the etiology of severe retardation differs from the rest of the distribution. The mean IQ difference between the siblings of severely retarded probands and the unselected population is 3 (i.e. $103 - 100$). Selected probands had IQs less than 50. Assuming an average IQ of 40 for the probands, the difference between the probands and the unselected population is -60 (i.e. $40 - 100$). Group familiality is thus -0.05 (i.e. the ratio of 3 to -60).

Power of estimating group and individual familiality

Group familiality can be detected with considerable power because it is based on a comparison of means. In contrast, power to detect individual familiality is much lower. For this reason, samples of unselected siblings must be about twice as large as samples of diagnosed probands and their siblings if individual familiality is to be estimated with power

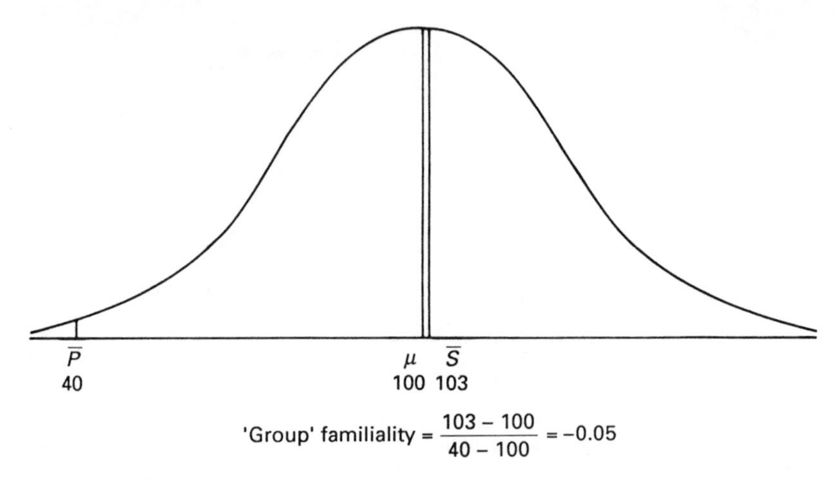

Figure 5.3. Severe retardation: IQ means for severely-retarded probands, their siblings, and the population. (Data from Nichols, 1984).

comparable to estimates of group familiality. For example, 80 pairs of probands and their siblings and 160 pairs of unselected siblings yield 80% power ($p < 0.05$, one-tailed) to detect group and individual familialities as low as 20% (Cohen, 1988).

Detecting significant differences between group familiality and individual familiality requires much larger sample sizes. To get a rough idea of the needed sample sizes to detect differences between group and individual familiality, if group and individual familiality were considered as correlations, samples of the above size can only detect differences larger than 0.25 as significant (i.e. 50% power if $p < 0.05$, two-tailed). That is, if individual familiality were 25%, group familiality would need to be zero to detect a significant difference. Differences between group and individual familialities on the order of 0.15 would require samples of about 160 pairs of probands and their siblings and 350 pairs of unselected siblings to identify differences of this magnitude as significant.

Individual and group heritability: reading disability

Twins or adoptees are needed to establish that familiality in such sibling analyses is due to heredity rather than environment shared by twins. Group heritability (h_g^2) indicates the proportion of the difference between the probands and the unselected population that is due to genetic differences. It is based on the differential regression to the mean for co-twins of MZ and DZ probands. That is, h_g^2 is zero if MZ and DZ co-twins regress to the population mean to the same extent. In contrast,

h_g^2 is 1.0 if MZ co-twins do not regress to the mean and if DZ co-twins regress halfway back to the mean.

In the first explicit analysis comparing h_g^2 and individual heritability (h^2), DeFries & Fulker (1985) employed a continuous measure of reading ability for probands diagnosed as reading disabled and their co-twins. The continuous measure was a discriminant function score whose weights were obtained from a battery of reading, perceptual speed and memory tests in samples of 140 reading-disabled and 140 control non-twin children. The twin analysis of h_g^2 included 64 pairs of identical twins and 55 pairs of fraternal twins in which at least one member of the pair met criteria for a diagnosis of reading disability.

Results of the study are depicted in Figure 5.4. The data are expressed as standardized deviations from control means. The mean discriminant function score for probands is 2.8 standard deviations lower than the control means for the discriminant function score, which is not surprising because the probands were diagnosed in part on the basis of low discriminant function socres. It can be seen that DZ co-twins regress to the mean more than MZ co-twins, which suggests some genetic influence on the difference between the probands and the population mean. It should also be noted that neither MZ nor DZ co-twins regress very far to the population mean. This suggests that shared environmental influences are also in part responsible for the difference between the probands and the population mean.

As in the case of h^2, h_g^2 can be estimated by doubling the difference between MZ and DZ resemblance, in this case, MZ and DZ group familiality. Group familiality (denoted as MZ r_g and DZ r_g) can be

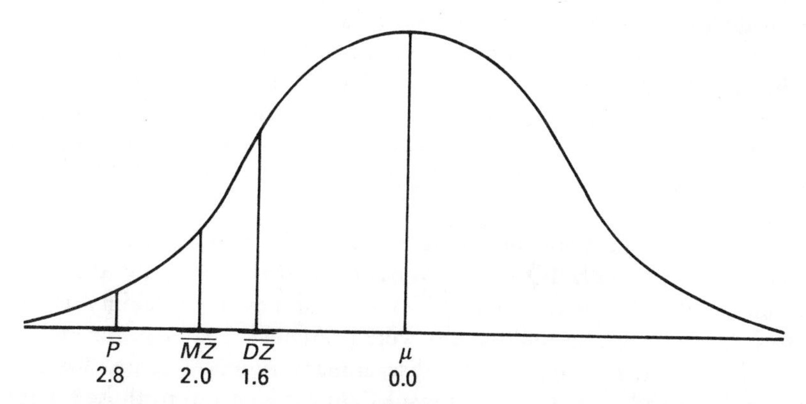

Figure 5.4. Group heritability for reading disability: discriminant function score means for reading-disabled probands, MZ and DZ co-twins of the probands and the population. Group familiality for MZ twins (MZ r_g) = 0.71 and DZ r_g = 0.57. Group heritability (h_g^2) = 2(MZ r_g − DZ r_g) = 2(0.71 − 0.57) = 0.28. Group shared environment (c_g^2) is estimated as MZ $r_g - h_g^2$ = 0.71 − 0.28 = 0.43.

estimated from these data as 0.71 for MZ twins and 0.57 for DZ twins. Doubling the difference between MZ r_g and DZ r_g estimates h_g^2 as $2(0.71 - 0.57) = 0.28$. In other words, less than a third of the mean difference between the probands and the population is due to genetic factors. In twin analyses, shared environment (c^2) is estimated as the extent to which twin resemblance cannot be explained by heredity. In the case of group parameters, c_g^2 is the difference between MZ r_g and h_g^2, $0.71 - 0.28 = 0.43$. In other words, the mean difference between probands and the population is due 28% to genetic factors and 43% to shared environment. The remainder of the difference, 29%, is ascribed to nonshared environment (e_g^2).

No unselected twin population is available to estimate individual heritability for the reading discriminant function score. However, h^2 of reading scores is generally quite substantial, in the range of 0.50. The comparison between h_g^2 of about 0.25 and h^2 of about 0.50 suggests that the etiology of reading disability is different genetically from the normal distribution of reading ability. Another etiological difference between reading disability and ability is also suggested by these data. Although environmental factors shared by children growing up in the same family are important for reading scores, estimates of c^2 are usually less than 0.30. The c_g^2 estimate of 0.43 suggests that the mean difference between reading-disabled probands and the population may be disproportionately due to shared environmental factors.

DeFries & Fulker (1985, 1988) offer a multiple regression approach to the estimation of h_g^2 and its standard error. Their approach yields a significant estimate of 0.29 ± 0.10 for these data (DeFries *et al.*, 1987a), which is similar to the above estimate of 0.28. DeFries & Fulker also provide an approach to estimate individual heritability from a selected sample and to test the significance of the difference between h_g^2 and h^2. Although their estimate of h_g^2 was less than h^2, the difference in the two heritabilities was not significant. However, estimating h^2 from small selected samples of probands is hazardous in contrast to using estimates from a large sample of unselected twins which was not available in this study.

Two other aspects of these data are especially noteworthy. First, the analyses rerun with IQ as a covariate yielded essentially the same results, indicating that group heritability of reading disability is not attributable to IQ. Second, results were presented separately for each of the six tests that comprise the discriminant function score. Reading recognition and spelling yielded results almost identical to those for the discriminant function score: h_g^2 is about 0.30 and c_g^2 is about 0.40. Reading comprehension, however, suggested lower h_g^2 (0.18) and higher c_g^2 (0.54). This finding suggests that, compared to reading recognition and spelling, reading comprehension contributes to reading disability more for reasons of shared environment than heredity.

Coding produced odd results – MZ familiality of 0.98 and DZ familiality of 0.80, suggesting estimates of 0.36 for h_g^2 and 0.62 for c_g^2. However, coding scores were less than a standard deviation different for probands and controls. This result illustrates an important point. In quantitative genetic analyses of covariance between traits, when there is little pheonotypic covariance between traits, estimates of genetic and environmental contributions to the covariance are not powerful. Analyses of h_g^2 and c_g^2 can be viewed as multivariate analyses of the covariance between a diagnosis and continuous measures of dimensions that are presumably related to the diagnosis. If there is little covariance between a diagnosis and a dimension (that is, probands do not differ much from the population mean), estimates of h_g^2 and c_g^2 are unreliable. This problem might also account for the results of the remaining two tests – another perceptual speed test and digit span – for which the differences between probands and controls were approximately one standard devation. For the perceptual speed measure, h_g^2 was high, 0.68, and c_g^2 was low, 0.12. For digit span, just the reverse findings emerged: h_g^2 was 0.04 and c_g^2 was 0.82.

Other analyses of reading data from the Colorado group yield what may be a critically important finding concerning reading disability (Olson *et al.*, 1989). Probands' scores on PIAT Reading Recognition, the key element in the discriminant function score used to diagnose reading disability, were compared to their twins' scores on a different dimension, phonological coding, which is a measure of speed and accuracy in pronouncing one- and two-syllable nonwords such as 'ter' and 'tegwop'. Phonological coding shows a group heritability of nearly unity; MZ and DZ twin group correlations can be computed as 0.81 and 0.34, respectively. PIAT Reading Recognition yields a group heritability of 0.40 based on MZ and DZ twin group correlations of 0.67 and 0.47. However, when phonological coding is partialled from PIAT Reading Recognition, group heritability for PIAT Reading Recognition is nearly zero – group correlations are 0.54 for both MZ and DZ twins. This finding suggests that phonological coding may be a key genetic element in the genetics of reading disability.

Liability correlations

Before describing other data relevant to the estimation of h_g^2 and c_g^2, liability correlations should be considered. Recognizing the need to take into account a continuous distribution of genetic and environmental risk underlying dichotomous measures, geneticists typically convert concordances for family members into so-called liability correlations (Falconer, 1965; Smith, 1974). Liability correlations are nothing more than tetrachoric correlations routinely computed for data in which continuous, normally-distributed data have been reduced artificially to two categories. As mentioned earlier, rather than assessing discontinuous diagnoses and assuming continuous dimensions, it is far better to study continuous dimensions directly and to consider diagnoses in the context of continua of variability. A critical point often overlooked in the use of liability correlations is that they do not refer to the disorder as diagnosed but rather to a hypothetical construct of continuous liability. For this reason, heritability computed from liability correlations does not refer to heritability of the disorder as diagnosed but rather to heritability of a hypothetical construct of continuous liability to the disorder.

For example, the most recent twin study of schizophrenia mentioned earlier yielded MZ annd DZ twin concordances of 30.9% and 6.5% (Kendler & Robinette, 1983). Assuming a population incidence of 1%, these concordances convert to liability correlations of 0.75 and 0.33. Doubling the difference between the liability correlations for MZ and DZ twins suggests a heritability of liability of 84% (which is too high because it exceeds the liability correlation for MZ twins). In other words, the heritability of the construct of liability to schizophrenia is extremely high even though genetically identical twins are much more often discordant than concordant for schizophrenia.

The formula for the liability correlation is conceptually the same as group familiality. Although the equation for the tetrachoric (liability) correlation is complicated, Smith (1974) noted that an approximation of the liability correlation is:

$$r_t = \frac{x - x_R}{b}$$

where x is the threshold (i.e. diagnostic cut-off), x_R is the difference between the threshold and the mean liability for relatives, and b is the mean difference between the probands and the population. (See Figure 5.5) Thus, b is the same as the denominator in the computation of group familiality. Although the numerator appears complicated, it is in fact the same as the numerator used in the computation of group familiality, the mean difference between the relatives and the population. Smith's equation depends on the use of standard scores so that the threshold is the same as the difference between the threshold and the population mean. The numerator in Smith's equation is the threshold minus the difference between the threshold and the mean of the relatives. This is equivalent to the difference between the mean of the relatives and the population mean, as illustrated in Figure 5.5.

Thus, the liability correlation is conceptually the same as group familiality, but there is a critical difference: the liability correlation

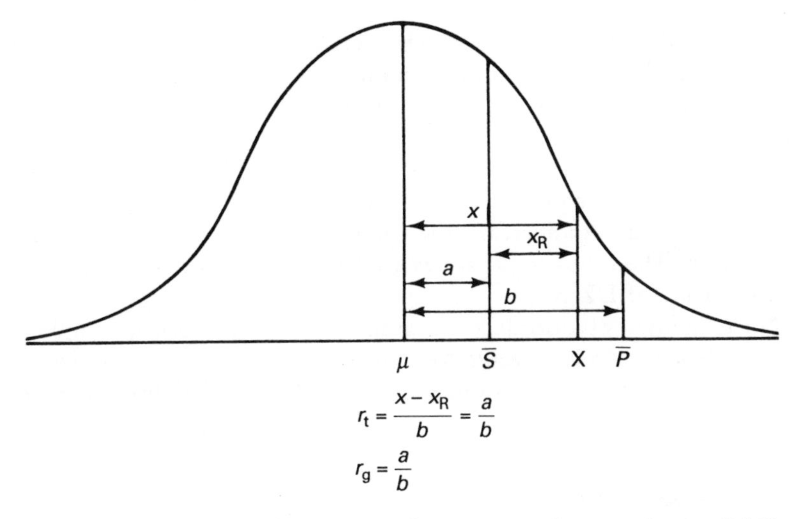

$$r_t = \frac{x - x_R}{b} = \frac{a}{b}$$

$$r_g = \frac{a}{b}$$

Figure 5.5. Group familiality (r_g) is the same as the tetrachoric (liability) correlation (r_t), except that group familiality is derived empirically from continuous data whereas the liability correlation is used to assume an underlying continuous distribution from discontinuous data. *X* denotes the threshold value assumed in the computation of a liability correlation.

assumes an underlying continuous distribution based on dichotomous data, whereas group familiality is based on an empirical assessment of continuous data for probands and their relatives. None-the-less, if the assumptions that underlie the computation of the liability correlation from dichotomous data are correct, the liability correlation should be similar to group familiality computed empirically from quantitative measures. Explicit comparisons between liability correlations and group familiality are presented later.

SATSA comparisons between group and individual heritability

If liability correlations computed for categorical diagnostic data accurately estimate group familiality based on analyses of quantitative measures, comparisons between group and individual familiality/heritability ought to be available from the literature on psychosocial disorders. As indicated earlier, however, such comparisons are hampered by the lack of comparability of measures of diagnosed disorders and measures of individual differences in the normal range.

Because so few data are available that permit comparisons between group and individual heritability, data from the Swedish Twin/Adoption Study of Aging (SATSA) were analyzed from this perspective. SATSA is a study of middle-aged adult twins reared apart and matched twins reared together, derived from the Swedish Twin Registry which contains information on both members of nearly 25 000 pairs of like-sexed twins (McClearn *et al.*, 1991). Because virtually no evidence is found for shared rearing environment as assessed directly by comparisons between twins reared apart and twins reared together, twins reared apart and twins reared together were combined in these analyses in order to increase the sample size for analyses of group heritability. The following analyses are based on 259 pairs of MZ twins and 441 pairs of DZ twins.

No diagnoses of disorders are available for this normal sample of twins. However, it is possible to compare group heritability estimated by selecting extreme individuals to individual heritability estimated from the entire sample.

Neuroticism

Results for neuroticism are illustrated in Figure 5.6. Neuroticism was assessed in SATSA using a short form of the Eysenck measure (Pedersen *et al.*, 1988). As indicated in Figure 5.6, neuroticism is skewed towards high neuroticism. A cut-off of 6 was used that captured the skewed tail of the distribution, with 14.6% of the sample thus selected as probands. MZ r_g is 0.38 and DZ r_g is 0.26. Thus, h_g^2 is 0.24,

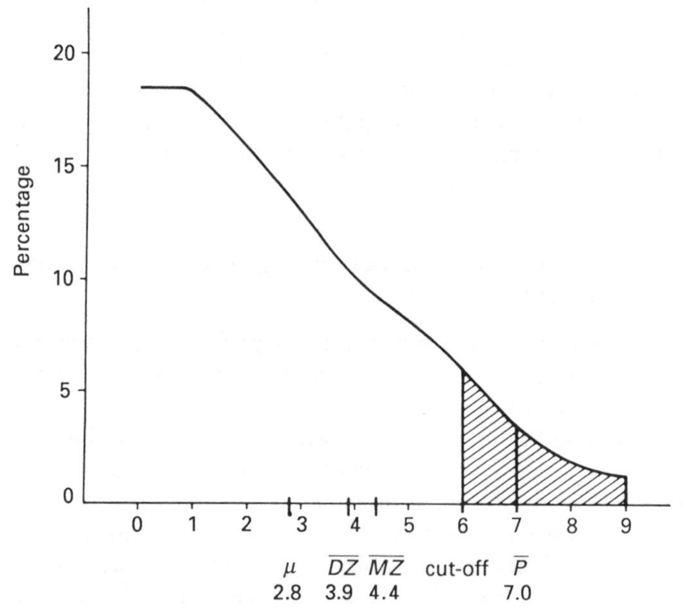

Figure 5.6. Group heritability for extreme scores of self-reported neuroticism in a normal sample. MZ $r_g = 0.38$; DZ $r_g = 0.26$; $h_g^2 = 0.24$; $c_g^2 = 0.14$.

c_g^2 is 0.14, and e_g^2 which includes error of measurement is 0.62. The multiple regression approach of DeFries & Fulker (1985) indicates that h_g^2 is significant and yields an estimate of 0.23.

How do these group parameter estimates compare to individual parameters? MZ and DZ correlations for the entire sample (0.38 and 0.28, respectively) are similar to the group correlations. Thus, individual parameter estimates based on these correlations are similar to the group parameter estimates: 0.20 for h^2, 0.18 for c^2, and 0.62 for e^2. Applying DeFries & Fulker's (1985) multiple regression model yields the following parameter estimates: 0.21 ± 0.11 for h^2, 0.17 ± 0.08 for c^2 and 0.62 for e^2.

In summary, the results for neuroticism are consistent with the hypothesis that the most neurotic individuals in the SATSA sample score highly for the same genetic and environmental reasons as individuals in the middle of the distribution. In other words, the skewed tail representing high neuroticism may be, etiologically, just the high end of the distribution of individual differences in neuroticism. It should be emphasized, however, that SATSA is a normal sample and even its most neurotic individuals might not show clinically-relevant levels of emotional instability.

These data can also be employed to explore the empirical relationship between group correlations that utilize continuous data and liability correlations that assume a continuous distribution from dichotomous data. Probandwise concordances were 40% for MZ twins and 30% for DZ twins, using the same cut-off of 6 for the neuroticism scale. With an incidence of 14.6%, these concordances convert to liability correlations of 0.53 and 0.35, respectively. Thus, liability correlations that assume that a continuous distribution underlies dichotomous concordance data are substantially different in magnitude from the group correlations derived from the continuous data.

Depression

Analyses of other SATSA measures such as somatic complaints and life satisfaction yielded similar results suggesting that the high extreme of somatic complaints and the low extreme of life satisfaction are etiologically just the extreme of the distribution of individual differences. One possible exception involves a measure of depression. The depression scale from the OARS (Older Americans Resources and Services; Gatz *et al.*, 1987) was employed. Seven per cent of the SATSA population reported scores of 4 or 5 on this scale which ranged from 0 to 5. As illustrated in Figure 5.7, the distribution of scores on this scale are highly skewed towards the depressed end of the scale.

The means shown in Figure 5.7 indicate that group correlations for

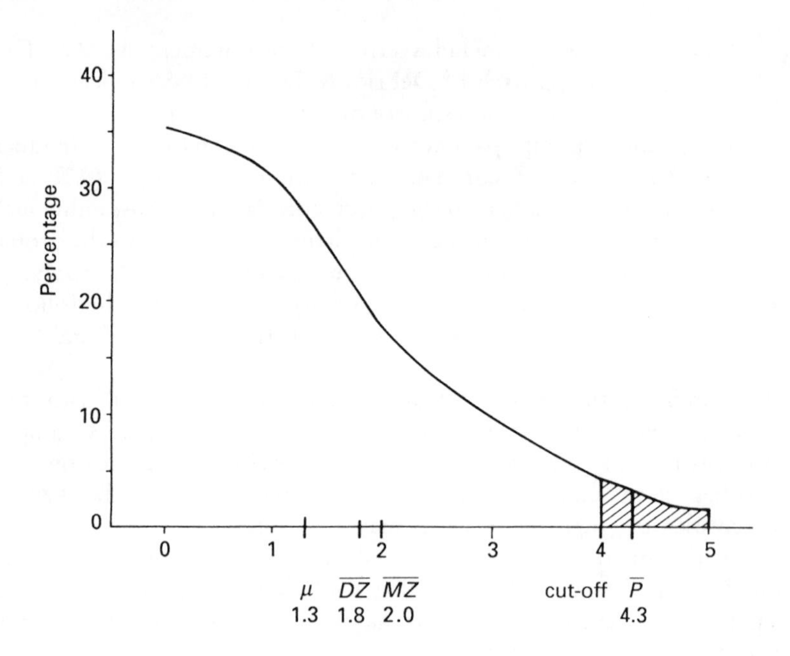

Figure 5.7. Group heritability for extreme scores of self-reported depression in a normal sample. MZ $r_g = 0.23$; DZ $r_g = 0.17$; $h_g^2 = 0.12$; $c_g^2 = 0.11$.

both MZ and DZ twins are quite low, suggesting little genetic influence or shared environmental influence on these extreme scores. MZ and DZ r_g estimates are 0.23 and 0.17, respectively, which yield the following group parameter estimates: $h_g^2 = 0.12$, $c_g^2 = 0.11$, and $e_g^2 = 0.77$. In contrast, for the entire SATSA sample, MZ and DZ correlations are 0.31 and 0.19, respectively, for this measure. Doubling the difference between the MZ and DZ correlations yields a heritability estimate 0.24, which is the same as the model-fitting estimate of 0.24 ± 0.13. Thus, individual heritability appears to be about twice as great as group heritability for this depression measure, suggesting that genetic factors may be less important for extreme depression scores than for the rest of the distribution. Diagnoses of clinically depressed individuals could, of course, yield different results. Indeed, extant data reviewed earlier suggest that extreme depression shows substantial genetic influence, although published data do not yield a clear estimate of the magnitude of genetic influence.

Liability correlations were also calculated for these depression data. Unlike neuroticism, liability correlations for depression were similar to group correlations. Probandwise concordances were 17% for MZ twins and 15% for DZ twins. With an incidence of 7%, these concordances convert to liability correlations of 0.29 and 0.25, for MZ and DZ twins, respectively. Thus, unlike neuroticism, liability correlations for depression are somewhat similar to the group correlations of 0.23 and 0.17.

Criteria for research on group and individual heritability

These SATSA data merely illustrate the interesting results that could emerge from analyses of group and individual heritability of psychosocial disorders. The SATSA examples are quite limited in that the probands were not diagnosed for psychopathology. An ideal study would include a large sample of siblings or twins carefully diagnosed for a disorder and an even larger sample of comparable unselected siblings or twins. An ideal but practically impossible design is one that obtains a sample of unselected siblings large enough to yield large numbers of individuals who meet diagnostic criteria for a disorder. A more feasible strategy is to estimate group familiality/heritability from selected probands, who meet diagnostic criteria, and their siblings. Individual familiality/heritability can be estimated separately from a large sample of unselected siblings comparable to the sample of selected siblings. All siblings need to be administered disorder-relevant quantitative measures that are sensitive to variability both in the normal range and at the extreme. This criterion is easier to meet for some dimensions and disorders than for others. Often there are obvious parallels between overt disorders and variations within the normal range: for example, delinquency, conduct disturbance, anxiety disorders and unipolar depression. For some disorders, especially rare ones, dimensional parallels are less clear. For example, for bipolar manic-depression, is a dimension of mood swings related? Is dissatisfaction with body shape a dimension related to anorexia? Autism and schizophrenia have no obvious dimensional equivalent.

Comparisons between group and individual heritability may be valuable in identifying etiological thresholds for disorders. That is, do estimates of h_g^2 differ from h^2 when different cut-offs are employed? In addition, a multivariate extension of the univariate approach described in this chapter will be valuable in analyzing heterogeneity and comorbidity of disorders. The analysis described above relating reading disability to phonological coding is a good example of the possible pay-offs of this approach (Olson *et al.*, 1989). For this reason, an additional criterion of an ideal study is the inclusion of continuous measures of several facets of a disorder and of related disorders.

CONCLUSIONS

The goal of this chapter is to begin to build a bridge between the study of individual differences in the normal range and the study of abnormal behavior. A new reason for rapprochement between research on the normal and abnormal ranges of behavior is the development of quantitative genetic techniques that can provide an answer to the perennial question concerning the distinction between the normal and abnormal. Specifically, comparisons between group familiality/heritability and individual familiality/heritability indicate the extent to which abnormal behavior is etiologically part of the normal distribution. So far, the bits of available data indicate that some disorders such as mild mental retardation and high scores on neuroticism may be part of the normal continuum of variability whereas other disorders such as severe mental retardation, reading disability and high scores on depression are etiologically distinct.

The implications of these concepts and methods are far reaching. If it is found that psychosocial disorders are etiologically part of the normal continuum, as in the case of mild mental retardation, then causes and possibly cures can be sought in factors that affect the entire range of individual differences. Conversely, special factors unique to psychosocial disorder are not likely to explain the disorder. On the other hand, if a psychosocial disorder is found to be etiologically distinct from individual differences in the normal range, as in the case of severe retardation, factors that affect variability in the normal range are not likely to explain the disorder. Although cures need not be related to causes, understanding the extent to which disorders are etiologically part of the normal continuum of variability is surely relevant to the goal of predicting and preventing disorders.

ACKNOWLEDGEMENTS

Preparation of this chapter was supported in part by grants from the US National Science Foundation (BNS-8806589), the US National Institute of Child Health and Human Development (HD-10333 and HD-18426) and the US National Institute of Mental Health (MH-43373 and MH-43899).

REFERENCES

Bakwin, H. (1970) Sleepwalking in twins. *The Lancet*, **2**, 446–7.

Bakwin, H. (1973) The genetics of bedwetting. In Kolvin, I., MacKeith, R. & Meadow, S. R. (eds.) *Bladder control and enuresis (Clinics in Developmental Medicine, Nos. 48/49)*. London: Heinemann.

Bergeman, C. S., Chipuer, H. M., Plomin, R., Pedersen, N. L., McClearn, G. E., Nesselroade, J. R., Costa, P., Jr & McCrae, R. R. (1991) *Openness to experience, agreeableness, and conscientiousness assessed separately by age and gender: an adoption/twin study*. Manuscript submitted for publication.

Bertelsen, A., Harvald, B. & Hauge, M. (1977) A Danish study of manic-depressive disorders. *British Journal of Psychiatry*, **130**, 330–51.
Bohman, M. (1971) A comparative study of adopted children, foster children and children in their biological environment born after undesired pregnancies. *Acta Paediatrica Scandinavica*, Supplement 221.
Bohman, M. (1972) The study of adopted children, their background, environment and adjustment. *Acta Paediatrica Scandinavica*, **61**, 90–7.
Bohman, M., Cloninger, C. R., Sigvardsson, S. & von Knorring, A.-L. (1987) The genetics of alcoholism and related disorders. *Journal of Psychiatric Research*, **21**, 447–52.
Bohman, M., Cloninger, C. R., von Knorring, A.-L. & Sigvardsson, S. (1984) An adoption study of somatoform disorders. III. Cross-fostering analysis and genetic relationship to alcoholism and criminality. *Archives of General Psychiatry*, **41**, 872–8.
Bouchard, T. J., Jr & McGue, M. (1981) Familial studies of intelligence: a review. *Science*, **212**, 1055–9.
Buss, A. H. & Plomin, R. (1984) *Temperament: early developing personality traits.* Hillsdale, NJ: Erlbaum.
Cadoret, R. J. (1978) Evidence for genetic inheritance of primary affective disorder in adoptees. *American Journal of Psychiatry*, **133**, 463–6.
Cadoret, R. J., Troughton, E., O'Gorman, T. W. & Heywood, M. A. (1986) An adoption study of genetic and environmental factors in drug abuse. *Archives of General Psychiatry*, **43**, 1131–6.
Chipuer, H. M., Rovine, M. & Plomin, R. (1990) LISREL Modelling: genetic and environmental influences on IQ revisited. *Intelligence*, **14**, 11–29.
Clifford, C. A., Fulker, D. W. & Murray, R. M. (1981) A genetic and environmental analysis of obsessionality in normal twins. In Gedda, L., Parisi, P. & Nance W. E. (eds.) *Twin research 3, part B: intelligence, personality, and development.* New York: Liss, pp. 163–8.
Cloninger, C. R. & Gottesman, I. I. (1987) Genetic and environmental factors in antisocial behavior disorders. In Mednick, S., Moffit, T. & Stack, S. (eds.) *The causes of crime.* New York: Cambridge University Press, pp. 92–109.
Cloninger, C. R., Martin, R. J., Guze, S. B. & Clayton, P. J. (1986) A prospective follow-up and family study of somatization in men and women. *American Journal of Psychiatry*, **143**, 873–8.
Cohen, J. (1988) *Statistical power analysis for the behavioral sciences.* Hillsdale, NJ: Erlbaum.
Costa, P. T., Jr, Zonderman, A. B., McCrae, R. R. & Williams, R. B., Jr (1985) Content and comprehensiveness in the MMPI: an item factor analysis in a normal adult sample. *Journal of Personality and Social Psychology*, **48**, 925–33.
Crowe, R. R., Noyes, R., Pauls, D. L. & Slyman, D. (1983) A family study of panic disorder. *Archives of General Psychiatry*, **40**, 1065–9.
DeFries, J. C. & Fulker, D. W. (1985) Multiple regression analysis of twin data. *Behavior Genetics*, **15**, 467–73.
DeFries, J. C. & Fulker, D. W. (1988) Multiple regression analysis of twin data: etiology of deviant scores versus individual differences. *Acta Geneticae Medicae et Gemellologiae*, **37**, 205–16.

DeFries, J. C., Fulker, D. W. & LaBuda, M. C. (1987a) Evidence for a genetic aetiology in reading disability in twins. *Nature*, **329**, 537–9.

DeFries, J. C., Plomin, R. & LaBuda, M. C. (1987b) Genetic stability of cognitive development from childhood to adulthood. *Developmental Psychology*, **57**, 348–56.

DeFries, J. C., Vogler, G. P. & LaBuda, M. C. (1986) Colorado family reading study: an overview. In Fuller, J. L. & Simmel, E. C. (eds.) *Perspectives in behavior genetics*, pp. 29–56. Hillsdale, NJ: Erlbaum.

DeLisi, L. E., Mirsky, A. F., Buchsbaum, M. S., van Kammen, D. P. & Berman, K. F. (1984) The Genain quadruplets 25 years later: diagnostic and biochemical followup. *Psychiatric Research*, **13**, 59–76.

Detera-Wadleigh, S. D., Berrettini, W. H., Goldin, L. R., Boorman, D., Anderson, S. & Gershon, E. S. (1987) Close linkage of c-harvey-ras-1 and the insulin gene to affective disorder is ruled out in three North American pedigrees. *Nature*, **325**, 806–8.

Detera-Wadleigh, S. D., Goldin, L. R., Sherrington, R., Encio, I., de Miguel, C., Berrettini, W., Gurling, H. & Gershon, E. S. (1989) Exclusion of linkage of 5q11–13 in families with schizophrenia and other psychiatric disorders. *Sciences*, **340**, 391–3.

Digman, J. M. (1990) Personality structure: emergence of the five-factor model. *Annual Review of Psychology*, **41**, 417–40.

DiLalla, L. F., Thompson, L. A., Plomin, R., Phillips, K., Fagan, J. F., Haith, M. M., Cyphers, L. H. & Fulker, D. W. (1990) Infant predictors of preschool and adult IQ: a study of infant twins and their parents. *Developmental Psychology*, **26**, 759–69.

Edwards, M. D., Stuber, C. W. & Wendel, J. F. (1987) Molecular-marker-facilitated investigations of quantitative-trait loci in maize. I. Numbers, genomic distribution and types of gene action. *Geneticae*, **116**, 113–25.

Egeland, J. A., Gerhard, D. S., Pauls, D. L., Sussex, J. N. & Kidd, K. K. (1987) Bipolar affective disorders linked to DNA markers on chromosome 11. *Nature*, **325**, 783–7.

Falconer, D. S. (1965) The inheritance of liability to diseases, estimated from the incidence among relatives. *Annals of Human Genetics*, **29**, 51–76.

Farmer, A. E., McGuffin, P. & Gottesman, I. I. (1984) Searching for the split in schizophrenia: a twin study perspective. *Psychiatric Research*, **13**, 109–18.

Folstein, S. & Rutter, M. (1977) Infantile autism: a genetic study of 21 twin pairs. *Journal of Child Psychology and Psychiatry*, **18**, 297–332.

Fulker, D. W., DeFries, J. C. & Plomin, R. (1988) Genetic influence on general mental ability increases between infancy and middle childhood. *Nature*, **336**, 767–9.

Galton, F. (1875) The history of twins as a criterion of the relative powers of nature and nurture. *Journal of the Anthropological Institute*, **6**, 391–406.

Gatz, M., Pedersen, N. L. & Harris, J. (1987) Measurement characteristics of the mental health scale from the OARS. *Journal of Gerontology*, **42**, 332–5.

Gill, M., McKeon, P. & Humphries, P. (1988) Linkage analysis of manic depression in an Irish family using H-ras A and INS DNA markers. *Journal of Medical Genetics*, **25**, 634–7.

Goodman, R. & Stevenson, J. (1989a) A twin study of hyperactivity: I. an examination of hyperactivity scores and categories derived from Rutter teacher and parent questionnaires. *Journal of Child Psychology and Psychiatry*, **30**, 671–89.

Goodman, R. & Stevenson, J. (1989b) A twin study of hyperactivity: II. the aetiological role of genes, family relationships and perinatal adversity. *Journal of Child Psychology and Psychiatry*, **30**, 691–709.

Goodwin, D. W. (1979) Alcoholism and heredity. *Archives of General Psychiatry*, **36**, 57–61.

Gottesman, I. I. (1963) Heritability of personality: a demonstration. *Psychology Monographs*, **77** (Whole No. 572).

Gottesman, I. I. (1965) Personality and natural selection. Vandenberg, S. G. (ed.) *Methods and goals in human behavior genetics* New York: Academic Press, pp. 63–80.

Gottesman, I. I. & Bertelsen, A. (1989) Confirming unexpressed genotypes for schizophrenia. *Archives of General Psychiatry*, **46**, 867–72.

Gottesman, I. I., Carey, G. & Hanson, D. R. (1983) Pearls and perils in epigenetic psychopathology. In Guze, S. B., Earls, E. J. & Barrett, J. E. (eds.) *Childhood psychopathology and development* New York: Raven Press, pp. 287–300.

Gottesman, I. I. & Shields, J. (1982) *Schizophrenia: the epigenetic puzzle.* Cambridge: Cambridge University Press.

Guze, S. B., Cloninger, C. R., Martin, R. L. & Clayton, B. J. (1986) A follow-up and family study of Briquet's syndrome. *British Journal of Psychiatry*, **149**, 17–23.

Hanson, D. R. & Gottesman, I. I. (1976) The genetics, if any, of infantile autism and childhood schizophrenia. *Journal of Autism and Developmental Disorders*, **6**, 209–34.

Henderson, N. D. (1982) Human behavior genetics. *Annual Review of Psychology*, **33**, 403–40.

Hodgkinson, S., Sherrington, R., Gurling, H., Marchbanks, R. & Reeders, S. (1987) Molecular genetic evidence for heterogeneity in manic depression. *Nature*, **325**, 805–6.

Holland, A. J., Hall, A., Murray, R., Russell, G. F. M. & Crisp, A. H. (1984) Anorexia nervosa: a study of 34 twin pairs and one set of triplets. *British Journal of Psychiatry*, **145**, 414–9.

Howie, P. M. (1981) Intrapair similarity in frequency of disfluency in monozygotic and dizygotic twin pairs containing stutterers. *Behavior Genetics*, **11**, 227–38.

Jary, M. L. & Stewart, M. A. (1985) Psychiatric disorder in the parents of adopted children with aggressive conduct disorder. *Neuropsychobiology*, **13**, 7–11.

Johnson, C. A., Ahern, F. M. & Johnson, R. C. (1976) Level of functioning of siblings and parents of probands of varying degrees of retardation. *Behavior Genetics*, **6**, 473–7.

Kamin, L. (1974) *The science and politics of I.Q.* New York: Wiley.

Kelsoe, J., Ginns, E. I., Egeland, J. A., Gerhard, D. S., Goldstein, A. M., Bale, S. J., Pauls, D. L., Long, R. T., Kidd, K. K., Conte, G., Housman, D. E. & Paul, S. M. (1989) Re-evaluation of the linkage relationship between chromosome 11p loci and the gene for bipolar affective disorder in the Old Order Amish. *Nature*, **342**, 238–43.

Kendler, K. S. & Gruenberg, A. M. (1984) An independent analysis of the Danish Adoption Study of Schizophrenia. *Archives of General Psychiatry*, **41**, 555–64.

Kendler, K. S., Heath, A., Martin, N. G. & Eaves, L. J. (1986) Symptoms of anxiety and depression in a volunteer twin population. *Archives of General Psychiatry*, **43**, 213–21.

Kendler, K. S. & Robinette, C. D. (1983) Schizophrenia in the National Academy of Sciences–National Research Council twin registry: a 16-year update. *American Journal of Psychiatry*, **140**, 1551–63.

Kennedy, J. L., Giuffra, L. A., Moises, H. W., Cavalli-Sforza, L., Pakstis, A. J., Kidd, J. R., Castiglione, C. M., Sjogren, B., Wetterberg, L. & Kidd, K. K. (1988) Evidence against linkage of schizophrenia to markers on chromosome 5 in a northern Swedish pedigree. *Nature*, **336**, 167–70.

Kety, S. S. (1987) The significance of genetic factors in the etiology of schizophrenia: results from the national study of adoptees in Denmark. *Journal of Psychiatric Research*, **21**, 423–9.

Kety, S. S., Rosenthal, D. & Wender, P. H. (1978) Genetic relationships with the schizophrenia spectrum: evidence from adoption studies. In Spitzer, R. L. & Klein, D. F. (eds.) *Critical issues in psychiatric diagnosis*. NY: Raven Press, pp. 213–23.

Kimberling, W. J., Fain, P. R., Ing, P. S., Smith, S. D. & Pennington, B. F. (1985) Linkage analysis of reading disability with chromosome 15. *Behavior Genetics*, **15**, 597–8.

Le Couteur, A., Bailey, A., Rutter, M. & Gottesman, I. (1989) Epidemiologically-based twin study of autism. Paper presented at the *First World Congress on Psychiatric Genetics*, Churchill College, Cambridge, August 1989.

Loehlin, J. C. (1982) Are personality traits differentially heritable? *Behavior Genetics*, **12**, 417–28.

Loehlin, J. C. (1989) Partitioning environmental and genetic contributions to behavioral development. *American Psychologist*, **44**, 1285–92.

Loehlin, J. C., Willerman, L. & Horn, J. M. (1982) Personality resemblances between unwed mothers and their adopted-away offspring. *Journal of Personality and Social Psychology*, **42**, 1089–99.

Loehlin, J. C., Willerman, L. & Horn, J. M. (1985) Personality resemblance in adoptive families when the children are late adolescents and adults. *Journal of Personality and Social Psychology*, **48**, 376–92.

Loehlin, J. C., Willerman, L. & Horn, J. M. (1988) Human behavior genetics. *Annual Review of Psychology*, **38**, 101–33.

Martin, N. G. & Jardine, R. (1986) Eysenck's contributions to behavior genetics. In Modgil, S. & Modgil, C. (eds.) *Hans Eysenck: consensus and controversy*. Philadelphia: Falmer, pp. 13–27.

McClearn, G. E., Pedersen, N. L., Plomin, R., Nesselroade, J. R. & Friberg, L. (1991) *Age and gender effects for individual differences in behavioral aging: the Swedish Adoption/Twin Study on Aging*. Manuscript submitted for publication.

McCrae, R. R. & Costa, P. T., Jr (1987) Validation of the five-factor model of personality across instruments and observers. *Journal of Personality and Social Psychology*, **52**, 81–90.

McGue, M. & Bouchard, T. J., Jr (1990) Genetic and environmental determinants of information processing and special mental abilities: a twin analysis. In Sternberg, R. J. (ed.) *Advances in the psychology of human intelligence*, Vol. 5, pp. 7–45. Hillsdale, NJ: Erlbaum.

McGuffin, P. (1987) The new genetics and childhood psychiatric disorder. *Journal of Child Psychology and Psychiatry*, **28**, 215–22.

McGuffin, P. & Gottesman, I. I. (1985) Genetic influences on normal and abnormal development. In Rutter, M. & Hersov, L. (eds.) *Child and adolescent psychiatry: modern approaches*, 2nd edn. Oxford: Blackwell Scientific, pp. 17–33.

McKusick, V. A. (1988) *Mendelian inheritance in man*, 8th edn. Baltimore: Johns Hopkins University Press.

Mednick, S. A., Gabrielli, W. F., Jr & Hutchings, B. (1984) Genetic influences in criminal convictions: evidence from an adoption cohort. *Science*, **224**, 891–4.

Mednick, S. A., Moffitt, T. E. & Stack, S. (1987) *The causes of crime: new biological approaches.* New York: Cambridge University Press.

Montgomery, M. A., Clayton, P. J. & Friedhoff, A. J. (1982) Psychiatric illness in Tourette's syndrome patients and first-degree relatives. In Friedhoff, A. J. & Chase, T. N. (eds.) *Gilles de la Tourette Syndrome.* New York: Raven Press, pp. 335–9.

Nichols, P. L. (1984) Familial mental retardation. *Behavior Genetics*, **14**, 161–70.

Norman, W. T. (1963) Toward an adequate taxonomy of personality attributes: replicated factor structure in peer nomination personality ratings. *Journal of Abnormal and Social Psychology*, **66**, 574–83.

O'Connor, M., Foch, T., Sherry, T. & Plomin, R. (1980) A twin study of specific behavioral problems of socialization as viewed by parents. *Journal of Abnormal Child Psychology*, **8**, 189–99.

Olson, R., Wise, B., Conners, F., Rack, J. & Fulker, D. (1989) Specific deficits in component reading and language skills: genetic and environmental influences. *Journal of Learning Disabilities*, **22**, 339–48.

Pauls, D. L., Cohen, D. J., Heimbuch, R., Detlor, J. & Kidd, K. K. (1981) Familial pattern and transmission of Gilles de la Tourette syndrome and multiple tics. *Archives of General Psychiatry*, **38**, 1091–3.

Pauls, D. L., Towbin, K. E., Leckman, J. F., Zahner, G. E. P. & Cohen, D. J. (1986) Evidence supporting a genetic relationship between Gilles de la Tourette's syndrome and obsessive compulsive disorder. *Archives of General Psychiatry*, **43**, 1180–2.

Pedersen, N. L., Plomin, R., McClearn, G. E. & Friberg, L. (1988) Neuroticism, extraversion, and related traits in adult twins reared apart and reared together. *Journal of Personality and Social Psychology*, **55**, 950–7.

Peele, S. (1986) The implications and limitations of genetic models of alcoholism and other addictions. *Journal of Studies on Alcohol*, **47**, 63–73.

Plomin, R. (1986a) *Development, genetics, and psychology.* Hillsdale, NJ: Erlbaum.

Plomin, R. (1986b) Multivariate analysis and developmental behavioral genetics: developmental change as well as continuity. *Behavior Genetics*, **16**, 25–44.

Plomin, R. (1988) The nature and nurture of cognitive abilities. In Sternberg, R. J. (ed.) *Advances in the psychology of human intelligence*, Vol. 4. Hillsdale, NJ: Erlbaum, pp. 1–33.

Plomin, R. (1990) The role of inheritance in behavior. *Science*, **248**, 183–8.

Plomin, R., Chipuer, H. & Loehlin, J. C. (1990c) Behavioral genetics and personality. In Pervin, L. A. (ed.) *Handbook of personality theory and research*. New York: Guilford, pp. 225–43.

Plomin, R., DeFries, J. C. & Fulker, D. W. (1988a) *Nature and nurture during infancy and early childhood*. New York: Cambridge University Press.

Plomin, R., DeFries, J. C. & McClearn, G. E. (1990a). *Behavioral genetics: A primer*, 2nd edn. New York: W. H. Freeman.

Plomin, R. & Nesselroade, J. R. (1990) Behavioral genetics and personality change. *Journal of Personality*, **58**, 191–220.

Plomin, R., Nitz, K. & Rowe, D. C. (1990b) Behavioral genetics and aggressive behavior in childhood. In Lewis, M. & Miller, S. M. (eds.) *Handbook of developmental psychopathology*. New York: Plenum, pp. 119–133.

Plomin, R., Pedersen, N. L., McClearn, G. E., Nesselroade, J. R. & Bergeman, C. S. (1988b) EAS temperaments during the last half of the life span: twins reared apart and twins reared together. *Psychology and Aging*, **3**, 43–50.

Pogue–Geile, M. F. & Rose, R. J. (1985) Developmental genetic studies of adult personality. *Developmental Psychology*, **21**, 547–57.

Price, R. A., Kidd, K. K., Cohen, D. J., Pauls, D. L. & Leckman, J. F. (1985) A twin study of Tourette syndrome. *Archives of General Psychiatry*, **43**, 815–20.

Reed, T. E. (1989) Correlations between information processing and intelligence: current research. Nineteenth Annual Meeting of the Behavior Genetics Association. Charlottesville, Virginia, June 8–11.

Reich, T., Van Eerdewegh, P., Rice, J., Mullaney, J., Endicott, J. & Klerman, G. L. (1987) The familial transmission of primary major depressive disorder. *Journal of Psychiatric Research*, **21**, 613–24.

Reznikoff, M. G. & Honeyman, M. S. (1967) MMPI profiles of monozygotic and dizygotic twin pairs. *Journal of Consulting Psychology*, **31**, 100–10.

Rice, J. P., Reich, T., Andreasen, N. C., Endicott, J., Van Eerdewegh, M., Fishman, A., Hirschfield, R. M. A. & Klerman, G. L. (1987) The familial transmission of bipolar illness. *Archives of General Psychiatry*, **41**, 441–7.

Roberts, J. A. F. (1952) The genetics of mental deficiency. *Eugenics Review*, **44**, 71–83.

Rose, R. J. (1988) Genetic and environmental variance in content dimensions of the MMPI. *Journal of Personality and Social Psychology*, **55**, 302–11.

Rose, R. J. & Ditto, W. B. (1983) A developmental-genetic analysis of common fears from early adolescence to early adulthood. *Child Development*, **54**, 361–8.

Rowe, D. C. (1983) Biometrical genetic models of self-reported delinquent behavior: twin study. *Behavior Genetics*, **13**, 473–89.

Rowe, D. C. (1986) Genetic and environmental components of antisocial behavior: a study of 265 twin pairs. *Criminology*, **24**, 513–32.

Rutter, M. (1988) Epidemiological approaches to developmental psychopathology. *Archives of General Psychiatry*, **45**, 486–95.
Rutter, M., Macdonald, H., Le Couteur, A., Harrington, R., Bolton, P. & Bailey, A. (1990) Genetic factors in child psychiatric disorders: II. empirical findings. *Journal of Child Psychology and Psychiatry*, **31**, 39–83.
Scarr, S., Webber, P. I., Weinberg, R. A. & Wittig, M. A. (1981) Personality resemblance among adolescents and their parents in biologically related and adoptive families. *Journal of Personality and Social Psychology*, **40**, 885–98.
Searles, J. S. (1988) The role of genetics in the pathogenesis of alcoholism. *Journal of Abnormal Psychology*, **97**, 153–67.
Sherrington, R., Brynjolfsson, J., Petursson, H., Potter, M., Dudleston, K., Barraclough, B., Wasmuth, J., Dobbs, M. & Gurling, H. (1988) Localization of a susceptibility locus for schizophrenia on chromosome 5. *Nature*, **336**, 164–7.
Smalley, S. L., Asarnow, R. F. & Spence, M. A. (1988) Autism and genetics. *Archives of General Psychiatry*, **45**, 953–61.
Smith, C. (1974) Concordance in twins: methods and interpretation. *American Journal of Human Genetics*, **26**, 454–66.
Smith, S. D., Kimberling, W. J., Pennington, B. F. & Lubs, H. A. (1983) Specific reading disability: identification of an inherited form through linkage analysis. *Science*, **219**, 1345–7.
Smith, S. D., Pennington, B. F., Kimberling, W. J. & Ing, P. S. (1990) Familial dyslexia: use of genetic linkage data to define subtypes. *Journal of the American Academy of Child Psychiatry*, **29**, 204–13.
St. Clair, D., Blackwood, D., Muir, W., Baillie, D., Hubbard, A., Wright, A. & Evans, H. J. (1989) No linkage of chromosome 5q11–q13 markers to schizophrenia in Scottish families. *Nature*, **339**, 305–8.
Stevenson, J. & Graham, P. (1988) Behavioral deviance in 13-year-old twins: an item analysis. *Journal of the American Academy of Child and Adolescent Psychiatry*, **27**, 791–7.
Stevenson, J., Graham, P., Fredman, G. & McLoughlin, V. (1987) A twin study of genetic influences on reading and spelling ability and disability. *Journal of Child Psychology and Psychiatry*, **28**, 229–47.
Tellegen, A., Lykken, D. T., Bouchard, T. J., Wilcox, K., Segal, N. & Rich, S. (1988) Personality similarity in twins reared apart and together. *Journal of Personality and Social Psychology*, **54**, 1031–9.
Torgersen, S. (1983) Genetic factors in anxiety disorders. *Archives of General Psychiatry*, **40**, 1085–9.
Vandenberg, S. G. (1967) Hereditary factors in normal personality traits (as measured by inventories). In Wortis, J. (ed.) *Recent advances in biological psychiatry* New York: Plenum, pp. 65–104.
Vandenberg, S. G., Sisnger, S. M. & Pauls, D. L. (1986) *The heredity of behavior disorders in adults and children.* New York: Plenum.
Waller, N. G., Kojetin, B. A., Bouchard, T. J., Lykken, D. T. & Tellegen, A. (1990) Genetic and environmental influences on religious interest, attitudes, and values: a study of twins reared apart and together. *Psychological Science*, **1**, 138–42
Welsh, G. S. (1956) Factor dimensions A and R. In Welsh, G. S. & Dahlstrom,

W. G. (eds.) *Basic readings on the MMPI in psychology and medicine.* Minneapolis: University of Minnesota Press.

Wender, P. H., Kety, S. S., Rosenthal, D., Schulsinger, F., Ortmann, J., *et al.* (1986) Psychiatric disorders in the biological and adoptive families of adopted individuals with affective disorders. *Archives of General Psychiatry*, **43**, 923–9.

Wierzbicki, M. (1987) Similarity of monozygotic and dizygotic child twins in level and lability of subclinically depressed mood. *American Journal of Orthopsychiatry*, **57**, 33–40.

Wiggins, J. S. (1966) Substantive dimensions of self-report in the MMPI item pool. *Psychological Monographs.* (Whole No. 630).

Wilde, G. J. S. (1964) Inheritance of personality traits: an investigation into the hereditary determination of neurotic instability, extroversion, and other personality traits by means of a questionnaire administered to twins. *Acta Psychologica*, **22**, 37–51.

6 Prenatal and perinatal risk factors for psychosocial development

PAUL CASAER, LINDA DE VRIES AND NEIL MARLOW

INTRODUCTION

On the basis of a series of detailed clinical observations, Little (1862), Freud (1897) and Osler (1889) postulated a possible causal relation between perinatal or prenatal hazards and subsequent developmental disabilities, including cerebral palsy. During the century since these classical papers, the nature and extent of this causal relation has remained a topic of debate. In this chapter we review the empirical findings selectively in order to illustrate the various approaches used in recent years to answer the questions raised by Little, Freud and Osler.

What is the present evidence that prenatal and perinatal complications result in abnormal outcome? What is the place of neonatal clinical assessment in detecting those infants who will show later developmental disabilities? What is the impact of non-invasive brain-imaging techniques on our understanding of these relationships? What is the evidence that genetic make up before, and environmental differences after, the accidents to the brain explain the observed differences in outcome? Special attention will be paid in this review to psychosocial sequelae in the absence of gross neurological handicap and to the strength of longitudinal research strategies in answering these questions.

STUDIES OF NORMAL INFANTS

A first approach, the study of normal infants, was proposed by Prechtl and his research group in Groningen (Prechtl, 1980). They undertook a prospective longitudinal study of a population of several hundreds of normal or near-normal newborns. They asked the following question: is there any relation between a series of optimal obstetric and perinatal factors (the optimality score) and the neonatal neurological clinical examination? If a relation could be demonstrated in the near normal, a similar approach should be applicable in disease states.

Prechtl proposed an optimality score, each point representing a well-defined optimal condition that carried the least risk for mortality and morbidity. A comprehensive list of optimality criteria was compiled covering: 11 factors related to maternal and obstetrical history including social factors, 11 pregnancy factors, 10 factors related to parturition, 10 perinatal factors and 10 postnatal factors related to the infant. In a series of elegant studies, the relation between 'obstetric' optimality score and neonatal neurological optimal examination was established by Prechtl, Beintema, Touwen and Kalverboer (see Prechtl, 1980).

The next step was to study in this near-normal population the relation between neonatal neurological status and subsequent neurological and behavioural performances. This was the topic of a prospective longitudinal study on 150 children. The surprising result was not that a strong relation was found between social class and later outcome but that a weak but significant relation was found between the neurological status in newborns and the neurological status of children up to the age of two years. Furthermore preschool and school age children, rank-ordered along their neurological optimality, showed different behavioural performances in various experimental conditions (Kalverboer, 1975).

Optimality scores, for both prenatal and perinatal factors and the neurodevelopmental examination of infants should remain useful instruments. Optimality scores avoid the overestimation of one clinical symptom or one clinical risk factor in the study of causal relationships and outcome. Furthermore they constitute tools to compare populations from different hospitals and to evaluate changes over time in a population under study (Casaer & Eggermont, 1985).

MULTICENTRE STUDIES

A second approach is provided by multicentre studies. Perinatal and follow-up data at specific ages have been collected from large groups of newborns, born in many centres, in an attempt to obtain social, obstetric, and perinatal risk factors predicting cerebral palsy or other adverse outcomes. Classical examples are the National Institute of Health (NIH) collaborative study in the USA (see Nelson & Ellenberg, 1986) and the British national perinatal study (Butler & Bonham, 1969).

It is obvious from these studies that socio-economic and maternal factors are more important than perinatal factors in predicting intelligence. These studies once and for all have taken away the hope that one or a few clinical factors could predict global outcome. Besides birth weight and gestational age, the two factors that are regarded as important predictors of cerebral palsy are abruptio placenta and neonatal convulsions. The first one is a strong clinical indicator of a circulatory collapse resulting in hypoperfusion of the baby's brain. The second is a sign, but not an explanation, of severe dysfunctioning of the neonatal nervous system.

The Apgar score (Apgar, 1953) deserves a comment. The score was proposed and proved to be an excellent indicator for the assessment of babies immediately after birth. But as a predictor of later outcome, the Apgar score is weak. In the study on more than 40 000 newborns by Nelson & Ellenberg (1981), an Apgar score of 0–3 persisting for more than 15 or 20 minutes was associated with a risk of death only during the first year of life. The same study demonstrated that a low (0–3) score at 15 minutes was associated with only a 10% increased risk for later cerebral palsy. More than 9 out of 10 (93%) infants with scores of 0–3 at 5 and 10 minutes were later neurologically normal (Thompson *et al.*, 1977). Recent changes in postnatal care, such as preventive respiratory assistance in newborns with a high risk for subsequent respiratory difficulties have been associated with even weaker predictions from the Apgar score in recent prospective studies (Apgar, 1953; *Lancet*, 1989). The better the perinatal care the weaker will be perinatal risk predictors from single symptoms or conditions, because the neonatal physician is able to correct most of them efficiently and without a long delay.

EPIDEMIOLOGICAL STUDIES

Epidemiological studies that monitor prevalences of cerebral palsies, sensory deficits and (a more difficult issue) mental retardation, longitudinally over years in a given population constitute a third approach. The Swedish population studies by Hagberg & Hagberg (1984) and the Australian studies by Stanley & Alberman (1984) are classics in this group.

One important finding is that severe mental retardation (IQ < 50), with a prevalence of 3 per 1000, can be explained by perinatal causes in only 13% of cases; mild mental retardation (50 < IQ < 70), with a prevalence of 24 per 1000 is explained by perinatal causes in only 18% of cases. The most important origins of mental retardation have thus to be found in genetic and early gestational abnormalities.

Recent surveys indicate that, although the chance of survival of premature infants has dramatically increased between 1960 and 1985, there has been no significant increase in the prevalence of cerebral palsy at school age in those birth cohorts; it remains at 2 per 1000 live-born newborns. There has been almost no effect of improved perinatal care on the prevalence of cerebral palsy in the group of infants born at term. Unexpected asphyxia remains the most difficult perinatal condition to influence, with an incidence of 6 per 1000 infants resulting in a rate of moderate to severe post-asphyxial encephalopathy of 1.1 per 1000 (Levene *et al.*, 1985). There has been a decrease in cerebral palsy in the preterm population born between 30 and 37 weeks but there has been a small increase in the number of cerebral palsies in infants born at a gestational age of 30 weeks or younger, and in infants born with a birth weight less than 1000 g (see Stanley & Alberman, 1984).

These last results have been frequently misquoted as: 'the introduction of intensive neonatal care increased the prevalence of cerebral palsy'. The only appropriate way to look at this issue is to compare the gains with the losses. In Australia, the rate of survivors in neonates with a birth weight below 2000 g increased from 598 per 1000 in 1968 to 704 per 1000 live-born newborns in 1975. The prevalence of cerebral palsy in those birth cohorts rose from 18 per 1000 to 23 per 1000; for a gain of 106 survivors a price of 5 children with cerebral palsy had to be paid (Stanley & Atkinson, 1981). In Sweden, the gain for a population cohort including all birth weight categories was 3.2 per 1000 live-born newborns between 1966 and 1974; the losses were an increase in cerebral palsies of 0.1 per 1000 live-born newborns (Hagberg *et al.*, 1982). In our study in Leuven the chance of survival increased between 1955 and 1987 in the following way: for newborns with a birth weight less than 1000 g from 13 to 35%, for the group between 1000 and 1499 g, from 32 to 74% and for the group between 1500 and 1999 g, from 75 to 91%. Eggermont (1988) plotted for 704 consecutively born neonates with a birth weight less than 2000 g the percentage of normal survivors against the percentage of survivors. Taking different gestational and weight categories the values do not fall on the diagonal line, this would indicate that all survivors are normal, but on a level of 10 to 12% below the diagonal.

However, recently Hagberg *et al.* (1989) have shown that the prevalence of cerebral palsy in the birth-cohorts 1979–82 is greater than it was in the 1970s and the 1960s. The rise is especially marked in those with a birth weight less than 1500 g and what is most troublesome is that it applies particularly to severe forms of cerebral palsy. Besides cerebral palsy, these very low birth weight children are at risk for mental retardation (frequently associated with hydrocephalus) and visual impairment and epilepsy.

Cerebral palsy is used to monitor perinatal changes, the main reason being that cerebral palsy is a relatively clear-cut clinical condition that can be monitored already at the age of 2 years and certainly by the age of 4 years, allowing an early feedback to the perinatal physicians. More subtle motor, cognitive and emotional disturbances have to wait until school age for their detection (see below).

In a recent review on 'kernicterus and the yellow brains in 1988', we stressed the value of longitudinal epidemiological studies (Casaer, 1989). Owing to an active medical management of perinatal hyperbilirubinemia, kernicterus and its related mortality has almost disappeared in modern neonatology. The main aspects of management are summarized in Table 6.1.

Table 6.1. *Management of neonatal hyperbilirubinemia*

Prevention
Maternal utilization of anti-Rh immunoglobulin and fetal blood transfusion
Surveillance and early detection
Diagnostic work-up and specific therapy
Exchange transfusion
Phototherapy

Table 6.2. *Prevalence of choreoathetosis in Western-Australia, birth years* 1956–1975

	n	Rate per 10 000 live-births
1956–60	13	1.54
1961–65	15	1.80
1966–70	11	1.15
1971–75	3	0.29

Stanley & Alberman (1984).

When studying the birth-cohorts between 1960 and 1975, the cerebral palsy syndrome of choreoathetosis and deafness progressively decreased (Hagberg *et al.*, 1975; Kearn, 1978; Cussen *et al.*, 1978; Glenting, 1982.) Stanley & Alberman (1984) reported a more than sixfold decrease in the prevalence of choreoathetosis for the birth-cohorts 1956–1975 (see Table 6.2).

For a good understanding of the disappearance of choreoathetosis due to bilirubin toxicity, a distinction should be made between the clinical syndrome of choreoathetosis due to kernicterus and the syndrome of spastic quadriplegia with athetotic features that can be the result of severe asphyxia in term infants (Kyllerman, 1982; Marquis *et al.*, 1982).

Although longitudinal epidemiological monitoring is a strong research tool, its findings need to be considered together with other scientific evidence before final conclusions are drawn. The clinical picture of kernicterus disappeared in recent years but not the pathological finding of yellow brains. The postmortem finding is not disappearing at all in the premature infant; thus our attention to the problem of bilirubin toxicity should remain but shift towards the preterm infant (Casaer, 1989). In a recent study, of all newborns born with a birth weight less than 1500 g in 1983 in the Netherlands, autopsy findings changed the neonatal diagnosis or the understanding of pathophysiological mechanisms in 15% of cases (Verloove-van Horick & Verwey, 1988).

DETAILED LONGITUDINAL STUDIES

Detailed longitudinal studies based on individual perinatal centres are mandatory for the provision of clinical feedback to the perinatal team on the development of the children treated there. In our own Developmental Neurology Research project, we study cohorts of about one hundred consecutively-born infants. In each study a series of fixed variables are scored in the neonatal and follow-up studies, but each study also attempts to answer a specific question (Casaer & Eggermont, 1985; Casaer *et al.*, 1986).

A first example of this approach is a detailed study on feeding behaviour in preterm infants with a birth weight of less than 2000 g. Using a longitudinal approach in the neonatal period a clear 'learning' effect was found in feeding efficiency and feeding posture. This result never could have been found if cross-sectional data collection had been used (Casaer *et al.*, 1987). Ultrasound studies of prenatal behaviour demonstrated that sucking, swallowing and thoracic and diaphragm movements already emerge in utero between the tenth and the twentieth week of fetal development (de Vries *et al.*, 1984); the 'learning' of postnatal feeding is thus the integration of prenatal behavioural subprogrammes into a goal-directed postnatal task. Such age-appropriate tasks seem to be good indicators of nervous system integrity. In a subsequent longitudinal study, feeding behaviour turned out to be a good predictor of the neurological status before discharge at 36–40 weeks and of the mental development at the end of the first year of life (Casaer *et al.*, 1982, 1987). This postnatal 'learning' or postnatal 'tuning' of mechanisms or subsystems already available before birth deserves more attention and needs a longitudinal approach.

In a recent study in our department on postnatal adaptation using somatosensory-evoked responses, Pierrat *et al.* (1990) showed a dramatic change in amplitude and latencies of the evoked responses during the first week of life, following which the latencies followed the normal data obtained by cross-sectional data collection. This postnatal adaptation could be an important indication of the success in the programming of the transition of prenatal to postnatal life by the central nervous system and of the required neurometabolic and neuroendocrine adaptations.

For the study of the impact of disease states and of the possible effect of treatment and their outcome, this longitudinal approach is much more sensitive than comparing one or two measurements on cross-sectional reference data. Recently de Vries *et al.* (1990) demonstrated the negative effect of intracranial hypertension on the somatosensory-evoked potentials, and their quick normalization after adequate treatment.

A third example of a useful longitudinal neonatal strategy is the day-by-day description of the clinical status of newborns during their stay in the unit or during a critical period or condition. In our unit, the neonatal special care score was developed to quantify the course of neonatal events better during the stay in the unit (Casaer & Eggermont, 1985). The items include major vital functions such as respiration and circulation, metabolic homeostasis, neurological condition, method of feeding and level of care required for the baby. The higher the score (with a maximum of 30) the higher is the intensity of care needed. The interscorer reliability calculated on 160 daily scores was 0.89 (Casaer *et al.*, 1982). The percentiles of the scores have been longitudinally plotted for various neonatal populations. The impact of a given problem (e.g. hypothyroidism and its treatment in the preterm, or an intracranial bleed) on the neonatal course of an individual baby or of a group of babies could be studied (Casaer & Eggermont, 1985; Kalubi, 1989).

In follow-up studies, the surface underneath the curve showed a stronger correlation with mental and motor outcome at the age of two, than did the initial value of the score (Daniels *et al.*, 1989). The same applies to other scores describing specific neonatal conditions such as perinatal asphyxia. The time course of the Sarnat score and of the Levene score are much stronger predictors of survival and outcome than the Apgar score describing the initial state of the infant (Sarnat & Sarnat, 1976; Levene *et al.*, 1986). A recent study in Leuven on 21 fullterm infants with perinatal asphyxia showed that the change over time in the asphyxia score between day 1 and 6 was the strongest indicator for the further evolution during the first months of life (T. Minami, V. Pierrat, L. de Vries & P. Casaer, unpublished data).

It is obvious that those studies should be interpreted with care. In particular, generalizations regarding the total population of newborns in a given area need to be based on information concerning referred and non-referred infants in that area during the study period (Kollee *et al.*, 1988). These hospital-based studies have the strength that detailed longitudinal descriptions of the population can be performed by a small group of researchers. Such studies are valuable for the evaluation of new diagnostic instruments and therapeutic interventions. Hypotheses formulated in such smaller studies should be tested in larger projects, or at least in another hospital-based population. Results obtained from regional population studies can be studied in detail to determine the underlying mechanisms in these smaller hospital-based studies.

NEUROIMAGING

Neuroimaging has greatly increased the potential to understand the processes involved in prenatal and perinatal damage. The nervous system in perinatal distress is not just a structure with a certain degree of damage. The nervous system develops from a series of regional specializations and hence being able to see where lesions have affected the nervous system really changed our strategies for neonatal and developmental neurological research.

The brain of the neonate, who was nursed in the intensive care unit, was considered as a 'black box' until the late seventies. Only at autopsy did we discover what happened to the brain during life. Intraventricular haemorrhages were a common finding in preterm infants with hyaline membrane disease and survival of infants with large bleeds was considered unlikely. The early imaging studies, first with computerized tomography (CT) (Burstein *et al.*, 1979) and shortly thereafter with ultrasound (Pape *et al.*, 1979), made it clear that intraventricular haemorrhages were very common in the very low birthweight infant and that survival was very well possible. As ultrasound is considered to be a technique without biological hazard and as it is very easy to bring the ultrasound equipment into the neonatal unit, this technique is now widely used in most neonatal intensive care units and we have been able to obtain an enormous amount of useful information in both the preterm and full-term infant.

Germinal matrix and intraventricular haemorrhage (GMH–IVH)

The early ultrasound studies mainly dealt with haemorrhagic lesions in the premature infant. Recognition of the lesion and the comparison with postmortem and computed tomography findings were studied by several groups showing that the correlation was good (Pape *et al.*, 1983). Ninety per cent of these haemorrhages occur into the germinal matrix at the head of the caudate nucleus adjacent to the foramen of Monro. Blood may extend into the ventricular system and sometimes spread into the brain parenchyma. This spread into the parenchyma used to be interpreted as a true extension. Recent studies have pointed out that the spread may be due to a venous infarction or to bleeding into an area of ischaemia. Although the shape of the parenchymal spread may be different it is usually not possible to make a distinction on the basis of ultrasound only.

To classify these lesions, the grading system of Papile (Table 6.3) is most commonly used (Papile *et al.*, 1978). By performing scans at regular intervals information has been obtained about timing of the lesion and possible risk factors (Levene *et al.*, 1982; Szymonowicz *et al.*, 1984).

Time of onset

Germinal matrix and/or intraventricular haemorrhages (GMH–IVH) are rarely present at birth, but tend to develop during the first few days

Table 6.3. *Grading system for the extent of GMH-IVH*

Grade I: Isolated germinal matrix haemorrhage
Grade II: Rupture of haemorrhage into the ventricle but without ventricular dilatation
Grade III: Rupture of haemorrhage into the ventricle with ventricular distension in the acute phase
Grade IV: Intraventricular haemorrhage with parenchymal involvement

Papile *et al.*, 1978.

of life and rarely beyond the end of the first week (Levene *et al.*, 1982). The presence of blood in the ventricles or ventricular dilatation is sometimes picked up by an antenatal ultrasound examination (McGahan *et al.*, 1983). The aetiology of these prenatal bleeds often remains unknown, but a careful clotting study should always be performed as some form of coagulopathy has been found in some of these children (de Vries *et al.*, 1988b). Maternal trauma, even when not very severe, has also been associated with antenatal haemorrhage or infarction (Larroche, 1977; Larroche, 1986). The antenatal death of one of monozygotic twins also carries a high risk of haemorrhage, usually combined with ischaemic lesions in the surviving twin (Szymonowicz *et al.*, 1986). It is of interest that the infant may have recovered from this insult in utero and thus show very few abnormal neurological signs at birth.

Risk factors

Several groups have tried to identify the risk factors for GMH–IVH (Levene *et al.*, 1982; Thorburn *et al.*, 1982; Szymonowicz *et al.*, 1984) and in fact similar risk factors have been identified. Obstetric factors appear to play only a minor role. Children born elsewhere, who need to be transported to an intensive care unit appear to be at risk but these children are highly selected (Levene *et al.*, 1982). Other factors such as mode of delivery, caesarean versus vaginal and vertex versus breech, and antepartum haemorrhage do not appear to be relevant.

The less mature the infant, the greater the risk of GMH–IVH. This fits in well with the maturational changes observed in the vascular rete, known as the germinal matrix, located at the head of the caudate nucleus (Wigglesworth & Pape, 1978; Pape & Wigglesworth, 1979). Respiratory distress syndrome (RDS) is the most commonly recognized risk factor. RDS, however, does not appear to have a causal relationship to GMH–IVH, but complications such as acidosis or hypercarbia are commonly encountered in this condition. Levene *et al.* (1982) found that 81% of low birth weight infants with both hypercarbia ($P_{CO_2} >$ 6 kPa) and severe acidosis (pH < 7.10) developed GMH–IVH and over 50% of these infants had moderate or severe degrees of haemorrhage.

Fluctuations in blood pressure have also been reported as a risk factor for GMH–IVH. Perlman *et al.* (1983) showed a correlation between fluctuations in blood pressure in infants ventilated for RDS and the occurrence of GMH–IVH. A reduction in the incidence of GMH–IVH was found when these fluctuations were abolished following neuromuscular relaxation (Perlman *et al.*, 1985). These findings were not supported by Miall-Allen *et al.* (1989), possibly because the fluctuations of the blood pressure were not as pronounced in their group of infants. Other factors, such as pneumothorax, coagulopathy, the use of bicarbonate and the presence of a persistent ductus arteriosus have been identified as risk factors by some groups but not by others.

Leukomalacia

With the linear-array ultrasound equipment used in the late 1970s; the ventricles could be well visualized, but the periventricular white matter escaped the view of the examiner. Following the introduction of the mechanical sector scanner and the high resolution transducer (7.5 MHz), leukomalacia could also be diagnosed using this technique (Hill *et al.*, 1982).

Cystic periventricular leukomalacia

When the infants are not scanned beyond the first week of life, it is unlikely that the diagnosis of cystic leukomalacia will be made. Several stages can be identified (See Figure 6.1): (a) the acute echogenic phase, when areas of increased echogenicity can be recognized; (b) the cystic

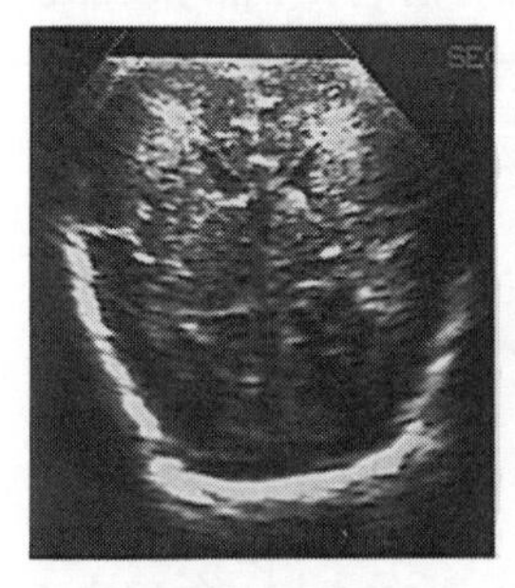
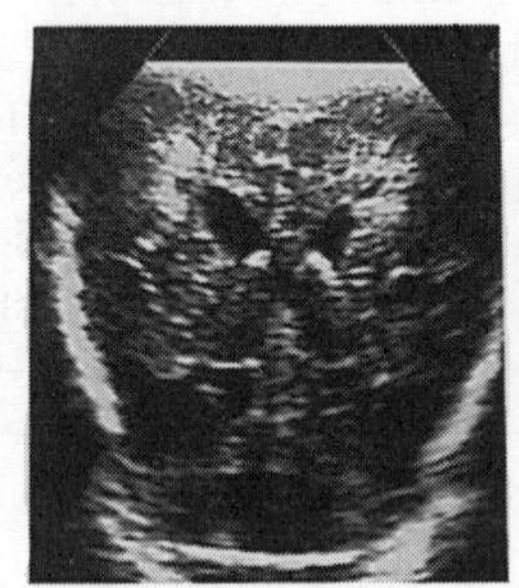
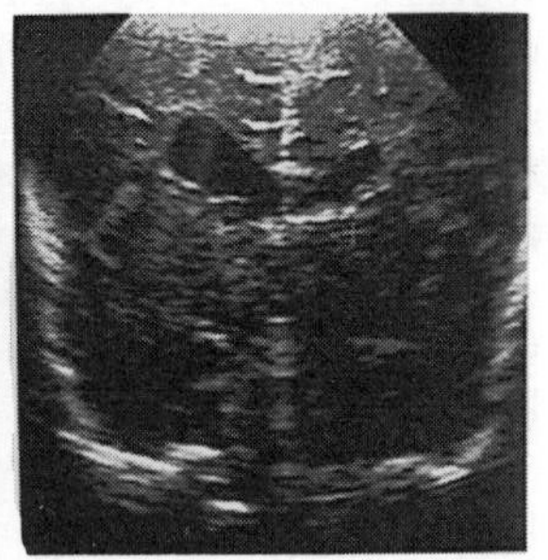

Figure 6.1. Cystic periventricular leucomalacia; on coronal ultrasound scans the 3 subsequent stages described in the text can be seen from left to right: (a) increased echodensity; (b) cystic lesions; and (c) ventricular dilatation.

Table 6.4. *Grading system for the severity of leukomalacia*

Grade I: Transient densities
Grade II: Periventricular densities evolving into localized cystic lesions at the external angle of the lateral ventricle
Grade III: Periventricular cystic lesions in the frontal, parietal and/or occipital regions
Grade IV: Subcortical cystic lesions

de Vries *et al.*, 1988a.

phase, when cystic lesions develop 2–4 weeks later in the previously echogenic areas; and (c) the late phase, when the cysts can no longer be identified but when ventricular dilatation is usually present, due to atrophy of the periventricular white matter.

Transient densities

Areas of increased echogenicity may be present for several days or weeks and subsequently resolve without the evolution into cystic lesions. These areas of increased echogenicity are referred to in the literature as 'flares' (Trounce & Levene, 1985) or 'transient densities' (de Vries *et al.*, 1988a). From correlation with postmorten findings it would appear that these densities represent a milder degree of leukomalacia (de Vries *et al.*, 1988a) (Table 6.4).

Subcortical leukomalacia

In some infants, the densities are seen further away from the ventricles and large cystic lesions are identified 2–3 weeks later in the subcortical white matter (Trounce & Levene, 1985; de Vries *et al.*, 1987). These lesions are referred to as subcortical leukomalacia. The cysts tend to persist and, using ultrasound, the diagnosis can be made as long as the fontanelle can be used as an acoustic window. Correlation with postmortem findings has shown that white matter destruction can be detected rather well using ultrasound, while selective neuronal necrosis is usually also present in these more mature infants, which cannot, however, be identified using ultrasound (Trounce *et al.*, 1986).

Time of onset

The onset of the condition occurs over a very wide range of time. In almost 25% of our cases the onset was antenatal. The majority of the infants developed leukomalacia during the first week of life, but any acute clinical deterioration, such as sepsis or necrotizing enterocolitis could still lead to the development of this condition up to 40 weeks postmenstrual age (de Vries *et al.*, 1986).

Risk factors

As the incidence of cystic leukomalacia is considerably lower than that of GMH–IVH, it has been more difficult to collect adequate numbers to study the possible risk factors. In contrast to the risk factors identified for GMH–IVH, there is no good agreement between the risk factors identified by the six studies performed so far. This might be due to (a) the small number of infants available in four of the six studies, and (b) the way the children were selected. In some studies only the infants with extensive cystic lesions were included, while in other studies infants with densities without subsequent evolution into cystic lesions were included as well as children who had large associated haemorrhages.

A few risk factors tend to recur in most of these studies and are of interest. Antepartum haemorrhage was regarded as being of importance in three studies (Sinha *et al.*, 1985; Weindling *et al.*, 1985; Calvert *et al.*, 1987). Hypocarbia was shown to be of significance in the study of Calvert *et al.* (1987), while this almost reached significance in the study of Ikoonen *et al.* (1988). This item was not studied by the other groups, but as hypocarbia is known to cause vasoconstriction, this factor should be studied further. While some of the risk factors shown by Sinha *et al.* (1985) are often associated with hypotension, hypotension was not identified as a risk factor in any of the other studies (Trounce *et al.*, 1988; de Vries *et al.*, 1988a). de Vries *et al.* (1988a) excluded infants with associated large haemorrhages and matched their infants with normal controls and with infants who suffered a large haemorrhage. No differences in neonatal risk factors could be identified when comparing the infants with extensive cystic lesions and those with large haemorrhages. It was, however, of interest to note that the gestational age was significantly higher in infants with cystic leukomalacia.

Neurological assessment in the neonatal period

Volpe (1987) described two clinical manifestations in children with large haemorrhages who usually died: (a) a rapid deterioration with coma and a decerebrate posture, and (b) a slower saltatory course – seizures and a bulging fontanelle were common features. Using a more comprehensive neurological assessment, Dubowitz *et al.* (1981) were able to correlate clinical signs with ultrasound findings. Three stages could be identified: (a) excessive mobility before the onset of the haemorrhage, (b) a tight popliteal angle, hypotonia and a decrease in mobility in the acute phase, and (c) poor visual orientation, with roving eye movements, but improvement of limb tone in the recovery phase.

On examination at 40 weeks postmenstrual age, infants who have suffered a haemorrhage still tend to show hypotonia. In infants with asymmetrical lesions, for example a porencephalic cyst, it is, however, usually possible to identify an asymmetry in tone at 40 weeks postmenstrual age, which relates well with the later development of a hemisyndrome or hemiplegia. The popliteal angle, plantar grasp reflex or placing reaction are all suitable tests to pick up this lateralization.

The clinical picture is different in the infants who develop severe cystic leukomalacia. In the early echogenic phase the infants tend to be hypotonic without any deviant signs. By the time they reach 40 weeks postmenstrual age, the picture has dramatically changed and many abnormal neurological signs can be identified in infants with marked cystic lesions. The tone pattern has changed and there is now marked arm flexion and leg extension. There is also abnormal finger and toe posturing, with flexion of the index finger and spontaneous extension of the big toe. The children are extremely irritable, but once settled, a tracking response to a bright red object can be elicited.

Follow-up during infancy

Being able to diagnose some brain lesions during life, we now have the opportunity to correlate early ultrasound findings with follow-up data. It should be stressed that in the early studies linear array equipment with low resolution transducers were commonly used and thus white matter lesions could not be diagnosed in those studies. In more recent studies, both haemorrhagic as well as ischaemic lesions could be recognized, but these intensive care graduates have not yet reached school age. The neonatal ultrasound data and, according to a few recent studies, especially ultrasound findings obtained at 40 weeks postmenstrual age (Nwasei *et al.*, 1988), have a strong predictive value as far as early neurodevelopmental outcome is concerned.

The following four conclusions can be drawn from most of the more recent studies:

(1) A small germinal layer haemorrhage or a small intraventricular haemorrhage with normal ultrasound at 40 weeks postmenstrual age is strongly predictive of a normal outcome at 1 year of age (Nwasei *et al.*, 1988). A similar conclusion was reached from the study in Leuven (Daniels *et al.*, 1989).

(2) Persistent posthaemorrhagic ventricular dilatation, with or without a unilateral porencephalic cyst carries a high risk for an abnormal outcome. In the experience of de Vries *et al.* (1985), infants with large haemorrhages without associated

ischaemic lesions tended to have a favourable outcome. Those with an unilateral porencephalic cyst usually did develop a hemiplegia, but had a normal developmental quotient at 3–5 years of age. Others, however, have not been able to support these findings (Cooke, 1985).

(3) Children with very extensive cystic leukomalacia invariably develop cerebral palsy. Those with periventricular leukomalacia tend to have a more favourable outcome (spastic diplegia, reasonable intellect, preservation of vision) than those with subcortical leukomalacia (quadriplegia, microcephaly, cortical blindness) (de Vries *et al.*, 1987). Seizures and, in particular, infantile spasms are unfortunately not uncommon, especially in the latter group.

(4) Children with a few cysts in the frontoparietal white matter or with transient densities without subsequent evolution into cystic lesions, tend to develop transient dystonia, but normalize between 12 and 18 months of age (de Vries *et al.*, 1988a). As these infants often tend to be hyperactive at 2 years of age, it is quite well possible that these children are at risk for school problems (see below).

Costello *et al.* (1988) looked at the correlation between neonatal ultrasound data and neurodevelopmental outcome at 4 years of age. The infants were born between 1979 and 1981, before the time that leukomalacia was diagnosed using ultrasound. The results broadly confirmed the associations between ultrasound appearances and neurodevelopmental outcome at 12–18 months, but the overall prevalence of impairments, both major and minor had increased from 20 to 29%, which was attributed to the presence of cognitive deficits that are not yet detectable at 18 months of age. This study stressed the importance of following the premature infants up until at least school age.

The more favourable outcome in children with haemorrhages compared to those with cystic leukomalacia may be attributed to two main factors. First, cystic leukomalacia invariably involves both hemispheres, while in children with haemorrhage commonly no parenchymal involvement is present, and if so, it can be restricted to one hemisphere (i.e. a porencephalic cyst). Second, children with haemorrhagic lesions tend to be less mature than infants with leukomalacia and the plasticity of the immature nervous system may be greater.

Postasphyxia encephalopathy (PAE)

So far we have been discussing the haemorrhagic and ischaemic lesions in the premature infant. The lesions seen in the full-term infant are not as clear cut and different conditions can develop in infants who suffer from apparently similar insults. Ultrasound studies may not always provide enough information and a combination of several imaging studies, ultrasound, CT and magnetic resonance imaging (MRI) may be necessary to better define the anatomical lesion.

During the first few days of life, areas of increased echogenicity are commonly present in the infant with PAE and this is usually interpreted as brain edema. In severe cases additional changes may be seen. Areas of increased echogenicity may develop in the thalami and basal ganglia (Voit *et al.*, 1987). When present early, haemorrhage is usually confirmed at CT or autopsy. In some cases thalamic densities first appear beyond the first week of life and late (haemorrhagic) necrosis or secondary capillary proliferation have been put forward as an explanation for these changes. Associated subcortical leukomalacia is often seen in these severe cases. In less severely affected children, the ultrasound changes are less specific and CT, especially when performed in the second week of life, may be of value to examine the preservation or loss of grey white matter contrast (Adsett *et al.*, 1985).

Other techniques such as continuous EEG recordings and Doppler ultrasound, may provide important additional information. The presence of persistent seizure activity, but especially abnormalities in background activity, are strongly predictive of a poor outcome. Archer *et al.* (1986) stressed the value of a low pulsatility index (PI) in children with PAE. All infants who had a PI less than 0.55 on more than one occasion either died or suffered from a major handicap. It is of interest that the low PI is usually not seen before 12–24 hours of age. This would be in agreement with nuclear magnetic resonance (NMR) spectroscopy findings where Pcr:Pi (phosphocreatine/inorganic orthophosphate) ratios first become abnormal after the first 24–48 hours of life (Hope *et al.*, 1984).

Neurological assessment

A careful neurological assessment is very important in the evaluation of newborns. In the acute stage it will help to assess the severity of the encephalopathy. Staging according to Sarnat & Sarnat (1976) or the simplified version of Levene *et al.*, (1985) will help to predict outcome. This staging also takes into account the rate of recovery, which should be within 48 hours for stage I and less than a week in stage II, according to Levene *et al.* (1985). A child who shows a quick recovery usually has a good chance of a normal outcome.

Which techniques to use and when to use them

For the low birthweight premature infant, cranial ultrasound is by far the best method of choice. It is important to do the scans on a regular basis. When the scans are not performed to identify risk factors, it will be sufficient to do examinations twice a week till discharge. A repeat ultrasound scan at 40 weeks postmenstrual age is important, as it is a good time to reassess the degree of ventricular dilatation in infants with posthaemorrhagic ventricular dilatation. Cystic lesions related to leukomalacia are usually still present, but may already be regressing and no longer provide an accurate picture of the maximal extent of the lesions. CT studies will not provide much additional information in this group of infants.

In the full-term asphyxiated infant, important lesions may be missed, if cranial ultrasound were the only imaging modality used. In the acute phase, CT may be important to visualize the convexity lesions (subarachnoid haemorrhage; subdural haematoma) and in the second week the CT will illustrate the preservation or loss of grey/white matter contrast. When available, MRI will provide additional information. Lesions in the thalami and/or basal ganglia are clearly seen using this technique, but are often missed using CT or ultrasound.

As the imaging techniques provide data only on structural changes of the brain, it is of importance to do additional investigations to test the functional integrity of the central nervous system. Continuous EEG recordings, auditory-, visual- and somatosensory-evoked responses have already been shown to be of predictive value. Continuous EEG recordings appear to provide most information when performed in the acute phase (Connell *et al.*, 1989). Evoked responses, however, appear to be more useful when used during the recovery phase to identify infants with persistent abnormalities (Klimack & Cooke, 1989).

NMR spectroscopy, near-infra-red spectroscopy and positron emission tomography (PET) are not yet widely used, but hopefully will provide information about metabolic and circulatory changes occurring in the neonatal brain (Hamilton *et al.*, 1986; Chugani & Phelps, 1986; Chugani *et al.*, 1987; Wyatt *et al.*, 1989).

INTERACTION BETWEEN GENETIC MAKE-UP AND PERINATAL RISK FACTORS

Even with brain imaging and with detailed assessments we cannot understand why a particular constellation of risk factors in a given pregnancy results in serious neonatal neurological problems in one infant and not in another. It is even more difficult to understand that a given neurological problem in the neonatal period does not always result in the same outcome. Before jumping too easily to explanations in terms of patterns of rearing on psychosocial circumstances we have to attempt to find underlying genetic differences in the infant and his parents.

A classical clinical example of a maternal genetic condition with an increased risk for perinatal asphyxia is the neuromuscular disorder known as Steinert's disease. The affected newborn has a much higher incidence of perinatal and postnatal respiratory difficulties; in unexplained perinatal respiratory depression in an infant, a close look at the mother is therefore indicated.

Hagberg & Hagberg (1984) demonstrated that simple ataxia is of early prenatal origin, and frequently of autosomal recessive or of dominant transmission, especially when associated with otherwise unexplained mental retardation.

The interaction between early gestational or genetic make-up, perinatal factors and socio-economic factors was elucidated in a recent elegant study (Largo *et al.*, 1989). The Zürich team studied those factors in relation to developmental outcome of preterm infants at the age of 5 to 7 years in two independent cohorts: a longitudinal study consisting of 97, and a cross-sectional study of 249 prematurely born infants with birthweight appropriate for gestational ages. Developmental assessment included Touwen's neurological examination, an intelligence test and a psycholinguistic test. Besides the classical prenatal, perinatal and postnatal factors, the authors paid detailed attention to minor congenital anomalies and to prenatal deformities. The number of minor congenital anomalies was negatively correlated with neurological outcome ($p <$ 0.001), but not with intellectual and language development; a similar relation was found with the prenatal deformity score. Although a significant relation was also found between prenatal anomalies and birthweight on gestational age, partial correlations for a given gestational age or birthweight categories remained significant.

This study is the first to disentangle the confounding variables of birthweight, gestational age and minor congenital anomalies with neurological and behavioural outcome, an association already proposed by Waldrop & Halverson in 1970 and further supported by Drillien *et al.* (1980) in their study of school age neurological and behavioural performances of low birthweight infants. In a recent Dutch study including all newborns with a birthweight less than 1500 g the incidence of congenital anomalies was 10.9%, of which 9.3% were severe in the group of small-for-dates (Verloove-van Horick & Verwey, 1988).

For a better understanding, a longitudinal linkage between perinatal registers and 'genetic registers' and refined studies of chromosomal anomalies, not only in abortions, but also in perinatal mortality and morbidity are indicated. This approach is particularly important now, since perinatal factors as such reduced in their importance owing to the improved perinatal care.

COMPENSATING ENVIRONMENTAL POSTNATAL MECHANISMS

Many follow-up studies have shown associations between socio-economic class and later behavioural and intellectual development. A few studies have looked into the positive effect of optimal rearing conditions on improvements in behavioural and intellectual outcome.

In a prospective longitudinal study, Beckwith & Parmelee (1986) studied sleep state organization and its EEG patterns at term in a group of 53 preterm infants, as an index of their neurophysiological maturity and integrity which might have implications for their later development. The rearing environments of the infants were also studied during home visits at 1, 8 and 24 months, with direct observations of caregiver–infant interaction. The children were assessed with the Gesell developmental scale at 4, 9 and 24 months and with intelligence tests at 5 and 8 years of age. In general the infants with less *407-traçé alternant* in non-rapid-eye-movement (non-REM) sleep had lower IQ scores beginning at 24 months and continuing to the age of 8 years, indicating a relation between neonatal neurophysiological variables and intelligence. There was an exception, however, for those children with less *407-traçé alternant* in non-REM sleep being reared in consistently attentive environments. By the age of 24 months and continuing until 8 years of age they had higher IQ scores, equal to those of children with better neonatal neurophysiological variables.

Largo *et al.* (1990) in a longitudinal study on the predictive value of infant tests on developmental outcome at school age showed the value of individual mental growth curves. These curves revealed that prediction from one age to the other could be hampered by dissociations in development and by subsequent organic impairment (epilepsy) and major life events (a negative influence of divorce and a positive effect of a new stable foster parents situation).

Early parent–infant interaction can be disturbed by the parent's anxiety for postneonatal mortality and for subsequent morbidity, especially for an adverse neurological outcome (Papousek & Papousek, 1984; Minde *et al.*, 1988). Therefore, it is important to take the burden of negative outcome away from the parents as soon as it is possible in high-risk infants. In our study on newborns with a birth weight less than 2000 g, we demonstrated that newborns with a normal examination at discharge, with a normal feeding behaviour and with normal ultrasound of the brain (excluding perinatal but also large antenatal developmental structural anomalies) had the same chances for normal development as their full-term control group (Daniels *et al.*, 1989). A similar result was reported by Amiel-Tison & Stewart (1989).

RELATION BETWEEN PERINATAL RISKS AND SUBSEQUENT PSYCHIATRIC DISORDERS

Relation between perinatal risks and schizophrenia

Schizophrenia is one of the most common causes of severe chronic handicap in adults, with a lifetime prevalence of 1% (Kendell, 1983). There has recently been increased interest in the hypothesis that complications of pregnancy and birth cause schizophrenia in some cases. This topic has been discussed in an excellent annotation by Goodman (1988). From family, twin and adoption studies there is compelling evidence for the importance of genetic factors in schizophrenia (McGuffin, 1984).

Genetic predisposition cannot be the whole story, however. Given a schizophrenic proband, only about 10% of first-degree relatives and fewer than 50% of monozygotic twins develop schizophrenia, suggesting an important role for non-genetic factors such as environmental factors and acquired brain-damage. Lesions of the temporal lobes or diencephalon, congenitally or postnatally acquired, are predisposing factors for schizophrenia (Davison & Bagley, 1969; Taylor, 1975). Although cases with a recognized 'organic' cause only account for a small proportion of schizophrenia they could be only the tip of an iceberg, if schizophrenia were commonly caused by early brain-damage due to pregnancy and birth complications (Goodman, 1988).

McNeil & Kaij (1978) reviewed a large number of early studies demonstrating that schizophrenics are more likely than matched controls to have experienced early brain-damage due to pregnancy and birth complications. The evidence of these studies is based on retrospective recall and this is an important limitation. In three recent Scandinavian studies, however, there is no problem of biased recall since the studies were based on contemporary birth-records. Comparisons of Danish schizophrenics with matched controls demonstrated that on average the schizophrenics had experienced more pregnancy and birth complications than matched controls (Jacobson & Kinney, 1980; Parnas *et al.*, 1982). A Swedish study based on hospital birth-records showed the same (McNeil & Kaij, 1978).

Goodman (1988) refuted two possible explanations for a link between pregnancy and birth complications and schizophrenia. There is no evidence for a genetic factor in the schizophrenic mother that predisposes her to more pregnancy and birth complications, since no increased rate of abnormal pregnancies and deliveries could be found in schizophrenic mothers when compared to matched controls. The hypothesis that pregnancy and birth complications might be due to psychosocial disadvantages of the mothers with schizophrenia can also be refuted.

Brain-imaging techniques have demonstrated abnormalities in roughly a third of schizophrenics (Parnas *et al.*, 1982; Schulsinger *et al.*, 1984; Pearlson *et al.*, 1985; Murray *et al.*, 1985; Wilcox & Nasrallah, 1987). The abnormal neuroradiological findings consist mainly of unusually large lateral and third ventricles, sometimes accompanied by the widening of the cortical sulci. Reveley *et al.* (1984) stressed that these findings are not a distinctive marker for the non-genetic subtype of schizophrenia. Both ventricular enlargement and an excess of pregnancy and birth complications occur in schizophrenics with a positive family history and in schizophrenics with a negative family history (Parnas *et al.*, 1982).

These studies are at present not conclusive. In the future not only the size of the ventricles but also the shape and irregularities of the ventricular wall should be studied in detail on CT scans. Even more interesting would be nuclear magnetic resonance studies, including the description of those periventricular and subcortical white matter and cortical lesions, which are at present known to be related to prenatal and perinatal developmental abnormalities or acquired damage.

A cautious conclusion at present would be that schizophrenia results probably from the combination of a genetic predisposition to a schizotypal personality disorder and an early brain-developmental abnormality. There is no compelling reason at present to conclude either that inadequate perinatal care causes schizophrenia or that improved perinatal care could prevent it (Goodman, 1988).

To improve our understanding in this field, follow-up studies on infants with a high risk for brain damage in perinatal life should continue until adulthood; there is a need for prospective longitudinal studies correlating perinatal clinical and neuroradiological findings with subsequent psychiatric development. The linking of perinatal registers with specific diagnostic registers in adult life would also be helpful but, of course, detailed attention would need to be paid to the protection of individual privacy.

Relation between perinatal events and learning difficulties and behavioural disturbances in childhood

Although there is little dispute that major perinatal events can result in major handicapping conditions for the child, it is less certain whether similar, but less severe, events may adversely affect performance in more subtle areas, and how perinatal influences interact with other external influences. The possible influence of perinatal events on performance in middle childhood is discussed with respect to four patient groups:

(1) children who have had significant perinatal asphyxia
(2) low birthweight children (<2500 g)

(3) small-for-dates children
(4) very preterm (<33 weeks gestation) or very low birthweight (<1501 g – VLBW) children without major impairment.

Studies of outcome in relation to clinical grades of perinatal asphyxia (Finer *et al.*, 1981; Levene *et al.*, 1986) indicate that children with mild encephalopathy (Sarnat & Sarnat, 1976) have little risk of major impairment, in contrast to those with severe encephalopathy who usually die or develop severe impairments. An intermediate group with moderate encephalopathy comprises a significant proportion of children who will develop major impairments, but a healthy or 'normal' outcome for the majority of children is traditionally predicted, based upon relatively short periods of follow-up.

In a recent report from Edmonton, Canada (Robertson *et al.*, 1989), children with clinical evidence of perinatal asphyxia were examined at 8 years of age. All 28 children with severe encephalopathy died or had severe impairments; in contrast none of the 56 children with mild encephalopathy developed later into children with a major impairment. Among the 84 with moderate encephalopathy the mean IQ, reading, spelling and mathematics scores were significantly lower than the peer group or those with a mild perinatal illness, even after allowing for confounding perinatal and demographic variables. These observations suggest a continuum of brain injury in asphyxia, rather than the 'all or none' concept which had previously prevailed, and clearly connects perinatal events to performance in middle-childhood outcome in this group.

Low birthweight, in contrast, has been known for some time to be a marker for later schooling difficulties and mild neurological and behavioural dysfunction in middle childhood. The nature of this relationship is, however, less clear. Low birthweight represents the end point of many preconceptional, antenatal and perinatal influences. In any individual, it is likely that different influences are active, the outcome for one child representing the complex social, environmental and genetic influences which determine ability for the majority of children, whilst the outcome for another child may be impaired as the result of biological factors operative during the pregnancy, delivery and neonatal period. Clearly such a mix of influences is likely to weaken any perinatal associations, which must be sought over a necessarily long period of time.

Many of the older studies which have followed low birthweight children prospectively have concentrated upon what today are considered 'low risk' children. The majority of children with birthweights 1501–2500 g have few postnatal complications, a low frequency of brain injuries detected by the techniques described previously and a low frequency of major handicapping conditions, compared with lighter birthweight groups. None-the-less the outcome for children in this birthweight category has been addressed in several prospective longitudinal studies which are of great interest (Francis-Williams & Davies, 1974; Neligan *et al.*, 1976; Illsley & Mitchell, 1984; Dunn *et al.*, 1986).

Common to these studies is the observation of population differences when compared with controls. Low birthweight populations have lower IQ scores, more motor difficulties, an excess of minor neurological signs and behavioural difficulties. In all such studies the lowest birthweight children perform least well. Few studies have, however, addressed the possibility of causation fully.

Epidemiological studies indicate that prematurity and low birthweights are features of poor social and environmental conditions. The extent that environmental factors determine outcome was addressed in a 10-year cohort study of 143 children with birthweights less than 2500 g born in Aberdeen in 1969–70. (Illsley & Mitchell, 1984). Controls were closely matched for maternal age, parity, smoking habit, height and social class. Despite this, the low birthweight group performed less well in the areas of IQ scores, perceptuomotor skills, behavioural traits and academic performance. Careful analysis revealed many adverse characteristics among the parents of low birthweight infants, who had poorer academic attainment and were likely to provide a less stimulating rearing environment compared with that provided by the ostensibly 'matched' control parents. Indeed these characteristics were better predictors of 10-year performance than birthweight – leading to the conclusion that a positive social environment can offset the disadvantage of low birthweight.

Whatever match is made on environmental terms, more subtle factors may be more powerful in the determination of outcome than the events surrounding low birthweight. Many studies, however, have pursued the subtle effects of 'prenatal' events without distinguishing a further set of environmental confounders (see discussion in Largo *et al.*, 1989).

Part of the 'preconceptional' determination of outcome must also result from genetic factors, rarely considered in low birthweight studies usually because of methodological difficulties. Several investigators have drawn attention to the increased frequency of 'minor dysmorphic features' among low birthweight populations and their association with adverse outcomes (Waldrop & Halverson, 1970; Drillien *et al.*, 1980; Largo *et al.*, 1989). Such signs are observed more frequently in children who are small-for-gestational age, as well as being independently associated with poor school performance (Drillien *et al.*, 1980). It is, however, unclear from current data whether minor dysmorphic features are the result of genetic or early antenatal insults from, for example, maternal alcohol abuse, use of drugs or medication, or infection.

The influence of inadequate intrauterine growth has been addressed in many studies. Poor weight for gestational age is the final common expression of many influences in pregnancy, both biological (e.g. pre-eclampsia) and environmental (e.g. substance abuse). The artificial definition of abnormal birthweight as being under the tenth percentile of birthweight for gestational age has resulted in conflicting results (reviewed by Allen, 1984), with indeterminate results for preterm small-for-gestational age children (Robertson *et al.*, 1990). Term small-for-gestational age children, in contrast, perform poorly compared with controls (Allen, 1984). Poor head growth in small-for-gestational age children may be a marker for poor IQ scores (Ounsted *et al.*, 1984; Dunn *et al.*, 1986) or developmental risk (Neligan *et al.*, 1976; Allen, 1984), but in a recent large study was associated with mild neurological dysfunction but no worsening of school performance or behaviour (Hadders-Algra & Touwen, 1990).

Better measures are required relating actual to optimal weight correcting for parental height, parity, race and multiple gestation. The ponderal index (Walther & Ramaekers, 1982) may prove one such useful measure. Growth failure may then be treated as a continuous variable using a standard deviation score or birthweight ratio (Morley *et al.*, 1990). If more extreme deviation of birthweight for gestational age is considered (below third percentile or −3 standard deviations (SD)) a clearer picture seems to emerge. Poor developmental (Marlow *et al.*, 1987) and neurological (Hadders-Algra *et al.*, 1988) performance parallels poor catch-up growth.

In contrast to infants of moderate birthweight or gestation, many very preterm children will be delivered because of biological risk factors which make continuation of pregnancy hazardous for either infant or mother. This intervention may alter the previous relation with socio-economic variables. Among 1034 children with birthweights less than 2001 g cared for in a regional referral unit in Manchester, UK, the distribution of socio-economic status (SEC) was similar to that of the local population, rather than showing the expected excess of disadvantage (Marlow, 1985). Similar results were observed in a geographically defined cohort of children of less than 33 weeks gestation born in the county of Avon (J. Emond, personal communication).

The association between preconceptional or antenatal influences and outcome is further complicated for very preterm or VLBW babies. As birthweight decreases below 1501 g the mortality and frequency of major impairments rises (Marlow & Chiswick, 1985). In this group a high frequency of brain lesions may be observed on sequential cerebral ultrasound scanning (Gowland & Chiswick, 1983; de Vries *et al.*, 1988a; Pidcock *et al.*, 1990). Ultrasound and clinical examination provide reasonable prediction of outcome in terms of major impairment (Stewart *et al.*, 1987) but in recent studies a significant proportion of children with abnormal late scans appear free of major problems at follow up (Cooke, 1988; Pidcock *et al.*, 1990; Bennett *et al.*, 1990). The relative influences of environment and perinatal events, expressed as brain injuries, are largely unexplored. The high frequency of major impairments in VLBW children may be expected to imply an excess of intermediate degrees of impairment, perhaps similar to that seen with perinatal asphyxia, within a continuum of 'reproductive casualty' (Sameroff & Chandler 1975). The observation that children with major impairments have a perinatal risk intermediate between children without disabilities and those who die in the neonatal period (Marlow *et al.*, 1988), and a differential association of perinatal variables with differing types of cerebral palsy (Marlow *et al.*, 1988; Powell *et al.*, 1988; Cooke, 1990) provide further impetus to search for perinatal associations within the continuum of impairment in this group.

Few studies have evaluated the performance of children who have been exposed to modern neonatal care and high resolution brain imaging through into junior school, as these graduates are as yet too young. Nickel *et al.* (1982) reported school performance for a group of children with birthweights of less than 1000 g born between 1960 and 1972. Of the small number of long-term survivors, 64% were considered to have failed at school. Vohr & Garcia Coll (1985) report that 54% of a cohort of VLBW (<1501 g) children born in 1975 needed special educational provision at 7 years. In contrast, subsequent reports suggest that over 90% of more recent populations are in mainstream education (Drillien *et al.*, 1980; Kitchen *et al.*, 1980). Fawer & Calame (1988, 1989) have estimated that 'minor developmental abnormalities' occur in 25–50% of school age VLBW children. School failure, which reflects intellectual, social and emotional maturity, is three times as frequent in this group compared with peers. In Leuven, 15% of children weighing less than 2000 g at birth fail to achieve grades during the first school year, compared with 6% for the general population (Daniels *et al.*, 1989).

Infant school outcome for a cohort of 53 Liverpool children with birthweights less than 1251 g, who were free of major impairments at six years, has recently been reported (Marlow *et al.*, 1989). These children had been followed prospectively and full perinatal and ultrasound scan data were available, births being between January 1980 and July 1981. Compared with age- and sex-matched classmates, the index group performed less well over a range of standard tests. Correlations with perinatal and environmental variables were sought. Considering index and control children, birthweight was the most powerful associate with motor and IQ scores, socio-environmental factors adding little to a multiple regression model. There was no relation between six-year performance in index children and appearances on neonatal ultrasound, but three perinatal factors (Apgar score at 5 minutes, positive blood culture and abnormal neurological behaviour) explained 32% of the variance in six-year motor scores, suggesting a significant association. Scanning was in its infancy in 1980 and poor definition together with a lack of sequential scans may have contributed to the lack of association noted.

These children have been re-examined at the age of 8 years, in junior school (B. L. Roberts, R. W. I. Cooke & N. Marlow, unpublished data). A range of educational, motor and behavioural measures were made, confirming the persistence of the differences noted at 6 years. Population scores differed mostly in terms of maths and spelling, but when dichotomized around the tenth percentile performance of the control group as a measure of poor classroom performance, 30% of the index group were failing in each of maths, spelling and reading. This confirms the earlier observations that performance was affected across the whole range of learning skills. One half of the preterm children were failing at one subject and 30% at two or more. The differences in motor scores between the two populations were less marked than at 6 years. Behaviour was assessed using the Rutter Scales. In contrast to the earlier study (using a different scale) parents now reported a similar frequency of problems to control parents. Teachers, however, identified psychiatric, (especially emotional), disorder more frequently among the preterm group. On a continuous performance test (similar to that of Taylor, 1986) the preterm children showed significantly more impulsivity, making more positive or negative errors.

The picture of school-age children with motor difficulties, an excess of minor neurological signs and a tendency to emotional problems (Hertzig, 1981; Hadders-Algra *et al.*, 1988; Marlow *et al.*, 1989) was evaluated by Shaffer *et al.* (1984) in a study unrelated to preterm birth. Seven-year-old children with an excess of 'soft signs', and evidence of emotional problems, were followed for 10 years. The presence of neurological abnormalities predicted psychiatric anxiety traits at 17 years. A similar progression was noted by Dunn *et al.* (1986) from 'minimal cerebral dysfunction' at 6 years to behavioural problems at 13 years in their population of low birthweight children. The current VLBW cohorts must be followed into adolescence in order to evaluate this further.

The spectrum of problems reported for the very preterm without major impairment closely mirrors that described in heavier infants born 20 years previously (Illsley & Mitchell, 1984; Dunn *et al.*, 1986). Is there evidence that this excess of late sequelae is caused by, rather than associated with, perinatal events?

Drillien *et al.* (1980) studied VLBW children from the first postnatal year through to school. Learning difficulties were related independently to social class, minor dysmorphic features with intrauterine growth retardation and transient neurological dysfunction (transient dystonia) observed during the first postnatal year. Children with transient dystonia were also noted to be inattentive and distractable when seen at 2 years. Recent observations by de Vries *et al.* (1988a) suggest that transient dystonia is related to the finding of prolonged periventricular echodensities (>10 days) on neonatal ultrasound scanning. Corroboration of the high frequency of attentional problems and the relation to IQ scores at 5 years in a population of VLBW babies was provided by Astbury *et al.* (1987).

The progression of intermediate degree of scan abnormality through transient dystonia in infancy, attentional defects as a toddler, motor delay in the preschool years to learning difficulties at school must as yet remain speculative.

There are no data to quantify longer term outcomes for the smallest survivors of modern intensive care as improvements in survival and the quality of neuroimaging have only occurred during the past decade.

Factors other than observable brain injuries may influence developmental outcome. Metabolic disturbances such as hyperphenylalaninaemia, hypoglycaemia or hypothyroidism may have longer-term effects on the child (see chapter 7, this volume). Although often unrecognized, all are observed to occur transiently in the sick preterm infant (Puntis *et al.*, 1986; Lucas *et al.*, 1988a; b). Kho *et al.* (1988) reported delayed nerve conduction velocities in children with marginal hypoglycaemia that persisted after correction of the metabolic defect. This suggests a prolonged effect from relatively mild hypoglycaemia. Although these data have not yet been confirmed (Greisen & Pryds, 1989) there is evidence that asymptomatic hypoglycaemia may have even longer-term effects. Re-analysis of data from the multicentre feeding trial (Lucas *et al.*, 1984) revealed that children with prolonged neonatal biochemical hypoglycaemia have a 13–14 point disadvantage at 18 months of age on testing with the Bayley scales compared with normoglycaemic study children (Lucas *et al.*, 1988a). This is a retrospective study with some inherent limitations but none-the-less it points to a potentially important and yet often ignored variable.

The quality of early neonatal nutrition has been emphasized in a multicentre feeding trial (Lucas *et al.*, 1989), where less rapid neonatal weight gain was associated with poorer developmental outcome at 18 months after correction for confounding variables.

The demonstration that these factors influencing the '*milieu interne*' determine developmental outcome has great implications for management in the newborn period, since in such instances prevention is possible.

CONCLUSIONS

With improving perinatal care the relationships between socio-economic, genetic and postnatal environmental factors became visible as being more important than the strict perinatal factors for later neurological and perhaps behavioural development. The neuroimaging studies convince us, however, of the utmost importance of keeping this perinatal care at the present high standard.

A clear 'dose–response relationship', described by Bradford Hill (1977) and proposed by Rutter (1988) as an essential prerequisite to accept causation, is present in the studies comparing the degree of damage as shown by imaging with the degree and the duration of neonatal neurologically abnormal behaviour and of neonatal neurophysiological dysfunctioning, and also with motor and mental abnormalities in the first years of life.

New prospective studies into the school-age period may well come to the same conclusion with respect to the severe and moderate structural changes. The effect of minor visible and not yet visible structural changes on minor developmental abnormalities, on school performance and on behavioural development is still an open question. Whether moderate and minor lesions will also show topographically specific disturbances is another key question for future studies.

A closer collaboration between scientists interested in behavioural and emotional development and those interested in neurological development is indicated if a better understanding of the nature–nurture problem has to be achieved; especially in the hope of stimulating the development of compensating mechanisms in both the child and his caregivers.

The value of longitudinal research in this field and the need to stay close to individual changes over time has been apparent in this review. For future studies, the various approaches should be more combined; clinical cohorts should be linked with pathology data and with population registers, after providing optimal guarantee for individual privacy.

ACKNOWLEDGEMENTS

This study is part of the Developmental Neurology Research Project, K. U. Leuven, Belgium. At present this research project is mainly supported by a grant of the Medical Research Council Belgium (FGWO) by a grant of 'Kind en Gezin' (Flemish Child Health Organization) and by a grant from Janssen Research Foundation, Beerse, Belgium.

REFERENCES

Adsett, D. B., Fitz, C. R. & Hill, A. (1985) Hypoxic ischaemic cerebral injury in the newborn: correlation of CT findings with neurological outcome. *Developmental Medicine and Child Neurology*, **27**, 155–60.

Allen, M. C. (1984) Developmental outcome and follow up of the small for gestational age infant. *Seminaries in Perinatology*, **9**, 123–56.

Amiel-Tison, C. & Stewart, A. (1989) Follow-up studies during the first five years of life: a pervasive assessment of neurological function. *Archives of Disease in Childhood*, **64**, 496–502.

Apgar, V. (1953) A proposal for a new method of evaluation of the newborn infant. *Anesthesia and analgesia*, **32**, 260–7.

Archer, L. N. J., Levene, M. I. & Evans, D. H. (1986) Cerebral artery Doppler ultrasonography for prediction of outcome after perinatal asphyxia. *Lancet*, **ii**, 1116–7.

Astbury, J., Orgill, A. & Bajuk, B. (1987) Relationship between two year behaviour and neurodevelopmental outcome at 5 years of very low birthweight infants. *Developmental Medicine and Child Neurology*, **29**, 370–9.

Beckwith, L. and Parmelee, A. H. (1986) EEG patterns of preterm infants, home environment and later IQ. *Child Development*, **57**, 777–89.

Bennett, F. C., Silver, G., Leung, E. J. & Mack, L. A. (1990) Periventricular echodensities detected by cranial ultrasonagraphy: usefulness in predicting neurological outcome in low-birth-weight, preterm infants. *Pediatrics*, **85**, 400–4.

Bradford Hill, A. (1977) *A short textbook of medical statistics*. London: Hodder and Stoughton.

Burstein, J., Papile, L. & Burstein, R. (1979) Intraventricular haemorrhage in premature newborns: a prospective study with CT. *American Journal of Roentgenology*, **132**, 631–5.

Butler, N. R. & Bonham, D. G. (1969) *Perinatal problems*. Edinburgh: Livingstone.

Calvert, S. A., Hoskins, E. M., Fong, K. W. & Forsyth, S. C. (1987) Etiological factors associated with the development of periventricular leukomalacia. *Acta Paediatrica Scandinavica*, **76**, 254–9.

Casaer, P. (1989) Kernicterus or yellow brains. In Duc, G. (ed.) *Controversial issues in neonatal interventions*. Berlin, New York: Springer Verlag, pp. 79–94.

Casaer, P. & Eggermont, E. (1985) Neonatal clinical neurological assessment. In Harel, S. (ed.) *The at risk infant*. New York: Paul Brooks, pp. 197–220.

Casaer, P., Eggermont, E. & Volpe, J. J. (1986) Neonatal clinical neurological assessment. In Robertson, N. C. R. (ed.) *Textbook of neonatology*. Edinburgh: Churchill Livingstone, pp. 527–32.

Casaer, P., Devlieger, H., Daniels, H. & Eggermont, E. (1987) Neural control of breathing and feeding in the preterm infant: a neurobehavioural and polygraphic study. In Kobayashi, A. (ed.) *Neonatal brain and behavior*. The University Press of Nagoya: pp. 183–92.

Casaer, P., Daniels, H., Devlieger, H., De Cock, P. & Eggermont, E. (1982)

Feeding behaviour in pre-term neonates. *Early Human Development*, **7**, 331–46.
Chugani, H. T. & Phelps, M. E. (1986) Maturational changes in cerebral function in infants determined by 18 FDG positron emission tomography. *Science*, **231**, 840–3.
Chugani, H. T., Phelps, M. E. & Mazziotta, J. C. (1987) Positron emission tomography of human brain functional development. *Annals of Neurology*, **22**, 487–97.
Connell, J., Oozeer, R., de Vries, L., Dubowitz, L. M. S. & Dubowitz, V. (1989) Continuous EEG monitoring of neonatal seizures: diagnostic and prognostic considerations. *Archives of Disease in Childhood*, **64**, 452–3.
Cooke, R. W. I. (1985) Neonatal cranial ultrasound and neurological development at follow-up. *Lancet*, **ii**, 494–5 (letter).
Cooke, R. W. I. (1988) Outcome and costs of care for the very immature infant. *British Medical Bulletin*, **44**, 1133–51.
Cooke, R. W. I. (1990) Cerebral palsy in very low birthweight infants. *Archives of Disease in Childhood*, **65**, 201–6.
Costello, A. M. de L., Hamilton, P. A., Baudin, J., Townsend, J., Bradford, B., Stewart, A. L. & Reynolds, E. O. R. (1988) Prediction of neurodevelopmental impairment at four years from brain ultrasound appearance of very preterm infants. *Developmental Medicine and Child Neurology*, **30**, 711–22.
Cussen, G. H., Barry, J. H., Maloney, A. M. & Buckley, N. M. (1978) Cerebral palsy: a regional study. *Journal of Irish Medical Association*, **71**, 568–72.
Daniels, H., De Cock, P., Casaer, P., Devlieger, H., Cornière, A., Van Brussel, J., Dammekens, K. & Eggermont, E. (1989) Resultaten van 8 jaar follow-up studie van prematuren met een geboortegewicht beneden de 2000 gram. *Info V.S.V.V.O.*, **2**, 11–9.
Davison, K. & Bagley, C. R. (1969) Schizophrenia-like psychoses associated with organic disorders of the central nervous system: a review of the literature. *British Journal of Psychiatry*, Special Publication, **4**, 113–84.
de Vries, J. I. P., Visser, G. H. A. & Prechtl, H. F. R. (1984) Fetal motility in the first half of pregnancy. In Prechtl, H. F. R. (ed.) *Continuity of neural functions from prenatal to postnatal life*. Clinics in Developmental Medicine no. 94. Oxford: S.I.M.P., Blackwell, pp. 46–55.
de Vries, L. S., Regev, R. & Dubowitz, L. M. S. (1986) Late onset leukomalacia. *Archives of Disease in Childhood*, **61**, 298–9.
de Vries, L. S., Regev, R., Wigglesworth, J. S. & Dubowitz, L. M. S. (1988a) Ultrasound evolution and later outcome of infants with periventricular densities. *Early Human Development*, **16**, 225–33.
de Vries, L. S., Connell, J., Bydders, G. M., Dubowitz, L. M. S., Rodeck, C. M., Mibashan, R. S. & Waters, A. H. (1988b) Recurrent intracranial haemorrhage in utero in an infant with allo-immune thrombocytopenia. *British Journal of Obstetrics and Gynaecology*, **95**, 299–302.
de Vries, L. S., Connell, J. C., Pennock, J. M., Oozeer, R. C., Dubowitz, L. M. S. & Dubowitz, V. (1987) Neurological, electrophysiological and MRI abnormalities in infants with extensive cystic leukomalacia. *Neuropediatrics*, **18**, 61–6.
de Vries, L. S., Smet, M., Ceulemans, B., Marchal, G., Wilms, G., Plets, C. &

Casaer, P. (1990) The role of high resolution ultrasound and MRI in the investigation of infants with macrocephaly. *Neuropediatrics*, **21**, 72–75.
de Vries, L. S., Dubowitz, L. M. S., Dubowitz, V., Kaiser, A., Lary, S., Silvermann, M., Whitelaw, A. & Wigglesworth, J. S. (1985) Predictive value of cranial ultrasound: a reappraisal. *Lancet*, **ii**, 137–40.
Drillien, C. M., Thomson, A. J. M. & Burgoyne, K. (1980) Low birthweight children at early school age: a longitudinal study. *Developmental Medicine and Child Neurology*, **22**, 26–47.
Dubowitz, L. M. S., Levene, M. I., Morante, A., Palmer, P. & Dubowitz, V. (1981) Neurological signs in newborns with intraventricular haemorrhage: a correlation with real-time ultrasound. *Journal of Pediatrics*, **99**, 127–33.
Dunn, H. G., Ho, H. H. & Schulzer, M. (1986) Minimal brain dysfunctions. In Dunn, H. G. (ed.) *Sequelae of low birthweight: the Vancouver study*. Oxford: MacKeith Press, pp. 97–113.
Eggermont, E. (1988) Voorstel van handelwijze bij een medisch uitzichtloze situatie bij de boorling. Verhandelingen Koninklijke Academic Geneeskunde. *Proceedings Royal Medical Academy Belgium*, **50**, 479–92.
Fawer, C. L. & Calame, A. (1988) Assessment of neurodevelopmental outcome. In Levene, M., Benett, M. J. & Punt, J. (eds.) *Fetal and neonatal neurology and neurosurgery*. London: Churchill Livingstone, pp. 71–88.
Fawer, C. L. & Calame, A. (1989) Prognosis of hypoxic-ischaemic lesions. In Duc, G. (ed.) *Controversial issues in neonatal interventiosn*. Stuttgart, New York: Georg Thième Verlag, pp. 193–202.
Finer, N. N., Richards, R. T. & Peters, K. L. (1981) Hypoxic-ischemic encephalopathy in term neonates: perinatal factors and outcome. *Journal of Pediatrics*, **98**, 112–7.
Francis-Williams, J. & Davies, P. A. (1974) Very low birthweight and later intelligence. *Developmental Medicine and Child Neurology*, **16**, 709–28.
Freud, S. (1897) *Infantile cerebrallähmung Nothnagel's specielle Pathologie und Therapie*, 9, Vol. 12, Vienna: A. Holder.
Glenting, P. (1982) Cerebral palsy in Eastern Denmark, 1965–1974. *Neuropediatrics*, **13**, 72–6.
Goodman, R. (1988) Are complications of pregnancy and birth causes of schizophrenia? *Developmental Medicine and Child Neurology*, **30**, 391–406.
Gowland, M. & Chiswick, M. L. (1983) Ultrasound imaging of the brain in the newborn. In Chiswick, M. L. (ed.) *Recent advances in perinatal medicine*. Edinburgh: Churchill Livingstone, pp. 209–28.
Greisen, G. & Pryds, O. (1989) Neonatal hypoglycaemia. *Lancet*, **i**, 1332.
Hadders-Algra, M., Huisjcs, H. J. & Touwen, B. C. L. (1988) Preterm or small for gestational age infants: neurological and behavioural development at the age of 6 years. *European Journal of Pediatrics*, **147**, 460–7.
Hadders-Algra, M. & Touwen, B. C. L. (1990) Body measurements, neurological and behavioural development in six-year-old children born preterm and/or small-for-gestational-age. *Early Human Development*, **22**, 1–13.
Hagberg, B. & Hagberg, G. (1984) Prenatal and perinatal risk factors in a survey of 681 Swedish cases. In Alberman, E. & Stanley, F. (eds.) *The epidemiology of cerebral palsy*. Clinics in Developmental Medicine no. 87. Oxford: S.I.M.P., Blackwell, pp. 116–35.

Hagberg, B., Hagberg, G. & Olow, I. (1975). The changing panorama of cerebral palsy. *Acta Paediatrica Scandinavica*, **73**, 433–40.

Hagberg, B., Hagberg, G. & Olow, I. (1982) Gains and hazards of intensive neonatal care: an analysis from Swedish cerebral palsy epidemiology. *Developmental Medicine and Child Neurology*, **24**, 13–9.

Hagberg, B., Hagberg, G., Olow, I. & von Wendt, L. (1989) The changing panorama of cerebral palsy in Sweden. *Acta Paediatrica Scandinavica*, **78**, 1–8.

Hamilton, P. A., Hope, P. L., Cady, E. B., Delpy, D. T., Wyatt, J. S. & Reynolds, E. O. R. (1986) Impaired energy metabolism in the brains of newborn infants with increased cerebral echodensities. *Lancet*, **i**, 1242–6.

Hertzig, M. E. (1981) Neurological 'soft' signs in low birthweight children. *Developmental Medicine and Child Neurology*, **23**, 778–91.

Hill, A., Melson, G. L., Clark, H. B. & Volpe, J. J. (1982) Haemorrhagic periventricular leukomalacia: diagnosis by real-time ultrasound and correlation with autopsy findings. *Pediatrics*, **69**, 282–4.

Hope, P. L., Costello, A. M. de L., Cady, E. B., Delpy, D. T. & Reynolds, E. O. R. (1984) Cerebral energy metabolism studied with NMR spectroscopy in normal and birth asphyxiated infants. *Lancet*, **ii**, 336–9.

Ikoonen, R. S., Kuusinen, E. J., Janas, M. O., Koivikko, M. J. & Sorto, A. E. (1988) Possible etiological factors in extensive periventricular leukomalacia of preterm infants. *Acta Paediatrica Scandinavica*, **77**, 489–95.

Illsley, R. & Mitchell, R. G. (1984) *Low birthweight: a medical psychological and social study*. Chichester: John Wiley.

Jacobson, B. & Kinney, D. K. (1980) Perinatal complications in adopted and non-adopted schizophrenics and their controls: preliminary results. *Acta Paediatrica Scandinavica*, **285**, 337–46.

Kalubi, M. (1989) *Hémorragie périventriculaire et intra-ventriculaire du nouveau-né. Etude clinique et ultrasonographique, thèse*. Leuven University Press.

Kalverboer, A. F. (1975) *A neurobehavioural study in pre-school children*. Clinics in Developmental Medicine no. 54. London: S.I.M.P., Heinemann.

Kearn, T. (1978) Congenital cerebral palsy. I, 1956–1973. *Danish Medical Bulletin*, **25**, 137.

Kendell, R. E. (1983) Schizophrenia. In Kendell, R. E. & Zealley, A. K. (eds.) *Companion to psychiatric studies*. Edinburgh: Churchill Livingstone.

Kho, T. H. H. G., Aynsley-Green, A., Tarbit, M. & Eyre, J. A. (1988) Neural dysfunction during hypoglycaemia. *Archives of Disease in Childhood*, **63**, 1353–8.

Kitchen, W. H., Ryan, M. M., Richards, A., McDougall, A. B., Billson, F. A., Keir, E. H. & Naylor, F. D. (1980) A longitudinal study of very low-birthweight infants. *Developmental Medicine and Child Neurology*, **22**, 172–8.

Klimack, V. J. & Cooke, R. W. I. (1989) Short-latency somatosensory evoked responses of preterm infants with ultrasound abnormalities of the brain. *Developmental Medicine and Child Neurology*, **30**, 215–21.

Kolee, L. A., Verloove-Van Horick, P., Verwey, R. A., Brand, R. & Ruys, J. H. (1988) Maternal and neonatal transport. *Obstetrics and Gynecology*, **72**, 729–32.

Kyllerman, M. (1982) Dyskinetic cerebral palsy. *Acta Paediatrica Scandinavica*, **71**, 551–8.

Lancet. The, (1989) Is the Apgar score outmoded? *Lancet*, **i**, 591–2.

Largo, R. H., Graf, S., Kundu, S., Hunziker, V. & Molinari, L. (1990) Predicting developmental outcome at school age from infant tests of normal, at-risk and retarded infants. *Developmental Medicine and Child Neurology*, **32**, 30–46.

Largo, R. H., Pfister, D., Molinari, L., Kundu, S., Lipp, A. & Duc, G. (1989) Significance of prenatal, perinatal and postnatal factors in the development of aga preterm infants at five to seven years. *Developmental Medicine and Child Neurology*, **31**, 440–56.

Larroche, J. C. (1977) *Developmental pathology of the neonate*. Amsterdam, New-York: Excerpta Medica, 1–445.

Larroche, J. C. (1986) Fetal encephalopathics of circulatory origin. *Biology of the Neonate*, **50**, 61–74.

Levene, M. I., Fawer, C. L. & Lamont, R. F. (1982) Risk factors in the development of intraventricular haemorrhage in the preterm neonate. *Archives of Disease in Childhood*, **57**, 410–7.

Levene, M. I., Kornberg, J. & Williams, H. C. (1985) The incidence and severity of post asphyxial encephalopathy in full term infants. *Early Human Development*, **11**, 21–8.

Levene, M. I., Sands, C., Grinoulis, H. & Moore, J. R. (1986) Comparison of two methods in predicting outcome in perinatal asphyxia. *Lancet*, **i**: 67–8.

Little, W. J. (1862) reprinted in *Cerebral Palsy Bulletin* (1958), **I**, 5–34.

Lucas, A., Gore, S. M. & Cole, T. (1984) Multicentre trial on feeding low birthweight infants: effects of diet on early growth. *Archives of Disease in Childhood*, **59**, 722–30.

Lucas, A., Morley, R. & Cole, T. J. (1988a) Adverse neurodevelopmental outcome of moderate neonatal hypoglycaemia. *British Medical Journal*, **297**, 1304–8.

Lucas, A., Morley, R., Cole, T. J. & Gore, T. J. (1989) Early diet in preterm babies and developmental status in infancy. *Archives of Disease in Childhood*, **64**, 1570–8.

Lucas, A., Rennie, J., Baker, B. A. & Morley, R. (1988b) Low plasma triiodothyronine concentrations and outcome in preterm infants. *Archives of Disease in Childhood*, **63**, 1201–6.

Marlow, N. (1985) Death and later disability in children of low birthweight (DM Thesis). Oxford Universtiy.

Marlow, N. & Chiswick, M. L. (1985) Neurodevelopmental outcome in extremely low birthweight survivors. In Chiswick, M. L. (ed.) *Recent advances in perinatal medicine*. Vol. II, Edinburgh: Churchill Livingstone, pp. 181–205.

Marlow, N., D'Souza, S. & Chiswick, M. L. (1987) Neurodevelopmental outcome in babies weighing less than 2001g at birth. *British Medical Journal*, **294**, 1582–6.

Marlow, N., Hunt, L. P. & Chiswick, M. L. (1988) Clinical factors associated with adverse outcome for babies weighing 2000 g or less at birt h. *Archives of Disease in Childhood*, **63**, 1131–6.

Marlow, N., Roberts, B. L. & Cooke, R. W. I. (1989) Motor skills in extremely low birthweight children at the age of 6 years. *Archives of Disease in Childhood*, **64**, 839–47.

Marquis, P., Palmar, F. B., Mahoney, W. J. & Capute, A. J. (1982) Extrapyramidal cerebral palsy: a changing view. *Journal of Developmental Behavioural Pediatrics*, **3**, 65–72.

McGahan, J. P., Haesslein, H. C., Meyers, M. & Ford, K. B. (1983) Sonographic recognition of in utero intraventricular haemorrhage. *American Journal of Radiology*, **142**, 171–4.

McGuffin, (1984) Genetic influences on personality, neurosis and psychosis. In McGuffin, P., Shanks, M. F. & Hodgson, P. (eds.) *Scientific principles of psychopathology*. London: Grune & Stratton.

McNeil, T. F. & Kaij, L. (1978) Obstetric factors in the development of schizophrenia: complications in the births of preschizophrenics and in reproduction by schizophrenic parents. In Wynne, L. C., Cromwell, R. L. & Matthysse, S. (eds.) *The nature of schizophrenia. New approaches to research and treatment*. New York: Wiley.

Miall-Allen, V., de Vries, L. S., Dubowitz, L. M. & Whitelaw, A. G. M. (1989) Blood pressure fluctuation and intraventricular haemorrhage in the preterm infant of less than 31 weeks gestation. *Pediatrics*, **83**, 657–61.

Minde, K., Perrotta, M. & Hellmann, J. (1988) Impact of delayed development in premature infants on mother–infant interaction: a prospective investigation. *Journal of Pediatrics*, **112**, 136–42.

Morley, R., Brooke, O. G., Cole, T. J. *et al.* (1990) Birthweight ratio and outcome in preterm infants. *Archives of Disease in Childhood*, **65**, 30–4.

Murray, R. M., Lewis, S. W. & Reveley, A. M. (1985) Towards an aetiological classification of schizophrenia. *Lancet*, **i**, 1023–6.

Neligan, G. A., Kolvin, J., Scott, D. M. & Gardide, R. F. (1976) *Born too small or born too soon, a follow-up study to seven years of age*. Clinics in Developmental Medicine no. 61. London: Spastics International.

Nelson, K. B. & Ellenberg, J. H. (1981) Apgar scores as predictors of chronic neurological disability. *Pediatrics*, **68**, 36–44.

Nelson, K. B. & Ellenberg, J. H. (1986) Antecedents of cerebral palsy: multivariate analysis of risk. *New England Journal of Medicine*, **315**, 81–6.

Nickel, R. E., Bennett, F. C. & Lamson, F. N. (1982) School performance of children with birthweights of 1000 g or less. *American Journal of Diseases of Children*, **136**, 105–110.

Nwasei, C. G., Allen, A., Vincar, M. J., Brow, St. J., Stinson, D. A., Evans, J. R. & Byrne, J. M. (1988) Effect of timing of cerebral ultrasonography on the prediction of later neurodevelopmental outcome in high risk preterm infants. *Journal of Pediatrics*, **112**, 970–5.

Osler, W. (1889) *The cerebral palsy of children*. London: H. K. Lewis.

Ounsted, M. K., Moar, V. A. & Scott, A. (1984) Children of deviant birthweight at the age of seven years: health, handicap, size and developmental status. *Early Human Development*, **9**, 323–40.

Pape, K. E. & Wigglesworth, J. S. (1979) *Haemorrhage, ischaemia and perinatal brain*. Clinics in Developmental Medicine no. 69/70. London: S.I.M.P., Heinemann.

Pape, K. E., Bennett-Britton, S., Scymonowicz, W., Martin, D. J., Fitz, C. R. & Becker, L. (1983) Diagnostic accuracy of neonatal brain imaging. A post-mortem correlation of computed tomography and ultrasound scans. *Journal of Pediatrics,* **102,** 275–80.

Pape, K. E., Blackwell, R. J., Cusick, G., Sherwood, A., Houang, M. T., Thorburn, R. & Reynolds, E. O. R. (1979) Ultrasound detection of brain damage in preterm infants. *Lancet,* **i:** 1261–4.

Papile, L. A., Burstein, J., Burstein, R. & Koffler, H. (1978) Incidence and evolution of subependymal and intraventricular hemorrhage. *Journal of Pediatrics,* **92,** 529–34.

Papousek, H. & Papousek, M. (1984) Qualitative transitions in integrative processes during the first trimester of human postpartum life. In Prechtl, H. F. R. (ed.) *Continuity of neural functions from prenatal to postnatal live.* CLinics in Developmental Medicine no. 94, Oxford: S.I.M.P., Blackwell, pp. 46–55.

Parnas, J., Schulsinger, F., Teasdale, T. W., Schulsinger, H., Feldman, P. M. & Mednick, S. A. (1982) Perinatal complications and clinical outcome within the schizophrenia spectrum. *British Journal of Psychiatry,* **140,** 416–20.

Pearlson, G. D., Garbacz, D. J., Moberg, P. J., Ahn, H. S. & de Paulo, J. R. (1985). Symptomatic, familial, perinatal and social correlates of computerized axial tomography changes in schizophrenics and bipolars. *Journal of Nervous and Mental Disease,* **173,** 42–50.

Perlman, J. M., McMenamin, J. B. & Volpe, J. J. (1983) Fluctuating cerebral blood flow velocity in respiratory distress syndrome: relation to the development of intraventricular haemorrhage. *New England Journal of Medicine,* **309,** 204–9.

Perlman, J. M., Goodman, S., Kreusser, K. L. & Volpe, J. J. (1985) Reduction in intraventricular haemorrhage by elimination of fluctuating cerebral blood flow velocity in preterm infants with respiratory distress syndrome. *New England Journal of Medicine,* **312,** 1353–7.

Pidcock, F. S., Graziani, L. J., Stanley, C., Mitchell, D. G. & Merton, D. (1990) Neurosonographic features of periventricular echodensities associated with cerebral palsy in preterm infants. *Journal of Paediatrics,* **116,** 417–22.

Pierrat, V., Casaer, P., de Vries, L. & Minami, T. (1990) Somatosensory evoked potentials and adaptation to extrauterine life: a longitudinal study. *Brain and Development,* **12,** 376–9.

Powell, T. G., Pharoh, P. O. D., Cooke, R. W. I. & Rosenbloom, L. (1988) Cerebral palsy in low birthweight infants, spastic diplegia: associated with fetal immaturity. *Developmental Medicine and Child Neurology,* **30,** 19–25.

Prechtl, H. F. R. (1980) The optimality concept. *Early Human Development,* **4,** 201–6.

Puntis, J. W. L., Edwards, M. A., Green, A., Morgan, I., Booth, I. W. & Ball, P. A. (1986) Hyperphenylalaninaemia in parenterally fed newborn babies. *Lancet,* **ii,** 1105–6.

Reveley, A. M., Reveley, M. A. & Murray, R. M. (1984) Cerebral ventricular enlargement in non-genetic schizophrenia: a controlled twin study. *British Journal of Psychiatry,* **144,** 89–93.

Robertson, C. M. T., Finer, N. N. & Grace, M. G. A. (1989) School performance of survivors of neonatal encephalopathy associated with birth asphyxia at term. *Pediatrics*, **76**, 753–60.

Robertson, C. M. T., Etches, P. C. & Kyle, J. M. (1990) Eight-year school performance and growth of preterm, small for gestational age infants: a comparative study with subjects matched for birth weight or for gestational age. *Journal of Paediatrics*, **116**, 19–26.

Rutter, M. (1988) Longitudinal data in the study of causal processes: some uses and pitfalls. In Rutter, M. (ed.) *Studies of psychosocial risk: the power of longitudinal data.* Cambridge: Cambridge University Press, pp. 1–28.

Sameroff, A. J. & Chandler, M. J. (1975) Reproductive risk and the continuum of caretaking casualty. In Horrowitz, F. D. (ed.) *Review of child development research.* Chicago: University of Chicago Press, pp. 187–244.

Sarnat, H. B. & Sarnat, M. S. (1976) Neonatal encephalopathy following fetal distress. *Archives of Neurology*, **33**, 696–705.

Schulsinger, F., Parnas, J., Peterson, E. T., Schulsinger, H., Teasdale, T. W., Mednick, S. A., Moller, l. & Silverton, L. (1984) Cerebral ventricular size in the offspring of schizophrenic mothers: a preliminary study. *Archives of General Psychiatry*, **41**, 602–6.

Shaffer, D., Schonfeld, I. & O'Connor, P. A. (1984) Neurological soft signs. *Archives of General Psychiatry*, **42**, 342–351.

Sinha, S. H., Davies, J. M., Sims, D. G. & Chiswick, M. L. (1985) Relation between periventricular haemorrhage and ischaemic brain lesions diagnosed by ultrasound in very preterm infants. *Lancet*, **ii:** 1154–6.

Stanley, F. & Alberman, E. (1984) *The Epidemiology of the Cerebral Palsies.* Clinics in Developmental Medicine no. 87, London: S.I.M.P., Blackwell.

Stanley, F. & Atkinson, S. (1981) Impact of neonatal intensive care on cerebral palsy of infants of very low birthweight. *Lancet*, **ii**, 1162.

Stewart, A. L., Reynolds, E. O. N., Hope, P. L. *et al.* (1987) Probability of neurodevelopmental disorders estimated from ultrasound appearance of brains of very preterm infants. *Developmental Medicine and Child Neurology*, **29**, 3–11.

Szymonowicz, W., Yu, V. Y. H. & Wilson, F. E. (1984) Antecedents of periventricular haemorrhage in infants weighing 1250 grams or less at birth. *Archives of Disease in Childhood*, **59**, 13–17.

Szymonowicz, W., Preston, H. & Yu, V. Y. H. (1986) The surviving monozygotic twin. *Archives of Disease in Childhood* **61**, 454–8.

Taylor, D. C. (1975). Factors influencing the occurrence of schizophrenia-like psychosis in patients with temporal lobe epilepsy. *Psychological Medicine*, **5**, 249–254.

Taylor, E. A. (1986) Attention deficit. In: Taylor, E. A. (Ed) *The overactive child.* Oxford, Blackwell Scientific, Chapter 4, pp. 73–106.

Thompson, A. J., Searle, M. & Russel, G. (1977) Quality of survival after severe birth asphyxia. *Archives of Disease in Childhood*, **52**, 620–6.

Thorburn, R. J., Lipscomb, A. P., Stewart, A. L., Reynolds, E. O. R. & Hope, P. L. (1982) Timing and antecedents of periventricular haemorrhage and of cerebral atrophy in very preterm infants.. *Early Human Development*, **7**, 221–38.

Trounce, J. Q. & Levene, M. I. (1985) Diagnosis and outcome of subcortical cystic leukomalacia. *Archives of Disease in Childhood*, **60**, 1041–4.

Trounce, J. Q., Fagau, D. & Levene, M. I. (1986) Intraventricular haemorrhage and periventricular leucomalacia: ultrasound and autopsy correlation. *Archives of Disease in Childhood*, **62**, 1203–7.

Trounce, J. Q., Shaw, D. E., Levene, M. I. & Rutter, N. (1988) Clinical risk factors and periventricular leukomalacia. *Archives of Disease in Childhood*, **63**, 17–23.

Verloove-van Horick, S. & Verwey, R. A. (1988) *Project on preterm and small for gestational age infants in the Netherlands 1983: a collaborative survey.* Ann Arbor, Michigan: U.M.I. Dissertation Information Service, pp. 1–378.

Vohr, B. R. & Garcia Coll, C. T. (1985) Neurodevelopmental and school performance of very low-birth-weight infants: a seven year longitudinal study. *Pediatrics*, **76**, 345–50.

Voit, T., Lemburg, P., Neuen, E., Lumenta, C. & Stark, W. (1987) Damage of thalamus and basal ganglia in asphyxiated full-term neonates. *Neuropediatrics*, **18**, 176–81.

Volpe, J. J. (1987) *Neurology of the Newborn*. Philadelphia: Saunders, pp. 1–386.

Waldrop, M. F. & Halverson, C. F. (1970) Minor physical anomalies and hyperactive behaviours in young children. In Hellmuth, J. (ed.) *Exceptional infant*, Vol. 2. Seattle: Special Child Publications.

Walther, F. J. & Ramaekers, L. H. J. (1982) The ponderal index as a measure of the nutritional status at birth and its relation to some aspects of neonatal morbidity. *Journal of Perinatal Medicine*, **10**, 42–7.

Weindling, A. M., Wilkinson, A. R., Cook, J., Calvert, S. A., Fok, T. F. & Rochefort, M. J. (1985) Perinatal events which precede periventricular haemorrhage and leukomalacia in the newborn. *British Journal of Obstetrics and Gynaecology*, **92**, 1218–23.

Wigglesworth, J. S. & Pape, K. E. (1978) An integrated model for haemorrhagic and ischaemic lesions in the newborn brain. *Early Human Development*, **2**, 179–99.

Wilcox, J. A. & Nasrallah, H. A. (1987) Perinatal distress and prognosis of psychotic illness. *Neuropsychology*, **17**, 173–5.

Wyatt, J. S., Edwards, A. D., Azzopardi, D. & Reynolds, E. O. R. (1989) Magnetic resonance and near infrared spectroscopy for the investigation of perinatal hypoxic-ischaemic brain injury. *Archives of Disease of Children*, **64**, 953–63.

7 Metabolic/endocrine disorders and psychological functioning

PETER FUGGLE AND PHILIP GRAHAM

INTRODUCTION

The mechanisms responsible for both continuity and discontinuity in psychological development are complex and influenced by a multitude of factors (Rutter, 1985). Study of the psychosocial aspects of treatable endocrine and metabolic disorders in childhood provides an opportunity to examine the role of specific biological influences in these processes.

In this chapter we will focus on three of the more common endocrine and metabolic disorders of childhood, namely: congenital hypothyroidism, phenylketonuria and childhood diabetes. These conditions share a number of common features. Firstly, biochemical abnormalities present before treatment have a direct action on the functioning and/or development of the central nervous system and, even with early diagnosis and treatment, may have permanent psychological effects. Secondly, these conditions all require the continuous monitoring and correction of dysfunctional biochemical processes, a task achieved with varying success in individual patients. Fluctuations of plasma levels outside the normal range may have transitory effects on psychological functioning which need to be distinguished from the effects of initial developmental damage. Thirdly, at present, the treatment of each condition is a continuous task throughout the life span. The demands of the treatment vary according to the specific condition, treatment for hypothyroidism being relatively undemanding whereas successful treatment of phenylketonuria and childhood diabetes is much more so. Successful treatment involves not only the effective maintenance of biochemical control but also the recognition of the emotional, behavioural and social aspects of any long-term treatment process. For childhood diabetes in particular, the behavioural demands on both child and family are highly significant if optimum treatment success is to be obtained. These behavioural demands need to be understood within the context of cognitive and emotional developmental processes along with family and social influences.

Two aspects of this need particular attention. It is important to distinguish between adaptive and maladaptive psychological processes or responses to a particular condition, the latter being more likely to be longer-term. In addition, from the perspective of the child (and the parents), there is always uncertainty on the extent to which such responses have a primary physiological basis. For example, how much is an adolescent's social anxiety a function of diabetes and to what extent does it arise independently of that condition? Both of these questions require longitudinal data in order to avoid overinclusive interpretation of the consequences of a particular condition.

Throughout this chapter early biological factors with a potentially enduring effect on development will be differentiated from those having more transitory psychological effects. This distinction mirrors comparable issues in all research into the continuity of psychological functioning in childhood. Is the continuity mediated by an unchanging environment or is it a lasting consequence of specific discrete events at an early stage of development? However, tidy conceptual alternatives of this kind are clearly an oversimplification. As Johnson (1988) has emphasized, conceptual models need to be complex and to recognize the two-way relationship between psychological and biological factors.

The achievement of optimum treatment for a child with chronic illness is the objective for both families and professionals alike. However, its achievement requires not only a clear understanding of the biochemical requirements of successful treatment but also the capacity to carry out treatment in a consistent and organized way. Both these aspects pose difficulties as uncertainties remain concerning optimum biochemical treatment for some conditions. However, in general, it is the behavioural aspects of treatment that may be most influential in the achievement or otherwise of effective treatment. Longitudinal studies with both biochemical and behavioural measures have an important role in obtaining more valid and precise measures of quality of treatment achieved over time.

This chapter is not intended as a comprehensive review of the psychosocial aspects of congenital hypothyroidism, phenylketonuria and childhood diabetes. Rather, the aim is:

(1) to examine the mechanisms (where known) that relate biological and psychological factors in these conditions; and
(2) to describe the contribution of longitudinal studies to our understanding of psychosocial aspects of these conditions and to highlight where this evidence has provided a different perspective from cross-sectional data. Particular attention will be given to the effects of quality of treatment on outcome.

PHYSIOLOGICAL BASIS OF DYSFUNCTION IN THE THREE CONDITIONS

In all forms of metabolic disorder arising from abnormalities of hormone secretion (as in congenital hypothyroidism and diabetes mellitus), or as a result of an enzymatic defect (as in phenylketonuria), interference with normal intra-cellular processes results in cellular changes which themselves lead to detectable neurochemical and neurophysiological disturbance, and sometimes to observable neuroanatomical damage. Such disturbance and damage underlies characteristic delays and deviations in neurological and behavioural development over time. Understanding the biological substrate of these delays and deviations not only helps to explain their clinical features, but may also clarify how environmental influences, including powerful medical interventions, can alter their nature and course over time.

Congenital hypothyroidism (CH)

The thyroid hormones, thyroxine (T_4) and triiodothyronine (T_3) have a wide range of actions. They influence cell multiplication, regulate enzyme activity and the synthesis of growth hormones (GH) and other substances necessary for growth, such as the somatomedins, growth hormone dependent peptides. They also stimulate the production of nerve growth factor (NGF), necessary for neuritic outgrowth in the embryo. At the intracellular level they probably influence both nuclear processes by stimulating the synthesis of proteins, and extra-nuclear structures, particularly the mitochondria (Walker, 1983). All of these processes affect brain development.

Fetal synthesis of T_4 and T_3 begins at the end of the first trimester. During the second trimester, the fetus is probably dependent for normal brain development partly on maternal thyroxine and partly on its own secretion. During the third trimester recent research has questioned previous studies (Dussault, 1983) which has suggested that there is little transfer of thyroid hormone during the later stages of pregnancy. Escobar *et al.* (1989) have reported evidence from animal studies indicating the transfer of maternal thyroxine late in gestation, and studies of thyroxine concentrations in human cord blood of athyroid neonates have also suggested continuing maternal transfer of thyroxine. After birth, even in the breastfed baby, the infant depends entirely on its own thyroid secretion. Brain development occurs most rapidly between the end of the first trimester and the first six months of postnatal life. However, the timing of events, including neuronal differentiation, the multiplication of glial cells, myelination, cell migration and the establishment of connections is different in different parts of the brain. In particular, the development of the cerebellum, of special significance in the control and coordination of movement, occurs later than in the rest of the brain, mainly in the postnatal period.

Evidence for the importance of serum thyroxine concentrations for neurological development during this period has been provided by observations of preterm infants with reduced thyroxine levels probably due to immaturity of the hypothalamic-pituitary-thyroid axis (Hadeed *et al.*, 1981). This thyroxine deficit usually normalizes spontaneously by the ninth week (Uhrmann *et al.*, 1981), but lower thyroxine levels during the first three weeks of life have been associated with reduced neural conduction velocity at 40 weeks postmenstrual age (De Vries, 1986). Whether this deficit indicates a short-term neurological immaturity or is an indication of more long-term sequelae remains to be established.

The effect of thyroid deficiency and thyroid replacement on brain development has been illuminated by experimental work with thyroidectomized rats (Escobar *et al.*, 1983). Permanent impairment of learning capacities dependent on the integrity of the cortex is produced if replacement treatment is delayed beyond 10 to 14 days after birth. Anatomical studies of the thyroidectomized rat reveal that cortical neurones are reduced in size, and there is a decrease in the length and branching of dendrites. A generalized reduction of axons and dendrites throughout the cortical mantle occurs, together with hypoplasia of the thalamo-cortical projection fibres. A marked decrease in total DNA in the somato-sensory area has been detected. Further, the degree of learning impairment has been correlated with neurohistological measures of brain damage. Early postnatal hypothyroidism in the rat also impairs normal maturation of the cerebellar cortex through damage to neuronal connectivity (Legrand, 1979). It has been shown in the tadpole that thyroxine plays an essential part in producing death of neuronal tissue necessary for normal modelling of the nervous structures. In the human it appears that most damage can be prevented if replacement treatment is commenced before 3 months of age, although psychomotor abnormalities, possibly due to cerebellar damage, may still occur. Such damage may be prevented if replacement treatment commences before 1 month of age.

Phenylketonuria (PKU)

In this condition an inherited deficiency of phenylalanine hydroxylase (PH) results in a failure of normal conversion of phenylalanine (PA), an essential amino acid, to tyrosine with resultant phenylalanine accumulation. There are other causes of hyper-phenylalaninaemia (HPA). These may be either inherited or acquired. The other main inherited cause, although much less common than PH deficiency, is tetrahydrobiopterin deficiency. Acquired causes include liver disease and drug effects.

HPA has a range of effects on brain metabolism, well described by Smith (1985) on whose account much of this section is based. In immature rats, experimental production of HPA produces a reduction in brain weight and myelin content. In vitro examination of the brains of rats treated in this way shows a low rate of utilization of cyclic AMP. Patients with classical PKU have low levels of the neurotransmitters, catecholamines and serotonin, and amine metabolites in the CNS due to reduced neurotransmitter amine synthesis.

The reasons for these changes in amine metabolism in classical PKU are not fully understood. It was thought at one stage that the excess of phenylketones, breakdown products of PA, produces the effect by inhibiting aromatic decarboxylases, but it is improbable that this is a major influence. It is now thought more likely that HPA competitively inhibits transport of tyrosine and tryptophan across the blood–brain barrier in both directions, and also directly inhibits tyrosine and tryptophan hydroxylation, together with the rate-limiting steps in amine synthesis (Piel *et al.*, 1982). This, along with the reduction of tryptophan and tyrosine in the intraneuronal substrate, then produces a reduction in the rate of dopamine and serotonin synthesis. Plasma amino acid concentrations normally affect the rate of serotonin and possibly dopamine synthesis in the CNS (Green, 1978). Thus, it is not surprising that high HPA levels have an important effect on both serotonin and catecholamine levels.

The changes described above in myelin, protein and amine metabolism are probably sufficient to explain the anatomical, neurochemical and clinical findings in untreated or inadequately treated patients. The fact that widespread, permanent damage occurs if the condition is untreated in the first two years of life, whereas adequate early treatment followed by later inadequate treatment has less devastating, though significant, effects probably reflects the fact that there is relatively slow brain-protein turnover after the first two years.

Through whatever precise mechanism its effects are produced, high plasma phenylalanine remains the best indicator of the likelihood of brain damage (Brunner *et al.*, 1983). The therapeutic range of plasma phenylalanine concentration is between 180 and 480 μmol/l (normal range 60–120 μmol/l). Patients with severe phenylalanine hydroxylase deficiency can usually tolerate up to 300 mg ingested phenylalanine per day without plasma concentrations going above this level. On a normal phenylalanine intake, their plasma concentrations rise to above 1200 μmol/l. Patients whose plasma concentrations remain below 1200 μmol/l have a mild form of the condition (Guttler, 1980).

There is uncertainty whether it is necessary to treat patients with plasma phenylalanine levels below 1200 μmol/l, but above 600 μmol/l. Most centres will treat patients with levels over 900 μmol/l. Certainly there are isolated examples of siblings in whom one is late treated and the other early treated, both with phenylalanine levels in the 900–1000 μmol/l range, where follow-up has shown that the early treated sibling has a considerable intellectual advantage (Smith, 1985).

Recent experimental studies of the relationship between concurrent phenylalanine levels and neuropsychological and behavioural functioning have shown significant deficits on cognitive vigilance and task persistence associated with higher concurrent phenylalanine levels (Lou *et al.*, 1987; Schor, 1983). In a well-designed double-blind cross-over study, Clarke (1987) showed that PKU adolescents not only had slower reaction times compared with controls matched for IQ but that reaction times significantly improved during the low phenylalanine phases of the study. This finding indicates that PKU children on unrestricted diets may have a cognitive deficit related to their current phenylalanine level that is independent of their overall intellectual functioning and that this may be partly reversible by return to stricter dietary control. These results indicate the value of including a blood test with routine cognitive assessments in children with PKU. Also, they suggest that cognitive deficits may be a consequence of a complex combination of permanent effects related to biochemical dysfunction in the prenatal and neonatal periods (see below) and transitory effects relating to concurrent phenylalanine levels.

Childhood diabetes (CD)

The insulin deficiency that occurs in diabetes mellitus results in numerous direct and indirect effects on glucose metabolism, well described in Shillitoe (1988) from which much of the following section is taken. Ingested glucose is stored as glycogen in the liver, or is converted into fat and stored as triglycerides. In the few hours following a meal, ingested glucose is the main source of energy. However, if insufficient food is ingested, liver glycogen is converted to glucose. In severe fasting fat triglyceride stores are mobilized through lipolysis, and ketone bodies, another source of energy, are produced.

Normally, the level of blood glucose is maintained within fairly narrow limits (3.5 and 8.0 mmol/l). If blood levels go above the upper limit of normal, insulin secretion occurs. This inhibits glycogen breakdown as well as gluconeogenesis. It stimulates the entry of glucose into cells and storage of glycogen and fat.

These anabolic actions are opposed by other, catabolic hormones, including glucagon, corticosteroids, and the catecholamines, adrenaline and noradrenaline. These either stimulate glycogen breakdown or indirectly increase available blood glucose by inhibiting insulin secretion. Catabolic hormone production increases considerably when subjects are stressed or physically traumatized. In contrast, parasympathetic innervation of the pancreas means that when the vagus nerve is stimulated, insulin production is increased. Stimulation of pancreatic islet cell beta-adrenergic receptors produces a similar result.

Lack of insulin in diabetes mellitus thus results in hyperglycaemia. This produces an increase in the osmotic pressure of extra-cellular fluid so that water is not recycled by the kidneys, producing dehydration and increased urination. Fat breakdown results in an increase in ketones with consequent ketoacidosis, producing gradual coma and death. Fluid replacement and insulin by injection can prevent this outcome.

It has been suggested that acute psychological stress is associated with disturbances of metabolic control in patients with insulin dependent (Type 1) diabetes (Baker *et al.*, 1969). In a carefully controlled experimental study, Kemmer *et al.* (1986) showed that exposure to stressful situations (public speaking and mental arithmetic) did result in marked cardiovascular responses and moderate elevations in plasma concentrations of catecholamines and cortisol, but this did not produce change in circulating levels of glucose, ketones or free fatty acids. This indicates that psychological stress does not increase the risk of hyperglycaemia resulting from lack of insulin.

Hypoglycaemia rarely occurs in normal individuals except after heavy, prolonged, physical exercise. It is however almost invariably experienced at times by patients with diabetes mellitus. It is usually produced by preventable causes, especially unsatisfactory matching of dietary intake with insulin. However, in some children and adolescents, it may occur as a result of impairment of other regulatory mechanisms or for reasons that are not fully understood.

Recent evidence (Lucas *et al.*, 1988) concerning the developmental significance of neonatal hypoglycaemia in preterm infants has indicated that the number of days on which moderate hypoglycaemia occurred during the first postnatal week was strongly related to reduced mental and motor development scores at 18 months even after adjustment for a wide range of factors known to influence development. Children where hypoglycaemia was recorded for more than five days showed a reduction of 14 DQ (Developmental Quotient) points compared with similar preterm infants with no recorded hypoglycaemia in the first week. Developmental assessments at 18 months remain only poorly predictive of longer-term cognitive functioning and longer follow-up will be needed in order to clarify whether the differences indicate a transient immaturity or a more permanent deficit.

A number of investigations have been carried out examining the effect of short-term variations of blood glucose level on cognitive functioning. Young adult diabetic males were found to have impaired performance on a complex reaction time task both with low (<3.3 mmol/l) and with high (>16.7 mmol/l) levels of blood glucose (Holmes, 1986; Holmes *et al.*, 1983). Performance was not impaired on simple reaction time or memory tasks. However Pramming *et al.* (1986) found impairment of attention, sequencing of information and short-term verbal memory at slightly lower levels of blood glucose (3.0 and 2.0 mmol/l). It is interesting that, although impairment was clearly evident to the outside observer, the subjects were often not aware that their performance was impaired, even at the lower level.

COGNITIVE DEVELOPMENT

Neonatal screening for phenylketonuria and hypothyroidism

Prior to the introduction of neonatal screening, both congenital hypothyroidism (CH) and phenylketonuria (PKU) usually resulted in moderate or severe mental retardation. For many years it has been recognized that CH children who were diagnosed at an early age tended to have a better psychological outcome than those diagnosed later. This observation was probably masked by the tendency of those CH children with a more severe form of the disorder to be diagnosed earlier. The introduction of screening programmes in most advanced industrialized societies during the last 20 years has resulted in the early diagnosis and treatment of these conditions. In general, the procedure is to obtain blood by heel prick between the fifth and tenth day of life although some countries (e.g. Finland) use cord blood. Confirmatory blood tests are performed on positive screening results and treatment initiated immediately. The screening programmes have been successful both in the efficiency of detecting new cases and also in obtaining earlier treatment and diagnosis. Recent evidence from a European collaborative study (Illig *et al.*, 1987) has shown that nearly 70% of all CH children are now started on treatment before the age of 1 month. This situation is similar for PKU children although earlier screening programmes which relied on urine testing as their method of detection tended to result in a later age of diagnosis compared with more recent procedures based on blood tests (Smith, 1985). In this respect, PKU children followed-up from early screening programmes may represent a different population of children from more recent cohorts. In general, the success of the screening programmes resulted in increased optimism about the longer-term outcome for children with both conditions. This optimism was supported by initial follow-up studies which tended to report IQ levels close to standardized population means for both conditions. Many of these follow-up studies reported results on children assessed during the preschool or primary age range. However, although these results clearly indicated a significant advance in comparison with the outcome of children prior to screening, it remained unclear whether there might nevertheless be evidence for a less severe cognitive impairment. Precise interpretation was hindered in many studies by the selected nature of samples, lack of appropriate controls and by increasing uncertainty regarding the calibration of the standardized IQ measures. In a comprehensive review of the longitudinal trends in IQ scores in both child and adult populations, Flynn (1984, 1987) has shown that there is a rise in IQ scores of about 0.3 points per year in children and adults from the time the test was standardized. This appears to be a remarkably consistent finding from European, North American and Japanese data and, unless this is taken into account when assessing the cognitive abilities of children with specific disorders, may lead to over-optimistic conclusions of their relative intellectual development.

Cognitive outcome in phenylketonuria

Outcome studies for PKU children have reported mean IQ scores that tend to be below the standardized mean for the population. For example, with assessments at 4 years of age the American Collaborative study with a sample of 111 PKU children reported a mean IQ of 93 points (Dobson *et al.*, 1977) and Smith *et al.* (1990) has reported a deficit of between 8 and 10 points on a large cohort of over 800 cases compared with the estimated mean for the general population adjusted to allow for an overall rise in IQ scores over time (Flynn, 1987). Comparisons with sibling controls also indicates some degree of cognitive impairment (Williamson *et al.*, 1981).

Treatment for PKU requires the affected child to eat a very restricted diet in which protein intake needs to be routinely measured and controlled. In order to avoid excessive phenylalanine intake, major sources of protein such as meat, fish, eggs and cheese need to be completely excluded and replaced by synthetic protein supplements. This dietary routine is very demanding for parents and often may become troublesome for PKU adolescents who become increasingly aware of wanting to join in ordinary activities with their peers. The quality of the treatment is also likely to be influenced by family characteristics such as cohesion and organization. Longitudinal studies that have continued follow-up into later childhood and adolescence have shown differential outcome depending on the continuation or discontinuation of dietary control after the preschool period. For example, Holtzman *et al.*, (1986) reported a difference of 11 IQ points at 10 years between PKU children who were still under dietary control and those whose dietary control had been relaxed at 6 years. Using a multiple regression analysis, age at which dietary control was lost was the only significant predictor of outcome at 10 years of age. PKU children who had maintained dietary control until 10 years of age showed no significant differences from sibling and parent controls. Similarly, data reported by Smith *et al.* (1978) described a decline in IQ associated with the age that dietary control was relaxed. The results of these longitudinal studies have influenced paediatricians and parents to continue dietary control throughout childhood.

Careful analysis of the effects of variations in dietary control on IQ has also been carried out by Smith *et al.* (1990) on a large cohort of PKU children during the first four years of life. IQ at 4 years was significantly and independently associated with average phenylalanine concentrations during treatment in an inverse direction (high phenylalanine levels with lower IQ scores). Of particular interest was the linear nature of this relationship indicating that relatively small differences in biochemical control had subtle but consistent effects. Children who had achieved optimum control showed no difference in IQ from the estimated population mean but had a mean IQ over one standard deviation higher than those children with least effective control. This treatment effect was independent of social class, which was also significantly related to IQ. It should be noted that, despite the large effect of dietary control on intellectual outcome, social class remained the single most influential variable on IQ. This study illustrates the value of longitudinal treatment data on a large cohort of children and suggests that differences within normal phenylalanine levels may be influential on longer-term outcome.

Conceptually this study is also significant in examining the relative contributions of specific biochemical measures and other variables, such as social class, known to be associated with cognitive outcome (Quinton, 1980). Although the mechanisms involved may be unclear, family factors such as birth order, number of siblings, marital conflict and father loss have all been shown to be associated with cognitive and educational attainment. The effects of birth order, for example, have been supported by a number of large cohort studies (see Hinde (1980) for review) but the effects, although statistically significant, remain small. There is a danger that the independent effects of a particular chronic disease on cognitive or behavioural functioning may be either minimized or exaggerated if not assessed against the background of well-researched psychosocial variables known to be associated with cognitive and behavioural measures. Three questions need to be addressed. Firstly, what are the independent effects of the initial pathology of the disorder prior to its diagnosis and the quality of treatment subsequently achieved over the longer term? Secondly, do these independent effects have an additive or interactional relationship with other variables known to be associated with either cognitive or behavioural outcomes? Thirdly, are these effects associated with specific developmental periods or independent of them? For example, to what extent are differences in dietary control related to variables, such as social class or family size, that are also associated with differences in IQ? At present, the evidence required to assess these complex relationships remains scarce.

Cognitive outcome in hypothyroidism

There are few outcome studies for CH children beyond the preschool and primary age, mainly because screening for CH was introduced later than for PKU. Nearly all the studies report mean IQ scores above 100 (range 97–109) with small deficits of between 0 and 5 points compared with controls. However, in several studies, it is unclear whether assessments at 5 years and older were representative of the original screened population as the number of children assessed at each age-level declined. Larger differences of 12 IQ points (patients 101, controls 113) as measured by the WPPSI (Wechsler Preschool and Primary Scale of Intelligence) at 5 years have been reported from an Australian follow-up study which had an extremely low attrition rate from the original screened population (Rickards *et al.*, 1989). The findings suggest significant remaining deficits approaching one standard deviation for CH children despite early treatment.

Research findings suggest that the initial severity of the condition, as measured by blood thyroxine levels at diagnosis, may influence cognitive outcome. The Toronto study (Rovet, 1986) reported a 10 point difference in favour of CH children with a milder form of the disorder and this was supported by assessment at both 3 years (Murphy *et al.*, 1986) and 5 years (Fuggle *et al.*, 1991) in the London study in which differences of 12 and 15 points respectively were reported. Assessment of initial severity can also be made according to physiological measures (e.g. position of the gland) or to indications of pre-diagnostic growth (e.g. bone surface of the knee) which tend to be significantly correlated. Letarte & La Franchi (1983) concluded that 'the intellectual performance of hypothyroid children was lower when they had clinical, biological or radiological features of a more intense thyroid deficit at the time of diagnosis'. However, some follow-up studies (New England Congenital Hypothyroidism Collaborative, 1984; Komianou *et al.*, 1988) have not found this association. The inconsistency of these findings may be related to differences in cognitive measures, age of the children at assessment or variations in the severity of hypothyroidism between samples. On balance, the evidence suggests that the severity of prenatal and short term neonatal hypothyroidism has long-term effects on cognitive functioning.

In comparison with the dietary changes required for PKU and CD, treatment of CH is far less invasive of family routines and is relatively undemanding. Daily oral administration of thyroxine medication is required along with out-patient attendance to review blood thyroxine levels and monitor growth measurements. Most follow-up studies have not found treatment variables to be predictive of cognitive functioning, although two studies (Rovet *et al.*, 1984; New England Congenital Hypothyroidism Collaborative, 1984) reported small groups of children in which poor cognitive functioning (mean IQ 87, both studies) was associated with undertreatment. The mean thyroxine (T_4) level for the undertreated group during the first year was at the lower end of the normal range but, although the difference from the total sample was statistically significant, it was not large (T_4: 111 nmol/l compared to 139 nmol/l). Such a large cognitive difference of nearly 20 IQ points suggests either an important threshold effect or the possibility that the measured differences in treatment may have been accompanied by additional factors influencing IQ. Recent preliminary data from Norway indicated that quality of treatment for all CH children during the first year may be associated with smaller yet significant differences in cognitive functioning at 6 years (S. Heyerdahl – personal communication). Fisher & Foley (1989) have suggested that the initial treatment period may require higher thyroxine (T_4) levels than previously considered. At present, as with PKU, there remains the possibility that variations of biochemical control within the therapeutic range, particularly during infancy, may be influential on long-term cognitive performance.

Cognitive outcome in childhood diabetes

By contrast with PKU and CH, childhood diabetes (CD) has not been associated historically with cognitive impairment. However, research findings (Ack *et al.*, 1961; Ryan *et al.*, 1984, 1985) suggest that cognitive deficits may be associated with the severity of the condition as measured by the age of initial onset of the condition; children diagnosed before 5 years showing both specific and general cognitive deficits. According to a recent epidemiological survey (Baum *et al.*, 1989) in the UK, this group represents 24% of the child diabetic population.

In their study of CD adolescents, Ryan *et al.* (1985) found no differences between later onset CD adolescents and matched sibling controls on a broad range of cognitive tasks. However, CD children diagnosed before 5 years showed statistically significant deficits compared with controls on predominantly visuospatial and memory tasks as well as on educational attainment such as reading (see also Gath *et al.*, 1980). 24% of the early onset group, but only 6% of the late onset group, scored at least two standard deviations below the mean of the healthy control group on three or more tests. In addition, duration of the disorder and age of onset had differential effects on outcome.

Children with diabetes diagnosed before 5 years were significantly more likely to show cognitive impairment in tasks requiring right-hemisphere functioning – e.g. visuo-constructional problem solving, recall of visual information and manipulation with the dominant hand. These deficits appear to be specific to effects on cognition during early development. The duration of diabetes during childhood and adolescence appears to have specific effects on left-hemisphere functioning, as assessed, for example, by verbal concept formation, reading and spelling skills. Rovet *et al.* (1987) noted that girls with longer-duration diabetes always showed this pattern, but longer-duration boys did so only when they had a history of hypoglycaemic convulsions. The effects of duration appear to be specific to childhood and adolescence because longitudinal studies of cognitive functioning in adults show that there is no increase in cognitive deterioration in later life specific to diabetes (Robertson-Tchabo *et al.*, 1986), indicating that cognitive deficits are not a consequence of long-term glycaemic dysfunction at all ages.

Treatment for Type 1 diabetes involves both dietary change and regular (usually twice daily) injections of insulin. The dietary regime typically divides food intake into small regular meals of known carbohydrate content. This traditional method may lead to unacceptably wide fluctuations of blood glucose but more determined attempts to achieve normal glucose levels (i.e. by having more frequent injections) may increase the risks of hypoglycaemic reactions. As already noted (Rovet *et al.*, 1987) such an increase may be linked to some deficits in cognitive functioning. Several studies have also suggested that better glycaemic control (as measured by lower glycosylated haemoglobin) may be associated with poorer adjustment and higher rates of disturbance. This issue will be considered more fully in the next section.

EMOTIONAL DEVELOPMENT AND BEHAVIOUR

Children suffering from chronic medical conditions have been recognized as being at risk from increased rates of psychological distress and disorder. However, chronic conditions vary considerably in terms of their experiential impact on the child, their prognosis and the amount of disruption of ordinary life consequent on successful treatment. Linkages between physical pathology and behaviour may reflect direct effects of the specific hormonal or neurological impairment or may indicate more indirect, probably multifactorial, consequences of the disorder. Recent research on a number of conditions (such as Williams syndrome, e.g. Udwin *et al.*, 1987) that result in moderate or severe mental handicap and which also have rather precise and consistent behavioural characteristics has led to increased interest in the idea of behavioural phenotypes. However, many behaviour problems may well be an understandable, indirect response to the difficulties of dealing with chronic physical disease and similarities between those with the same condition may be determined by the particular life-style restrictions inherent in the condition. There is no evidence that any of the three conditions described in this chapter have a particular behaviour pattern that is genetically determined. The processes that link behavioural disturbances with particular disorders may include many different factors ranging from the number of hospital visits, the type of treatment involved and varying degrees of stigmatization. Consideration of the behavioural outcome for children with metabolic/endocrine disorders will highlight some of these issues.

Phenylketonuria

Early-treated PKU children have a higher frequency of behaviour problems at 8 years than matched controls (Smith *et al.*, 1988; Stevenson *et al.*, 1979). Measured on the Rutter scale, 36% of PKU children compared with 19% matched classroom controls scored in the deviant range (>8 points). In particular, PKU children showed more mannerisms, fidgetiness, restlessness and poor attention as well as being more solitary, anxious and miserable. In general, problems tended to be emotional rather than anti-social and there was no difference from controls in terms of aggression and conduct disorder. Although anti-social disorders are more likely to show continuity into adulthood (Robins, 1978) evidence from the Isle of Wight study showed that 46% of 10-year-olds with emotional disorders still had important problems at 14 years (Graham & Rutter, 1973).

As has been found with other disorders, the frequency of behavioural deviance in PKU children is inversely related to IQ. Smith *et al.* (1988) reported that 14% of PKU children with an IQ greater than 110 had a deviant score compared with 31% of those with an average IQ (IQ 90–109) and 43% of those with a below average IQ (IQ 70–89). Several studies have reported higher rates of behavioural disturbance (Holtzman *et al.*, 1986; Smith *et al.*, 1988) and social impairment (Matthews *et al.*, 1986) for children with poorer dietary control. It is probable that this relationship is bi-directional, with behavioural difficulties increasing the likelihood of poor dietary control as well as being a consequence of it. In addition, the relationship is partially confounded by the effect of dietary control on IQ although experimental studies have indicated direct effects of concurrent phenylalanine levels on some aspects of behaviour particularly relevant to hyperactivity and attention (see above). It has been noted (Smith, 1985) that this pattern of behavioural difficulties is similar to, although milder than, the behaviour of PKU children prior to the introduction of early treatment and this specificity and consistency is suggestive of a neurological component to the impairment.

Studies of functioning in families with an early treated PKU child have not provided evidence of disturbance and suggest family resilience rather than disorder. Kazak *et al.* (1988) reported no differences with respect to parental stress and marital satisfaction compared with carefully matched controls but they did observe lower levels of adaptability and cohesion. In addition, there was no association between quality of dietary control and measures of family adjustment, stress or family interaction (Reber *et al.*, 1987).

Congenital hypothyroidism

Studies of CH children prior to the introduction of early detection and treatment have consistently shown high rates of behavioural deviance ranging from 20 to 50% (Hulse, 1984; Frost, 1986) compared with around 15% in the general population using similar measures. As with PKU children, increased severity and frequency of behavioural difficulties was inversely related to IQ and the pattern of presenting problems was more emotional than anti-social in kind, including poor attention span, fearfulness and toileting problems. Follow-up studies of CH children detected by screening have generally found no increased levels of behavioural disturbance compared with controls. In CH infants at 6 months there is some evidence for an increased frequency of 'difficult temperament' (Rovet *et al.*, 1983; Sorbara *et al.*, 1988) although there is only a low association with subsequent temperament scores at 3 years. Reduction in behavioural problems as a consequence of early treatment can be partly explained as a secondary effect of generally improved cognitive functioning. However, as with PKU children, the specific pattern of behavioural difficulties in late-treated CH children, particularly in relation to activity levels and attentional problems, is suggestive of specific effects of hormonal dysfunction. These difficulties are much less severe in early-treated children although parents may still report fluctuations in mood and activity level that are construed as being related to variations in thyroxine levels. Longitudinal data on the cognitive and behavioural progress of CH children through school is required in order to determine whether the increased educational and emotional demands of later schooling and adolescence are accompanied by behavioural or attentional difficulties not evident in early childhood.

Childhood diabetes

Emotional and behavioural aspects of childhood diabetes have been extensively investigated with some apparently conflicting findings. In particular, much research has been focused on psychological differences betweeen groups of diabetic children distinguished according to the quality of the treatment regime that they achieve. However, the measurement of quality of treatment over time presents a number of methodological and conceptual problems. As described earlier, successful treatment needs to be assessed in relation to both biochemical control and emotional, behavioural and social factors. Assumptions about the relationships between measures of these different aspects may lead to inappropriate conclusions. For example, it is important to separate measures of treatment compliance from measures of biochemical control. Several studies have shown that even when both variables are carefully measured, the relationship between them may be quite weak (Glasgow *et al.*, 1987). Despite this, there is a tendency for indications of poor biochemical control to be interpreted as showing poor treatment compliance.

Studies that have made direct comparisons between CD children as a whole and normal population controls have tended to describe less severe or prolonged psychological difficulties for the CD children compared with studies that focus on CD children with poor control. Lavigne *et al.* (1982) compared CD children with their siblings and with a group attending hospital for routine paediatric care. CD boys showed increased rates of psychiatric symptoms compared with both control groups, whereas CD girls showed no differences from controls. Behavioural symptoms tended to increase for males according to the length of illness. This contrasts with findings by Cassileth *et al.* (1984) in which improved mental health ratings were associated with increased length of time following diagnosis. This was interpreted as indicating a period of adjustment following an initial period of shock and distress. Both these studies were cross-sectional in design and their contradictory findings emphasize the risks of interpreting single-time measures in terms of longer-term developmental processes.

Evidence from longitudinal studies has tended to highlight processes of adaptation and resilience. Jacobson *et al.* (1986) compared CD children with a sample of children with a recent acute medical problem and found no differences between the two groups in terms of self-esteem, behavioural symptoms or social functioning. Within the CD group, adjustment to diabetes was strongly correlated with general personality and social functioning measures seen as reflecting pre-existing adaptation and development. Similar results were reported by Kovacs *et al.* (1985) who found that, although parents often experienced acute distress at the time of diagnosis, one year later most parents showed adaptive resilience to the new situation. In addition, they found no evidence for increased marital conflict. Family functioning was directly observed by Hauser *et al.* (1986) who compared CD children with acute-illness controls. The former group tended to carry out more 'enabling' interactions than controls, suggesting that a recently diagnosed chronic illness within the family did not reduce family communication. However, the validity of their family assessments remain uncertain and a non-paediatric control group would have been a valuable addition.

As already described, variations in the quality of treatment achieved by the child and family may have important effects on cognitive processing. Deficits from poor treatment may be transitory and partially reversible with improved biochemical control. Fluctuations in quality of treatment have also been associated with processes of adjustment and disturbance.

Effective treatment of diabetes requires regular monitoring of the patient's blood-sugar level and appropriate response to the information obtained. In his comprehensive review of new monitoring techniques Shillitoe (1988) emphasized that the treatment process is essentially a behavioural and cognitive task in which the foibles of human behaviour often appear to defeat improvements in technology. For example, in one study on the use of reflectance meters with a hidden memory chip it was shown that 40% of reported tests were not performed, 18% of tests were not reported and 27% of tests were unacceptably imprecise (Wilson & Endres, 1986). In conclusion Shillitoe stated: 'Previously, poor control could be blamed on inaccurate forms of assessment or limitations in conventional insulin delivery regimens. It is now clear that the patient is the major source of error'.

Many studies have been carried out in order to examine this 'source of error'. Typically, studies have divided CD children or adolescents into those who achieve good or poor control and look for psychological factors specific to each group. This methodology has produced some inconsistent findings. For example, Anderson *et al.* (1981) found that well-controlled adolescents had less anxiety, more positive self-image and better family relationships resulting in greater independence compared with those with poor control. The results contrast with other studies (Holstein *et al.* 1986; Simonds *et al.* 1981) that did not show significant differences between these groups.

Studies by Fonagy *et al.* (1987) and Sinzato *et al.* (1985) found that children with lower glycosylated haemoglobin (i.e. those with apparently better control) had *higher* rates of disturbance than those with apparently less good control. Perhaps 'good' control results in excessive rates of hypoglycaemic episodes with consequent neurological dysfunction and organically–determined behavioural disturbances. Coping strategies for the poor control group included neglect of medical procedures and the implicit denial of diabetes as central to their concerns. Similar findings were reported by Bouras & Delain (1987) in which the perceived concerns of CD adolescents were almost exclusively non-medical and unrelated to their condition. The majority of subjects in the study did not even mention diabetes as being a concern for them.

Psychological aspects of treatment for diabetes change in relation to developmental status and the duration of the illness. A large number of studies demonstrate that adherence to treatment is poor and deteriorates over time when the regimen is complicated and permanent (Haynes, 1979). Cross-sectional studies are likely to produce inconsistent findings unless both developmental level and duration of illness are adequately taken into account. Longitudinal studies are essential in order to gain a better understanding of the complex interaction of variables over time. Such studies need not encompass the entire life span in order to be fruitful. For example, Rose *et al.* (1983) carried out an intervention study using anxiety management techniques on five poorly controlled adolescents over a six-month period. Daily blood-sugar levels were obtained along with fortnightly measures of tension and anxiety. Although biochemical control improved, there was no change in perceived levels of anxiety. It would have been interesting to know whether this lack of dynchrony of effect persisted on longer follow-up.

CONCLUSIONS

Longitudinal study of the impact of congenital hypothyroidism (CH), phenylketonuria (PKU) and childhood diabetes (CD) on cognitive and behavioural development has revealed quite different patterns, but there are certain common lessons to be learned. First, the physiological basis of CH and PKU results in damage to the brain that is permanent if untreated in the first month or two of life. Early treatment in both conditions results in imperfect protection from impairment, though in mild forms of CH the protection afforded is probably virtually complete. In both CH and PKU, individual variations in the severity of the illness result in variations in outcome. In contrast, in CD, partly because it presents later and partly because the metabolic disturbances are episodic, permanent psychological impairment either does not occur or occurs in more subtle forms. Timing, however, may not be the sole reason for the differences here.

In all three conditions, concurrent variations in metabolic state may produce variations in cognitive performance and behaviour, so that psychological and psychiatric assessment requires awareness of current metabolic state if it is to have predictive value.

Although in CH and PKU there is a correlation between compliance with treatment and psychological outcome, findings in CD have been counter-intuitive with best control linked to less good behavioural development. This last finding calls into question current good practices in management.

Finally, in all these conditions, but particularly in CH and PKU, longitudinal comparisons with normal populations on cognitive performance have been made difficult by the steady secular rise in the IQ in the general population for each year since the test in question has been standardized.

REFERENCES

Ack, M., Miller, I. & Weil, W. B. (1961) Intelligence of children with diabetes mellitus. *Pediatrics*, **28**, 764–70.

Anderson, B. J., Miller, J. P., Auslander, W. F. & Santiago, J. V. (1981) Family characteristics of diabetic adolescents: relationship to metabolic control. *Diabetes Care*, **4**, 586–94.

Baker, L., Barcai, A., Kaye, R. & Hague, N. (1969) Beta adrenergic blockade and juvenile diabetes: acute studies and long term therapeutic trial. *Journal of Pediatrics*, **75**, 19–29.

Baum, J. D., Metcalf, M. A., Gale, E. A. M. & Jarrett, R. J. (1989) National survey of childhood onset diabetes. Paper presented at the British Paediatric Conference, York, England.

Bouras, M. & Delain, F. (1987) The child with diabetes and his illness. The place of diabetes in the psychological life of the child. *Archives Francaises de Pediatric (Paris)*, **44**, 51–5.

Brunner, R. L., Jordan, M. K. & Berry, H. K. (1983) Early treated phenylketonuria: neuropsychologic consequences. *Journal of Pediatrics*, **102**, 831–5.

Cassileth, B. R., Lusk, E. J., Strouse, T. B., Miller, D. S., Brown, L. L., Cross, P. A. & Tenaglia, A. N. (1984) Psychological status in chronic illness. A comparative analysis of six diagnostic groups. *New England Journal of Medicine*, **311**, 506–11.

Clarke, J. T., Gates, R. D., Hogan, S. E., Barrett, M. & MacDonald, G. W. (1987). Neuropsychological studies on adolescents with phenylketonuria returned to phenylalanine restricted diet. *American Journal of Mental Retardation*, **92**, 255–62.

de Vries, L. S., Heckmatt, J. Z., Burrin, J. M., Dubowitz, L. M. S. & Dubowitz, V. (1986) Low serum thyroxine concentrations and neural maturation in preterm infants. *Archives of Disease in Childhood*, **61**, 862–6.

Dobson, J. C., Williamson, M. L., Azen, C. & Koch, R. (1977) Intellectual assessment of 111 four-year old children with phenylketonuria. *Pediatrics*, **60**, 822–7.

Dussault, J. H. (1983) The developing fetal thyroid gland and the maternal fetal placental unit. In Dussault, J. H. & Walker, P. (eds.) *Cogenital hypothyroidism*. New York: Marcel Dekker, pp. 3–10.

Escobar, G. M., Obregon, M. J. & Escobar del Rey, F. (1989) Transfer of thyroid hormones from the mother to the fetus. In Delange, F., Fisher, D. A. & Glinoer, D. (eds.) *Research in congenital hypothyroidism*. New York: Plenum, pp. 15–28.

Escobar, G. M., Ruiz-Marcos, A. & Escobar del Rey, F. (1983) Thyroid hormone and the developing brain. In Dussault, J. H. & Walker, P. (eds.) *Congenital hypothyroidism*. New York: Marcel Dekker, pp. 85–126.

Fisher, D. A. & Foley, B. L. (1989) Early treatment of congenital hypothyroidism. *Pediatrics*, **83**, 785–9.

Flynn, J. R. (1984) The mean IQ of Americans: massive gains 1932–1978. *Psychological Bulletin*, **95**, 29–51.

Flynn, J. R. (1987) Massive IQ gains in 14 nations: what IQ tests really measure. *Psychological Bulletin*, **101**, 171–91.

Fonagy, P., Moran, G. S., Lindsay, M. K., Kurtz, A. B. & Brown, R. (1987) Psychological adjustment and diabetic control. *Archives of Disease in Childhood*, **62**, 1009–13.

Frost, G. J. (1986) Aspects of congenital hypothyroidism. *Child: Care, Health and Development*, **12**, 369–75.

Fuggle, P., Grant, D. B., Smith, I. & Murphy, G. (1991) Cognitive function at five years in early treated congenital hypothyroidism, in press.

Gath, A., Smith, M. A. & Baum, J. D. (1980) Emotional, behavioural and educational disorders in diabetic children. *Archives of Disease in Childhood*, **55**, 371–5.

Glasgow, R. E., McCaul, K. D. & Schafer, L. C. (1987) Self care behaviours and glycemic control in type 1 diabetes. *Journal of Chronic Disease*, **40**, 399–412.

Graham, P. & Rutter, M. (1973) Psychiatric disorder in the young adolescent: a follow-up study. *Proceedings of the Royal Society of Medicine*, **66**, 1226–9.

Green, A. E. (1978) The effects of dietary tryptophan and its peripheral metabolism on brain 5-hydroxytryptamine synthesis and function. In Youdim, M. B. H., Lovenberg. W., Shardan, D. F. & Lagrado, J. R. (eds) *Essays in neurochemistry and neuropharmacology. Vol. 3*. Chichester: John Wiley.

Guttler, F. (1980) Hyperphenylalaninaemia: diagnosis and classification of the various types of phenylalanine hydroxylase deficiency in childhood. *Acta Paediatrica Scandinavica Supplement*, **280**, 7–80.

Hadeed, A. J., Asay, L. M., Klein, A. H. & Fisher, D. A. (1981) Significance of transient postnatal hypothyroxinaemia in preterm infants with and without respiratory distress. *Pediatrics*, **68**, 494–8.

Hauser, S. T., Jacobson, A. M., Wertlieb, D., *et al.* (1986) Children with recently diagnosed diabetes: interactions within their families. *Health Psychology*, **5**, 273–96.

Haynes, R. B. (1979) Determinants of compliance: the disease and the mechanics of treatment. In Haynes, R. B., Taylor, D. W., & Sackett, D. L.

(eds.) *Compliance health care*. Baltimore, Maryland: John Hopkins University Press, pp. 49–62.
Hinde, R. A. (1980) Family influences. In Rutter, M. (ed.) *Scientific Foundations of Developmental Psychiatry*. London: Heinemann Medical, pp. 47–66.
Holmes, C. S., Hayford, J. T., Gonzalez, J. T. & Weydert, J. A. (1983) A survey of cognitive functioning at different glucose levels in diabetic persons. *Diabetes Care*, **6**, 180–5.
Holmes, D. M. (1986) The person and diabetes in psychosocial context. *Diabetes Care*, **9**, 194–206.
Holstein, B. E., Vesterdal-Jrgensen, H. & Sestoft, L. (1986) Illness behaviour, attitude and knowledge in newly diagnosed diabetics. *Danish Medical Bulletin*, **33**, 165–71.
Holtzman, N. A., Kronmal, R. A., Doorninck, W., Azen, C. & Koch, R. (1986) Effect of age at loss of dietary control on intellectual performance and behaviour of children with phenylketonuria. *New England Journal of Medicine*, **314**, 593–8.
Hulse, J. A. (1984) Outcome for congenital hypothyroidism. *Archires of Disease in Childhood*, **59**, 23–30.
Illig, R., Largo, R. H., Qin, Q., Torresani, T., Rochiccioli, P. & Larsson, A. (1987) Mental development in congenital hypothyroidism after neonatal screening. *Archives of Disease in Childhood*, **62**, 1050–5.
Jacobson, A. M., Hauser, S. T., Wertlieb, D. *et al.* (1986) Psychological adjustment of children with recently diagnosed diabetes mellitus. *Diabetes Care*, **9**, 323–9.
Johnson, S. B. (1988) Psychological aspects of childhood diabetes. *Journal of Child Psychology and Psychiatry*, **29**, 729–38.
Kazak, A. W., Reber, M. & Snitzer, L. (1988) Childhood chronic disease and family functioning: a study of phenylketonuria. *Pediatrics*, **81**, 224–30.
Kemmer, F. W., Bisping, R., Steingruber, H. J., Baar, H., Hardtmann, F., Schlaghecke, R. & Berger, M. (1986) Psychological stress and metabolic control in patients with type 1 diabetes mellitus. *New England Journal of Medicine*, **314**, 1078–84.
Komianou, F., Makaronis, G., Lambadaridis, J., Sarafidou, E., Vrachni, F., Mengreli, C. & Pantelakis, S. (1988) Psychomotor development in congenital hypothyroidism: the Greek screening programme. *European Journal of Paediatrics*, **147**, 275–8.
Kovacs, M., Finkelstein, R., Feinberg, T. L., Crouse-Novak, M., Paulauskas, S. & Pollock, M. (1985) Initial psychological responses of parents to the diagnosis of insulin-dependent diabetes mellitus in their children. *Diabetes Care*, **8**, 568–75.
Lavigne, J. V., Traisman, H. S., Marr, T. J. & Chasnoff, I. J. (1982) Parental perceptions of the psychological adjustment of children with diabetes and their children. *Diabetes Care*, **5**, 420–6.
Legrand, J. (1979). Morphogenetic action of thyroid hormones. *Trends in Neurosciences*, **2**, 234.
Letarte, J. & La Franchi, S. (1983) Clinical features of congenital hypothyroidism. In Dussault, J. H. & Walker, P. (eds.) *Congenital hypothyroidism*. New York: Marcel Dekker, pp. 351–84.
Lou, H. C., Lykkelund, C., Gerdes, A. M., Udesen, H. & Bruhn, P. (1987)

Increased vigilance and dopamine synthesis by large doses of tyrosine or phenylalanine restriction in phenylketonuria. *Acta Paediatrica Scandinavica*, **76**, 560–5.

Lucas, A., Morley, R. & Cole, T. J. (1988) Adverse neurodevelopmental outcome of moderate neonatal hypoglycaemia. *British Medical Journal*, **297**, 1304–8.

Matthews, W. S., Barabas, G., Cusack, E. & Ferrari, M. (1986) Social quotients of children with phenylketonuria before and after discontinuation of dietary therapy. *American Journal of Mental Deficiency*, **91**, 92–4.

Murphy, G., Hulse, J. A., Jackson, D., Tyrer, P. & Glossop, J. (1986) Early treated hypothyroidism: develoment at three years. *Archives of Disease in Childhood*, **61**, 671–5.

New England Congenital Hypothyroidism Collaborative (1984) Characteristics of infantile hypothyroidism discovered on neonatal screening. *Journal of Pediatrics*, **104**, 539–44.

Piel, N., Lane, J. T., Huether, G. & Neuhoff, V. (1982) Impaired permeability of the blood cerebro-spinal fluid barrier in hyperphenylalaninaemia. *Neuropadiatrie*, **13**, 88–92.

Pramming, S., Thorsteinsson, B., Theilgaard, A., Pinner, E. M. & Binder, C. (1986) Cognitive function during hypoglycaemia in Type 1 diabetes mellitus. *British Medical Journal*, **292**, 647–50.

Quinton, D. (1980) Cultural and community influences. In Rutter, M. (ed.) *Developmental Psychiatry*. London: Heinemann Medical, pp. 77–91.

Reber, M., Kazak, A. E. & Himmelberg, P. (1987) Phenylalanine control and family functioning in early treated phenylketonuria. *Journal of Developmental and Behavioral Pediatrics*, **8**, 311–7.

Rickards, A., Coakley, J., Francis, I., Armstrong, S. & Connelly, J. (1989) Results of follow-up at five years in a group of hypothyroid children detected by newborn screening. In Delange, F., Fisher, D. A. & Glinoer, D. (ed.) *Research in congential hypothyroidism*. New York: Plenum Press, p. 341.

Robertson-Tchabo, E. A., Arenberg, D., Tobin, J. D. & Plotz, J. B. (1986). A longitudinal study of cognitive performance in non-insulin dependent (type 2) diabetic men. *Experimental Gerontology*, **21**, 459–67.

Robins, L. N. (1978) Sturdy childhood predictors of adult antisocial behaviour: replications from longitudinal studies. *Psychological Medicine*, **8**, 611–22.

Rose, M. I., Firestone, P., Heick, H. M. C. & Faught, A. (1983) The effects of anxiety management training on the control of juvenile diabetes mellitus. *Journal of Behavioral Medicine*, **6**, 381–95.

Rovet, J. (1986) A prospective investigation of children with congenital hypothyroidism identified by neonatal screening in Ontario. *Canadian Journal of Public Health*, **77**, 164–73.

Rovet, J. F., Erlich, R. M., Westbrook, D. L. & Walfish, P. G. (1983) Intellectual and behavioural characteristics of children with congenital hypothyroidism detected by neonatal thyroid screening. *Pediatric Research*, **17**, 171A.

Rovet, J. F., Westbrook, D. & Ehrlich, R. M. (1984) Neonatal thyroid deficiency: early temperamental and cognitive characteristics. *Journal of the American Academy of Child and Adolescent*, **23**, 10–22.

Rovet, J. F., Ehrlich, R. M. & Hoppe, M. (1987) Intellectual deficits associated with early onset insulin-dependent diabetes mellitus in children. *Diabetes Care*, **10**, 510–5.

Rutter, M. (1985) Psychopathology and development: links between childhood and adult life. In Rutter, M. & Hersov, L. (eds.) *Child and adolescent psychiatry: modern approaches*. 2nd edn. Oxford: Blackwell Scientific Pub., pp. 720–39.

Ryan, C., Vega, A., Longstreet, C. & Drash, A. (1984) Neuropsychological changes in adolescents with insulin-dependent diabetes. *Journal of Consulting and Clinical Psychology*, **52**, 335–42.

Ryan, C., Vega, A. & Drash, A. (1985) Cognitive deficits in adolescents who developed diabetes early in life. *Pediatrics*, **75**, 921–7.

Schor, D. P. (1983) PKU and temperament. Rating children three through seven years old in PKU families. *Clinical Pediatrics*, **22**, 807–11.

Shillitoe, R. W. (1988) *Psychology and diabetes*. London: Chapman Hall.

Simonds, J., Goldstein, D., Walker, B. & Rawlings, S. (1981) The relationship between psychological factors and blood glucose regulation in insulin-dependent diabetic adolescents. *Diabetes Care*, **4**, 610–5.

Sinzato, R., Fukino, O., Tamai, H., Isizu, H., Nakagawa, T. & Ikemi, Y. (1985) Coping behaviors of severe diabetics. *Psychotherapy and Psychosomatics*, **43**, 219–26.

Smith, I. (1985) The hyperphenylalaninaemias. In Lloyd, J. K. & Scriver, C. R. (eds.) *Genetic and Metabolic Disease in Paediatrics*. London: Butterworths, pp. 166–210.

Smith, I., Lobascher, M. E., Stevenson, J. E., Wolff, O., Schmidt, H., Grubel-Kaiser, S. & Bickel, H. (1978) Effect of stopping low phenylalanine diet on intellectual progress of children with phenylketonuria. *British Medical Journal*, **2**, 723–6.

Smith, I., Beasley, M., Wolff, O. H. & Ades, A. E. (1988) Behavior disturbance in 8-year-old children with early treated phenylketonuria. *Journal of Pediatrics*, **112**, 403–8.

Smith, I., Beasley, M. G. & Ades, A. E. (1990) Intelligence and quality of dietary treatment in phenylketonuria. *Archives of Disease in Childhood*, **65**, 472–8.

Sorbara, D., Rovet, J. & Erlich, R. (1988) Early temperamental characteristics of neonatally identified hypothyroid children. In Delange, F., Fisher, D. A. & Glinoer, D. (eds.) *Research in congenital hypothyroidism*. New York: Plenum, p. 348.

Stevenson, J. E., Hawcroft, J., Lobascher, M., Smith, I., Wolff, O. & Graham, P. J. (1979). Behavioural deviance in children with early treated phenylketonuria. *Archives of Disease in Childhood*, **54**, 14–18.

Udwin, O., Yule, W. & Martin, N. (1987) Cognitive abilities and behavioural characteristics of children with idiopathic infantile hypercalcaemia, *Journal of Child Psychology and Psychiatry*, **28**, 2, 297–309.

Uhrmann, S., Marks, K. H., Maisels, M. J., Kulin, H. E., Kaplan, M. & Utiger, R. (1981) Frequency of transient hypothyroxinaemia in low birthweight infants. *Archives of Disease in Childhood*, **56**, 2147.

Walker, P. (1983) Developmental actions of thyroid hormones. In Dussault, J. H. & Walker, P. (ed.) *Congenital hypothyroidism*. New York: Marcel Dekker, pp. 63–84.

Williamson, M. L., Koch, R., Azen, C. & Chang, C. (1981) Correlates of intelligence test results in treated phenylketonuric children. *Pediatrics*, **68**, 161–7.

Wilson, D. P. & Endres, R. K. (1986) Compliance with blood glucose monitoring in children with Type 1 diabetes mellitus. *Journal of Pediatrics*, **108**, 1022–4.

8 Toxins and allergens

ERIC TAYLOR

Exogenous chemicals can damage brain function through a range of mechanisms. Neurological interest in the effects of toxins has increased greatly in the last few years because of the evidence for enduring and specific effects of exposure to chemicals in producing Parkinsonism, lathyrism and (arguably) the dementia–parkinsonism complex seen in Guam. These examples have added to the reasons for studying the actions of neurotoxins as causes of psychological disability. Chemical effects on behaviour and learning are also important because of the ubiquity of potential hazards and their public health significance.

There is nevertheless a reluctance among many scientists to get involved in the topic. This is a reaction to the excesses of fringe practitioners, misleading advertising by manufacturers of 'health products' and media hype. Excited claims are frequently made for dietary supplements that will treat previously unknown deficiencies and for this or that harmful substance that must be sedulously avoided. All the amino acids are promoted in this way, many minerals (boron, lithium, nickel, silica, silver, vanadium, zinc), all the known vitamins and a number of unknown ones (such as 'vitamins C3 and B15'). Parents are nagged by self-styled experts to avoid artificial colourings, to give evening primrose oil to their children, and either to avoid glutamate or to give large doses (there are two schools of thought here). It is small wonder that the subject has got a bad name.

Nevertheless, the chemical environment can affect the behaviour and learning of some children. Uncommon but severe events such as lead poisoning and neonatal hypoglycaemia carry major implications for later development. There is not enough scientific work on the nature of the abnormalities induced, nor on the determinants of recovery.

Understanding the developmental impact of intoxications, deficiencies and allergies is problematic. Not only might the impact vary at different ages, the pattern of exposure is different as children develop. Prenatally, the main toxic influences are considered to be alcohol and tobacco taken by the mother, and possibly lead from the mother's body (Taylor, 1986). The later stages of gestation and perinatal period are a time of particularly rapid brain growth, and it has often been supposed that it would also be a time of especial vulnerability to all forms of insult. This has not yet been shown unequivocally, though there is evidence in favour. The vulnerability of the neonate to hypoglycaemia is a striking example, with developmental impairment at 4 years being linearly related to the number of days in the neonatal period when glucose fell below threshold (Lucas *et al.*, 1988). But it remains possible that the same vulnerability would apply at later ages – although evidence from children with diabetes does not support the possibility (see chapter 7, this volume).

In the first year of life the child is a relatively passive recipient of chemical hazards. Lead in drinking water and dust, insecticides and other pollutants can all exert effects; as can poisons deliberately administered by caretakers. Through the toddler years, however, children are increasingly determining their own exposure. They ingest household chemicals, such as cleaners and polishes, and medications kept at home. As their diet expands, so they may come into contact with substances that provide allergic and other adverse reactions. Later still, as children age and become more independent, so their repertoire of self-injury increases. Self-administered solvents, alcohol and illegal drugs become added chemical hazards. The more that children determine their exposure, the harder it is to be clear of what is cause and what is effect.

The major current scientific issues in this area are still those of determining the degree of hazard associated with each substance. Most are of small effect in a population, and the detection of an increased risk is correspondingly difficult. This article will review the contrasting examples of lead, alcohol, micronutrient deficiency and food intolerance to point up where research has reached and where the next steps could go.

Chemical hazards can be those of global deficiency (malnutrition), selective deficiency, toxicity, or intolerance to aspects of the environment. There are several broad types of mechanism involved. The most direct is the *toxic*. The chemical involved causes direct disruption of tissue function and the prime determinant of damage is the degree and nature of exposure. The next type is the pattern of complex *hazard*, in which the chemical exerts tissue defects only if other factors are present too; and agents modifying the risk can be as important as the original risk factor itself. The third type, the least direct, is involved when the chemical is not hazardous to most people and an *altered response* of the individual is acquired for pathogenesis. This is the mechanism called 'idiosyncrasy' or 'intolerance'. The altered response may involve the immune system (*allergy*) but can also be a result of individual variation in levels of enzyme activity (such as deficiency of glucose 6 phosphate dehydrogenase) or cellular function (such as mast cell instability).

LEAD AND PSYCHOLOGICAL FUNCTION

Lead is a highly toxic element. The vast majority in the environment is the result of industrial activity, both in the mining and smelting of the mineral and from its manufactured forms (such as old water pipes, old paint and petrol vapour). It has a wide range of effects upon the body. Acute and chronic encephalopathies are a known result of high exposure.

The effects of low-level chronic exposure to lead are more controversial. The public importance of the question has led to a number of well-planned researches. As a result, knowledge is no longer restricted to the comparatively rare problem of severe intoxication. The general issue of community health can be addressed: the effect of levels of body lead burden that used to be considered as 'normal', corresponding to blood levels of less than 40 microgrammes per decilitre (μg/dl).

Lead and intelligence

It is now generally agreed that there is an association between IQ and body lead measured by levels in blood or tooth dentine. This was already the case ten years ago (Rutter, 1980) and nothing has appeared to alter the conclusion. It is not dependent upon referral bias to clinics, but appears clearly in representative samples from the general population. Table 8.1 sets out the general population studies and the size of the IQ differences between the highest and lowest lead groups in each study.

The meaning of the association is still argued about. It is consistent, but small in size by comparison with the effects of other factors determining intelligence, such as parental IQ and family circumstances. Biologically it is very plausible that a toxin known to have harmful effects upon the development of animals should also have effects upon humans; but there are marked differences between species and one must not make the direct jump from animal evidence to conclusions about humans.

Correlation does not prove causation. Both IQ and the burden of lead could be common results of some other cause. Psychosocial factors are known to be associated with IQ and school achievement as well as with lead exposure. White (1982) made a meta-analysis of some 200 studies relating academic achievement to socioeconomic status and showed that the most important social variables were childrearing practices and a home atmosphere conducive to learning, rather than those of resources available (such as income, housing and parental occupation). Parental IQ also has a well-known and strong association with IQ in children, and shares a good deal of variance with the quality of home environment.

Table 8.1. *Comparisons of high- and low-lead groups from epidemiological studies*

	n	uncorrected IQ difference (low-lead – high-lead)	lead level in high-lead group[c]	p (after adjustment for covariates)
General population				
Boston: Needleman *et al.* (1979)	158	+5	TL > 20	0.03
London: Yule *et al.* (1981)	168	+7	BL > 17	0.03
London: Smith *et al.* (1983)	403	+7	TL > 8	ns
London: Lansdown *et al.* (1986)	162	+2	BL > 13	ns
Christchurch: Fergusson *et al.* (1988)				
8-year-olds:	724	+4	TL > 12	<0.05
9-year-olds:	664	+5		<0.05
Aarhus: Hansen *et al.* (1988)	162	+6[a]	TL > 18	0.004
Heavily-exposed populations:				
El Paso: Landrigan *et al.* (1975)	124	+5	BL > 40	ns
McNeil & Ptasnik (1975)	138	+2	BL > 40	ns
Manchester: Ratcliffe (1977)	47	+6[b]	BL > 36	ns
Duisberg: Winneke *et al.* (1982)	52	+5	TL ≃ 9	ns
London: Hatzakis *et al.* (1988)	509	+11	BL > 45	<0.001

The table shows results of studies that compare high- and low-lead groups from population studies of children at elementary school and allow for psychosocial confounders. See text for studies using different methods of reporting and analysis. Wechsler intelligence scales used unless otherwise stated.

[a] High- and low-lead groups were matched for SES.

[b] Griffiths developmental scales used.

[c] Blood-lead levels (BL) are given in μg/dl, tooth-lead levels (TL) as μg/g, or parts per million.

Psychosocial factors such as these could be involved in the pathogenesis in several ways. First, they could be the entire cause of environmentally-determined cognitive impairment, with high lead being an epiphenomenon, associated with IQ only because of its independent relationship with social adversity. Second, psychosocial factors could be a main cause of exposure to lead and therefore could be exerting their action on IQ through neurotoxic effects. It is very plausible that, for example, a poor caregiving environment includes a lack of supervision of children and therefore a greater likelihood that they will ingest lead from the environment. Third, poor caretaking might be caused by the toxic effects of lead upon parents and other caregivers, who are presumably no less likely to be intoxicated than their children. Fourth, caretaking could modify the effects of lead intoxication. Lead, for example, might be a risk factor only in the presence of psychosocial adversity, as seems to be the case for gestational immaturity (Werner & Smith, 1977).

These are quite different forms of interaction. Different statistical and experimental approaches are needed to examine them, and it is conceptually and technically difficult to disentangle the effects of multiple interacting factors that are each of small effect. The first of the above hypotheses needs to be examined first, and if possible got out of the way: can the correlation between IQ and lead be wholly explained by a common association with the truly important environmental factors?

Multivariate statistics have been used to assess the size of the lead effect on IQ that is still present after allowing for factors that might be confounders because they are common associations of both. The exact factors vary from study to study: they usually include aspects of the social environment such as the occupational, educational and financial status of parents, family size and housing type; often include measures of family atmosphere and the quality of caregiving; and sometimes measures of parental intelligence. Analyses, too, vary. Table 8.1 shows the studies that have compared groups with the highest and lowest blood lead levels with IQ as dependent measure and adjusted for confounding variables by analysis of covariance. To be included, therefore, the studies had to have been based upon representative samples of children from the general population (to avoid referral artefacts) and to have allowed for psychosocial differences between groups. Most of the studies are therefore from the last few years; they have been divided into those from ordinary populations and those from populations at particularly high risk because of exposure to a smelter or other industrial source of lead.

Other studies have presented the relationship between lead and IQ as continuous variables over the whole range of scores, rather than comparing high- with low-lead groups. These are less easy to tabulate, but present similar findings. Silva *et al.* (1988) reported on a cohort of 579 11-year-old children from Dunedin: the correlation between Wechsler Intelligence Scale for Children (Revised) (WISC-R) full-scale IQ and blood lead was small and not significant ($r = -0.06$). Blood lead and social class were not themselves correlated in this study from the more egalitarian society of New Zealand. Studies from Birmingham reported correlation coefficients of −0.17 for a group of 133 children at 30 months of age (Harvey *et al.* 1984) and −0.01 for 177 children at 66 months (Harvey *et al.*, 1988). None of these findings was statistically significant once the effect of confounding variables had been partialled out. The correlation coefficients for a group of 237 children in Modena, Italy were −0.06 between IQ and blood lead, −0.22 between IQ and tooth lead ($p = 0.04$ for the latter finding) (Vivoli *et al.*, 1988).

A series of 501 children in Edinburgh was reported by Fulton *et al.* (1987). The regression coefficient of the logarithm (log) of blood-lead on the British Abilities Scale score was −3.79 ($p = 0.003$) after adjustment for confounding variables. This population was of relatively high social class, and the major source of lead was considered to be due to the combination of widespread lead plumbing and the plumbosolvency of the water; so exposure to lead may have been less confounded by social variables than in most areas.

For more heavily-exposed children, living close to polluting industrial plants, statistically significant relationships between lead and IQ have emerged from multiple regression and analyses in North Carolina (Hawk & Schroeder, 1983, $F = 7.7$, $p < 0.01$, in 104 children from mostly lower social classes; Schroeder *et al.*, 1985, $F < 1$, ns, in a 5-year follow-up of 50 of the same children; Hawk *et al.*, 1986, $F = 12.3$, $p < 0.0008$, in 75 black children from low-income families).

A multiple regression analysis has also been provided by Pocock *et al.* (1987) for the Institute of Child Health/Southampton study that was included in Table 8.1 (Smith *et al.*, 1983). As in the analysis of covariance, the association between tooth lead and IQ was no longer significant when confounding variables were allowed for. However, when boys and girls were compared, a difference appeared. For boys, the regression coefficient of log tooth-lead on IQ was −2.95 ($p = 0.01$); for girls it was +0.84 (n.s). One must be cautious of a significant finding appearing only in a subgroup, because a large number of subgroup analyses could be done. There was no prior hypothesis that only boys would be affected, and it is not a clear finding from other studies. Future work should examine the possibility of gender differences.

Significance of covariate analyses

The results of these nineteen carefully-planned epidemiological studies cannot be reduced to a single conclusion, and controversy still goes on about the meaning of the results so far. Nearly all find a relationship between high lead and lower IQ; none find the opposite relationship; nearly all find that the relationship is reduced in size, but the same in direction, after adjusting for possibly confounding variables. In some the relationship remains significant, in some it does not.

No obvious factor distinguishes the studies with positive findings from those without. Statistical significance is not a function of the choice of blood- or tooth-lead estimation, the number of subjects, or the stated source of exposure to lead. The actual blood levels are difficult to compare between studies: not only is there a good deal of disparity between studies but it is not at all clear that the results from different laboratories can be validly compared. Nevertheless, there is no sign of a threshold effect in most of the studies reporting the question: successively higher levels of lead are associated with successively lower mean IQs within individual studies. (The apparent exception is the study from Lavrion, where the lowest and second-lowest lead groups had equally high IQ; yet their second-lowest group was as high in lead as the highest-lead group from the London studies). Some of the studies giving non-significant results have had children with rather low lead levels (e.g. Lansdown *et al.*, 1986); on the other hand, some studies with equally low levels give positive findings (e.g. Fergusson *et al.*, 1988, Yule *et al.*, 1981). Lead level of the population does not seem to determine the presence of significant correlations within it.

One substantial methodological difference between studies is the exact measures of environmental confounding factors that are taken. The choice of measures can obviously make a great deal of difference. They are all rather indirect measures of the quality of caretaking, so it is possible that important variables have been missed and therefore the lead–IQ association is exaggerated because the confounders have not been sufficiently allowed for. On the other hand, there could be an over-correction. 'Confounding' variables could be strongly associated with lead – indeed, in some studies they were intended to be. The Boston study, for example, included an index of exposure to old lead-containing paint. It would therefore be possible to remove a true effect of lead by statistically correcting for the factors that determine lead level.

However, the basis on which covariates are chosen does not seem to determine results. Needleman *et al.*, (1979) for example, chose covariates if they were correlated with lead level. They might therefore have over-corrected, but in fact found that their correction did not abolish the statistical significance of their findings. By contrast, Smith *et al.* (1983) chose covariates only if they were correlated with IQ. The same reason to suspect over-correction was therefore not present in their study, yet they were one of the groups to find that statistical significance had disappeared after the correction process.

Since no obvious quality of the studies determines their results, it is reasonable to consider whether differences are due merely to random fluctuations between studies of which no one is large enough to be definitive. A rigorous meta-analysis is not possible, not least because of problems in the comparability of lead levels. However, I have made a rough calculation of effect size for each of the nineteen studies above. This is calculated either as the difference in IQ means (adjusted for covariate effects) between the highest and lowest reported lead groups (divided by the standard deviation (SD) of the least exposed group); or from the figures for the regression equation to estimate standardized difference between high and low lead groups (Cohen, 1988). This can only be a rather rough-and-ready procedure. It would be worthwhile for investigators to collaborate directly to develop a more satisfactory overall analysis. Nevertheless, results are interesting. No study finds IQ to be higher in the higher-lead group after correction. The adjusted effect size varies from 0 to 0.5, the mean being 0.22. In other words, the average member of a high-lead group has an IQ nearly one-quarter of a standard deviation below that of an average member of a low-lead group. Unfortunately, confidence intervals cannot always be determined. But, when the p values of all studies are converted to z values and combined, the overall level of significance for all studies together is less than 0.0001.

In short, it seems unlikely that all the effect of lead on IQ can be attributed to its prior association with qualities of the caretaking environment. There are some reservations still to be considered, not least the likely effects of measurement error. First, however, we should consider whether a similar conclusion can be drawn for the influence of lead upon the way children behave.

Lead and other psychological measures

The full-scale IQ has been used so far as the index of possible effects of lead. The score is a convenient summary of a range of abilities, is sufficiently standardized to be reasonably comparable between investigations, and has been used by nearly all investigators. Nevertheless the IQ score gives little evidence about the mechanism of effect and deeper neuropsychological analyses are now indicated.

Other psychometric tests have of course been used, but they vary a good deal from study to study. There is very little support for a specific action on any of the tests employed so far. Of course, one of the tests in any study has to be the most sensitive: Needleman *et al.* (1979) found particularly significant differences between groups with the highest and lowest lead levels on the Seashore Rhythm Test, McBride *et al.* (1982) on motor tests of tracking and balancing, Yule *et al.* (1981) on reading and spelling, Winneke *et al.* (1982, 1983) on the Bender Gestalt test. Though any one set of investigators may be tempted to emphasize the processes supposed to be involved in their 'best' test, the reviewer is struck chiefly by the variety of psychological tests that have been used and by the lack of consensus on the specific findings. It may well be that the effects of lead on cognition are rather broad (and possibly indirect) and that apparent differences between investigations are due to random variation.

Rating scales have been used extensively to obtain assessments of behaviour, and a few investigators have observed children's behaviour directly in standardized settings. Needleman *et al.* (1979) reported results from their own scale, rated by teachers, with significantly worse ratings found for a high-lead group ($p < 0.02$); Yule *et al.* (1984) used the same scale and found a similar trend ($p < 0.10$), with 4 of the 11 items significantly worse in high-lead groups; Lansdown *et al.* (1986) described non-significant analyses.

Rutter teacher and parent rating scales have been employed by several investigators: significant differences between groups with the highest and lowest lead levels were found by Yule *et al.* (1984), Silva *et al.* (1988), Fergusson *et al.* (1988) and Thomson *et al.* (1989); McBride *et al.* (1982) got non-significant results on teachers' and mothers' scale but the trend still favoured their low-lead group.

Conners' Classroom Rating Scale was used, and significantly differentiated between high- and low-lead groups, in the researches of Yule *et al.* (1984); it gave non-significant trends in the same direction in work by Smith *et al.* (1983), and Winneke *et al.* (1982, 1983).

Direct observation of behaviour was carried out by Harvey *et al.* (1984, 1988): they found no significant differences. Behavioural ratings during testing by Hansen *et al.* (1988) suggested impairment in the higher tooth-lead group.

It seems that behavioural measures are as likely to show impairments in association with lead exposure as are tests of intellectual performance. However, the causes of the association are much less clear than for IQ. I have not attempted a quantitative meta-analysis of corrected effect size, because of methodological problems. As with IQ, the influence of confounding psychosocial variables must be allowed for. However, deviant behaviour does not have the same psychosocial associations as low IQ. In most investigations, the psychosocial measures are well chosen for their ability to predict the lack of environmental stimulation that goes with intellectual impairment. They are much less satisfactory as the means of detecting the unhappy, tense and discordant family atmospheres that are the concomitants of psychiatric disorder and behavioural deviance. Accordingly, it is not possible to say whether the relation between lead and behaviour is independent of the other things in the child's environment that may be going wrong, nor to give a useful estimate of effect size.

Some of the most relevant measures of family mental health have been gathered by the Institute of Child Health – Southampton study (Smith *et al.*, 1983) and the Christchurch birth cohort study (Fergusson *et al.*, 1988). Parental mental health and marital quality were both estimated and allowed for statistically. The first study did not indicate a relationship between lead and behaviour, the second did.

One can only conclude that more research with adequate measures of relevant variables is called for. Of course, this may be an impractical request. Already the literature on lead is outstanding in developmental epidemiology for the quality of studies and the resources that have been afforded because of the public interest in the potential dangers of pollution. There is a real risk that a provisional conclusion (of a small effect on IQ) and a perceived solution (reduction of lead in petrol) will sate the public appetite and dry up the funds. The scientific interest of the questions raised by the work therefore needs to be underlined. Fuller analyses of the data already gathered on behaviour might well be helpful.

Effects on behaviour may be of more importance than IQ changes as effects upon later development. There is a strong association between IQ and some of the behavioural measures (e.g. the Needleman teacher scale). Sometimes this is taken to suggest that the behaviour problem is simply what is to be expected in people of lower IQ. The association is, of course, considerably richer than that. One of the next steps in investigation should be to determine whether the association between lead and behaviour is due to the prior relationship of lead and IQ. Indeed, reanalysis of data already gathered would probably help to answer the question. It should shed some light upon the mechanism of action of lead exposure.

Outstanding problems of method

As scientific studies proceed to investigate the mechanisms that give rise to the association, they are confronted by some unsolved questions that need advances in techniques of investigation.

The first is the possibility of *reverse causality*. While it is plausible that high lead may damage psychological function, the mechanism could work the other way round. It is equally plausible that children who are deviant in behaviour, disruptive and inattentive, may also bring themselves into closer contact with environmental lead. Pervasively hyperactive children may drink more water than controls, and therefore be more at risk from dissolved lead; or they may play in streets more and therefore inhale more petrol vapour.

Some analyses have tried to allow for this statistically. For example, Fergusson *et al.* (1988) used the symptom of pica as an index of self-exposure, and concluded that this pathway could not account for the whole of the lead–behaviour association. The argument, however, is not sufficient. Indiscriminate eating and mouthing are only one of the ways in which self-exposure might take place and cannot stand as a measure for all the others. Longitudinal studies are evidently necessary.

Cohort studies of the development of high-risk children have now been started, and are likely to give helpful information in due course. Preliminary results are available from Boston (Bellinger *et al.*, 1987), Cincinnati (Dietrich *et al.*, 1987), Cleveland (Ernhart *et al.*, 1987) and

Port Pirie (McMichael *et al.*, 1986). Lead is assayed in maternal blood in pregnancy or at delivery, or in cord blood, or in blood from the neonate, or in various combinations. The Boston and Cincinnati studies have both reported that blood-lead levels at birth predict the mental development index of the Bayley Scales in the first 2 years and even the first 6 months of life. This seems to make reverse causality less probable, though perhaps not to rule it out altogether. On the other hand, the Port Pirie results find that the mental development index at 2 years is predicted by blood lead at 6 months, not at birth; and the Cleveland data do not include developmental effects of lead once other sources of reproductive hazard (such as alcohol and cigarettes) have been allowed for. It is too early, and there is not yet enough detail in reports, to try to resolve them into a single conclusion. But the need to continue and develop longitudinal studies of population-based groups is very clear.

Another line of evidence makes reverse causality less likely as a sole mechanism for the association. David reported some time ago that children with hyperactivity of unknown cause had higher blood-lead levels than did those with a known physical cause for their behavioural disorder (David *et al.*, 1977). This needs to be studied again with the full methodology of assessing and allowing for psychosocial variables that has subsequently been developed. If still true, it implies of course that the increased lead burden is the cause rather than the consequence of hyperactive behaviour.

A second methodological problem that has not been fully resolved is the uncertainty associated with high levels of *measurement error*. This is a particular problem in needing to understand lead effects on behaviour. There is no question but that all the behavioural measures used are of relatively low generalizability. Questionnaire rating scales contain a large amount of variance attributable to the source of the rating, the rater and random fluctuation. Lead estimates themselves have similar problems. While lead at one point in time, and from one source of tissue, can be measured reliably within a single laboratory, levels still vary greatly according to when and where they are sampled.

Statistical methods have been used to try to make some allowance for this. Fergusson *et al.* (1988) applied modelling techniques to longitudinal data from a birth cohort study; previous analyses using this technique had indicated that only about 30% of the variance in scales of conduct disorder could be attributed to a persisting quality of the child's behaviour. The correlation between latent dimensions of behavioural disturbance and lead burden could therefore be estimated. It was increased by this procedure, as is of course to be expected when allowance is made for the low generalizability of the measure.

The same arguments apply, with at least equal force, to the

measurement of the psychosocial variables that might mediate the association. Family adverse factors are known to be linked to hyperactivity and to conduct disorder; and also to be commoner in the inner-city environments where lead is greatest. These factors are only approximately estimated by the measures used.

No investigators can truly be said to have allowed for the lack of generalizability of their measures of the psychosocial environment. The consequences are likely to be large but unpredictable. In general, measurement error is by definition unrelated to the trait being measured and can therefore be expected to reduce the degree of association with other important variables. The simple, uncorrected correlation between lead and behaviour (and, to a lesser extent, between lead and IQ) will therefore have been underestimated by most studies.

The effect of measurement error in variables treated as confounders is more complicated. For each variable considered singly, the effect of error will be an undercorrection for that variable. At the extreme, where the source of variance in a measure is almost all from error, there will be no effect of including that measure as a covariate and the result of an analysis of covariance will be the same as the simple analysis of variance between lead and behaviour or IQ. However, as considered above, some of the many covariates typically included in analyses of lead effects will be overcorrecting in effect, others undercorrecting. Measurement error in one undercorrecting variable only could therefore tip the balance towards overcorrecting variables that have been measured with greater precision. It is therefore possible to imagine circumstances in which the combined effects of measurement error and multiplicity of covariates are to underestimate the relationship between lead and its psychological effects. These circumstances are somewhat unlikely and should not be taken as an expectation. It is more probable that there is substantial error in all covariates, and therefore that the analyses have failed to correct completely for the power of psychological environmental variables.

The way forward must be in the direction of using more satisfactory means of assessment and more exploration of using analytic modelling techniques that can allow for the generalizability of the measures.

Analysis of behavioural changes in high-lead groups is another of the issues requiring some advances in methodology. If all kinds of behavioural change were combined into a single scale, then specific effects of lead upon particular types of behaviour might well be overlooked. A true effect could equally well be missed by an exclusive preoccupation with an irrelevant type of behaviour. The great majority of studies have concentrated on 'hyperactivity' as the relevant dimension of behaviour. This is not based upon sharp scientific knowledge but upon a tradition of investigation. One reason is that the early studies, which directed research attention to the effects of lead, were often based upon children referred to clinics with the problem of hyperactivity. Such a presenting problem, however, is so often accompanied by other types of morbidity that one must not conclude that the hyperactivity was responsible for the findings. Another reason for a focus on hyperactivity is even less satisfactory: a belief that hyperactive behaviour is particularly closely linked to organic brain dysfunction. While there is a little evidence that hyperactivity is associated with neurodevelopmental delay in childhood, the evidence comes from studies using much more restrictive definitions of hyperactivity than the dimensional scores on teachers' and parents' rating scales which have been the mainstay of the lead researchers (Taylor *et al.*, 1991).

Research emphasis has concentrated on reporting results for hyperactivity and there is little research describing the range of common behavioural problems in groups with high blood-lead levels. Needleman's scale gave emphasis to poor attention; many types of behaviour upset were not included; overactivity was not in fact associated with lead level (Needleman *et al.*, 1979). The Rutter and Conners scales are more broadly based. Thomson *et al.* (1989) found the aggressive and antisocial items of the Rutter scale to be the most clearly related to blood-lead levels. Hyperactivity was more weakly associated, while neurotic items were no different. Silva *et al.* (1988) stated that their behavioural rating scale of inattention and hyperactivity was more strongly associated with blood lead than were 'other behavioural items'. Unfortunately the comparison was only with the total Rutter scale scores, so the reader is left in uncertainty about what behavioural items were the most discriminative. Reanalyses of existing studies might well be helpful. For the moment, one should not be too swift to assume that the major behavioural effects of lead are exerted through mechanisms leading to hyperactivity. Non-hyperactive conduct disorder may be just as significant a problem.

Finally, methodology will be enhanced by a move towards *quasi-experimental designs.* Epidemiological surveys of naturally-occurring variations in lead levels are bound to leave some uncertainties about cause and pathogenesis. It is literally impossible to control, or make statistical allowance, for every possible confounding factor. It therefore becomes important that investigators should be opportunistic in seizing upon situations where a natural experiment has arisen. This might, for example, be a new source of lead pollution in which the differences between high-exposure and low-exposure are a matter of chance – rather than of social adversity or self-selection for exposure. Alternatively, the natural experiment could involve the tracking of changes after a source of lead pollution is removed or after individual treatment, as discussed below. Such interventions – e.g. urban renewal programmes to renew old water piping in an area – would ideally affect all families in an area in the same way.

Mechanisms of lead effects

This review of lead effects has had to be rather lengthy, and should have been lengthier still to give an adequate account of the researches so far. Methodological advances are required before one can be entirely confident even in the answer to the question: 'Does low-level lead exposure damage psychological development?'; let alone 'How?'. I believe nevertheless that the field is in the interesting position of having plausibly demonstrated small effects attributable to 'ordinary' levels of lead exposure; and of being able to move on to questions of mechanism.

One early question to be cleared up will have to be the timing of effects. A high lead level in childhood can be a problem in itself and also a marker to exposure in early development. The exact measure taken does not seem to be critical, for both tooth-lead and blood-lead levels give similar results. In theory, tooth-lead level should more closely reflect long-term exposure, but gives no further indication of the timing of exposure. What is the key associate of cognitive impairment? Is it the current level of exposure, or the peak level ever encountered, or the level encountered during brain growth in pregnancy and the neonatal period?

The issue of timing will have many implications as to whether we have to deal with a critical period for brain damage, the sequelae of an acute encephalopathy, a progressive effect upon neuronal functioning, or a reversible effect upon psychological activity. It will be important to find and study groups of children whose exposure to lead has changed at a definable point in time; adding emphasis to the recommendation above for quasi-experimental studies.

Epidemiological work is often a cumbersome approach to questions of pathogenesis. Animal experiments have emphasized how many toxic effects lead has upon different biochemical systems. Which ones predominate in compromising brain function, and how they interact, is likely to be hard to find out. It might be a better immediate goal to examine the final common pathways of the biochemical disturbances upon broad measures of cerebral physiology. It would then be possible to determine the more proximate causes of such change (e.g. abnormalities of calcium handling or the immune system).

Most physiological work in humans has centred upon the electrophysiological measures of sensory evoked potentials and event-related slow potentials. They have been reviewed by Otto (1988), drawing largely upon work from his own laboratory. Findings are neither simple nor unambiguous. The easiest to understand is probably the increased latency of brainstem auditory evoked potentials, since it can be immediately related to the poorer hearing of children with high lead levels. The more psychologically meaningful measures are harder to interpret. The late positive component of the auditory evoked potential has a shorter latency in children with higher blood-lead, and peripheral nerve conduction is apparently more rapid. (The results for latency of visual evoked potentials are quite contradictory). The surprising aspect of these findings is that they are usually associated with superior cognitive performance, not with impairment.

It is clear that we are a long way from understanding the brain reaction. The future seems to lie in simultaneous analyses of electrophysiological functioning and cognitive test performance; in designs that include psychosocial variables as potential confounders even of evoked potential measures. Neurotransmitter levels and metabolism should also be investigated as a function of lead exposure.

Other aspects of the pathogenesis of lead effects have been mentioned above. It is possible that the primary effect is upon behaviour and that inattentiveness to the environment leads to an impoverishment of cognitive development. It is also possible that behaviour change is the consequence of cognitive impairment, or that both are independent consequences of the underlying brain dysfunction. The nature of remedial action would depend upon which of these possibilities apply.

The role of the psychological environment will also have to be taken into account. The possibility that it is the whole reason for lead effects has been discounted. The opposite possibility – that the whole of the effect of the environment is attributable to lead – is also improbable. The size of the effects of psychosocial variables on IQ is much greater than that of lead in all the studies. The ability of the psychological environment to modify lead effects now needs to be examined. Comparing studies, there is little evidence for such an effect. Lead effects seem to be of a similar size in relatively advantaged populations (e.g. in Edinburgh) compared with most other areas. Nevertheless, this needs examining within studies, and physiological measures are likely to be particularly useful for this purpose.

Group findings and individual pathogenesis

The application of research findings to clinical practice is complex. Group findings need to be translated into individual terms, and fallacies can arise in the process.

The question of the existence of a threshold in the action of the lead is one such issue. It seems likely from the studies received that there is no population threshold for harmful effects, but a linear relationship between body burden and psychological impairment. This matters a lot at the level of the population, and rightly guides public health decisions about the need to reduce lead levels generally rather than only in very heavily exposed groups. However, the same conclusion of the absence of a threshold should not be automatically applied at the level of individual functioning (as it is when considering the mechanism of disorder). It would be quite possible for there to be a threshold for each individual, but for those thresholds to be continuously distributed in the population, so that groups show no discontinuity in lead effect with rising lead levels. We simply do not know the answer.

Another issue is that of the significance of lead burden in an individual. The same studies that indicate the 'lead effect' to be significant also show that it is small. But it is much less clear whether the smallness of the effect is a matter of a small change to many individuals or a large change for a few individuals. Needleman & Bellinger (1988) have argued theoretically and shown empirically that a small shift downwards in the population IQ mean entails a large proportionate increase in the numbers who are very far (e.g. 2 SD) below the mean. However, this is not to say that lead is therefore the dominating influence for the children at 2 SD below the mean. It does not imply that the removal of lead would have a large effect upon those individuals – only that it would have a large effect upon the numbers below a specific cutoff. Needleman's data imply that the effect of lead is similar in all IQ groups of children. It seems to follow that we should think of lead's effect as a small action upon each child.

When clinicians are making formulations about individual children with intellectual retardation or hyperactivity, they should not give excessive weight to a modestly elevated lead level, i.e. to a level above 20 but below 40 μg/dl. (Indeed, the reliability of estimation of such levels in routine clinical practice leaves a good deal to be desired at present and multiple estimates are advisable before any therapeutic decisions.) Such a finding should trigger a search for avoidable sources of exposure (including old paint, contaminated dust and lead water pipes). However, this should be planned only as one of several interventions.

FETAL EXPOSURE TO ALCOHOL

The study of the effects of a chemical hazard during embryonic life raises a different set of issues. Some of the methodological problems, that were noted in studying lead, become much less important: others look even larger.

The fetus is much more clearly a passive victim of exposure than the child. The question of 'reverse causality', discussed above, scarcely arises. Nevertheless, the psychological determinants of exposure are still important. The fetus is exposed to alcohol only because of the activities of the mother. Any positive findings between fetal alcohol exposure and later psychological problems could stem from a prior association between both these and the mother's personality, intelligence or social circumstances. Genetic factors may be involved in this inheritance of personality, given the known heritability of alcoholism itself.

The timing of exposure to alcohol in development is much more clear than was the case for lead. Alcohol intake is seldom significant in early childhood. By the same token, however, a substantial period of time passes between the exposure to alcohol and the point in childhood where disturbance of learning and behaviour become evident. Retrospective enquiry about parental drinking in pregnancy is notoriously prone to falsification. Prospective longitudinal studies are therefore required at an even earlier stage of scientific investigation than in a condition where markers of current exposure to a toxin are available. As we develop our knowledge about the learning and behaviour of the fetus, so it may become feasible to detect psychological effects prenatally. Even then, however, it will still be necessary to follow the development of affected babies to the age where psychiatric disability can arise.

The outstanding reason for the rapidity with which knowledge has developed about the effects of early alcohol exposure, is the existence of a specific marker to the effects of alcohol upon physical development. A set of dysmorphic features could be described in babies that constituted a specific 'fetal alcohol syndrome' (FAS) (Jones & Smith, 1973; Ouelette *et al.*, 1977). This has been the key to the recognition of the effects of alcohol in later childhood and to the suggestion that the fetal alcohol syndrome is now one of the commonest causes of mental handicap. For example, 'blind' assessments of the physical stigmata at the age of four are significantly related to measures of alcohol intake during pregnancy; they are still related after allowing for exposure to other substances such as cannabis and tobacco; and they are not related to the degree of exposure to substances other than alcohol (Graham *et al.*, 1988). The same dysmorphic features, assessed by the same group of investigators, showed a significant negative correlation with IQ (Streissguth *et al.*, 1978). The argument that IQ is lowered specifically by alcohol exposure can therefore be made, but is not sufficient. Even accepting the findings, it would still need to be shown that the dysmorphic features cannot be caused by other factors, and that the relation between alcohol and lowered IQ is not due to other mechanisms of association. Neither can be assumed. The dysmorphic features are often present in the offspring of mothers with no history of drinking alcohol. They are similar to the 'minor congenital anomalies' that probably have a mixed genetic and environmental origin (Rapoport & Quinn, 1975). Cognitive abnormalities are linked to paternal alcohol abuse as well as maternal (Tarter *et al.*, 1989). It is therefore necessary to examine the links between alcohol and psychological development with the same kind of methodology that has been used for the studies of lead.

The specificity of psychological effects needs more study. There are apparent effects upon behaviour and neurological status in infancy (Clarren & Smith, 1978). In later childhood, hypotonicity, hypoactivity, motor incoordination, stereotyped self-stimulating activity, and poor habituation have all been reported. Motor delay at age 4 years shows a dose–response relationship with mother's intake of alcohol during pregnancy – even allowing for intake of other drugs such as caffeine, tobacco and aspirin (Barr *et al.*, 1990). I am not myself convinced that a psychological syndrome specific to FAS has been found: rather the problems are those that would be seen in any group of cognitively disadvantaged children.

Several questions remain to be answered. What is the mechanism of development of psychological disorder? It has not been definitely established that physical injury to the brain is responsible, and there are many kinds of psychological stress that result from being the child of a parent who abuses alcohol. What is the range of behavioural effects? Clinical writers often seem to be straining after a specificity of effect that is not necessarily to be expected for biological reasons.

Does alcohol have an adverse effect in itself, after allowing for associated psychosocial adversity? Plant & Plant (1987, 1988) found alcohol to have only a minor impact on birth abnormality. On the other hand, Russell & Skinner (1988) have been able to find an effect on birth abnormalities using multiple regression techniques. If there is doubt on birth abnormalities considered as the outcome, there is all the more on later psychological deviance. Much more evidence is needed. Streissguth *et al.* (1984) described attention and reaction time abnormalities in a heavily-exposed group by comparison with a lightly-exposed group but were not able adequately to allow for the effects of general social adversity – let alone for the potentially more specific effects of parental intelligence and child-raising practices.

Is there a threshold? Evidence is somewhat contradictory. Some studies fail to find a dose–response relationship between alcohol and embryopathy even when studied at birth. Plant & Plant (1987), for instance, found no overall relationship between a modest alcohol intake by mothers (e.g., 3–4 units per week) and abnormalities at birth. They did, however, find more abnormalities in the children of heavily smoking and drinking mothers. Several other researchers have concluded that there is no evidence for a toxic effect of low-level alcohol intake (Kuzma & Sokol, 1982). On the other hand, all studies so far have had low power for the detection of the small degrees of risk that could be associated with low levels of intake. The question is too serious to be left in doubt, and large-scale surveys should be undertaken.

Micronutrient deficiencies

Selective nutritional deficiencies are conceivably causes of behaviour and learning problems, but in general the evidence is poor. In this instance, epidemiological studies scarcely contribute to the debate. There have of course been dietary analyses of populations, but all founder upon the inadequacy of methods used. Diet records are both inaccurate because of observer effects and imprecise because of day-to-day fluctuations in intake (Bingham, 1987). Even rigorously conducted studies with lengthy periods of recording may systematically underestimate the intake of nutrients because information about food taken is forgotten or suppressed. Since recording is considered to be especially poor by less well-educated subjects, the methods may be a strong confounding factor in studies of diet and intelligence.

The necessary methodology would therefore require blood tests for the concentrations of micronutrients, independent assessments of behaviour and intelligence, and measurement of the relevant factors in the psychosocial background: the same process through which the lead studies have evolved. Such studies have not yet begun. I believe none the less that there is a case for the work to go ahead.

The evidence for micronutrient deficiencies is not based upon survey data but upon controlled clinical trials. It is, of course, undisputed that severe vitamin deficiencies have neurological effects, just as severe lead intoxication causes an encephalopathy. The debate, as with lead, concerns the possibility that milder and commoner abnormalities play a substantial role for many cases of learning or behaviour impairment.

It has been known for a long time that a repetitive institutional diet may be low in B vitamins and indeed that thiamine has a greater effect than placebo upon the intelligence and visual acuity of children receiving such a diet (Harrell, 1946). Claims have been made that a 'normal' modern diet is comparably lacking in vitamins and minerals (Benton & Roberts, 1988). However, since these claims also are based upon the inadequate methodology of diet records by parents they are not worth lengthy consideration.

A recent trial, widely publicised in the UK, used double-blind methodology to compare the intellectual and behavioural development of ordinary schoolchildren given a vitamin/mineral supplement, a placebo, or no supplement at all (Benton & Roberts, 1988). There was a large rise in the non-verbal intelligence of the children given supplementary micronutrients – significantly greater than that of the placebo-treated group.

Much criticism has been levelled at this trial, not all of it deserved. One may, for instance, reasonably object that vitamin and mineral supplements should not be preferred to an adequate diet; but of course the purpose of the supplementation was to allow for a blind trial. One may with justification be irritated by the ammunition given to the exploitative industry of 'health foods'; but of course an idea should not be condemned because of its supporters. The statistical analysis of the trial was inadequate; but subsequent reanalyses improved matters (Benton, 1988). Many of the tests given did not change, so change might favour a single significant result out of many. All the same, the effect size was so very large – three-quarters of a standard deviation – that the demonstration was not dependent upon the particular analysis chosen. The test of non-verbal intelligence chosen, the Calvert test, is not widely used and the abilities required for it are unclear; but by the same token it may have been particularly sensitive to deficiencies and therefore give clues to the cognitive analysis of diet-induced changes. The double-blind may possibly have failed if the supplement coloured the children's urine, and any failure in the blinding process could introduce spurious findings.

Even if, technically, the trial were wholly satisfactory, and independently replicated, problems of interpretation would still arise. Treatments typically have multiple effects. It is hazardous to assume that the intended action is responsible for the final effect, but this assumption is a necessary part of the argument from treatment to mechanism. To take just one of many examples, the high amounts of folate contained in the supplementation could be psychoactive in themselves. Researches into the effects of folate on children with a fragile-X chromosome constitution have suggested that folate may have a stimulant-like effect. Indeed, the effect of folate does not seem to be contingent upon whether it reduces the rate of fragile X, and therefore might be seen in individuals with normal X chromosomes.

Similar arguments arise with respect to the effects of therapy in lead intoxication. David *et al.* (1976) reported a positive result from the use of penicillamine, a chelating agent, in the treatment of hyperactive children with modestly raised levels of lead. Penicillamine reduced hyperactivity more than a placebo. The difficulty arises when inferring that lead was therefore the cause of the hyperactivity. What else might penicillamine have done besides chelate lead? Could side-effects have broken the blind, or could the drug alter neurotransmitter balance? Either possibility could be responsible for the observation.

In all these examples of inferences from the effects of treatment, the argument would be greatly strengthened if investigators included measures of a range of possible actions of the treatment, not just the one in their hypothesis. If, for example, vitamin/mineral supplementation were shown to improve biochemical indices of vitamin depletion, and the extent to which this happened was correlated with the rise in IQ after treatment, then one would indeed have a persuasive argument. In the long run it could be even more important to know about mechanism than to have a partial therapy at hand.

Expediency and value-for-money guide the planning of research as well as strict scientific logic. It would not be desirable to test every commercially motivated claim with elaborate and publicly funded research. There are so many problems with the published trial of vitamin/mineral tablets that I for one would wish to see a confirmation that there is an effect to be studied before examining the reasons for it with detailed trials and adequate surveys. Naismith *et al.* (1988) have reported a failure to find any cognitive effects with a similar therapy. However, this work was not planned as a direct replication: different intellectual tests were used and the time scale was shorter. Replication should be attempted. Meanwhile the manufacturers' own lack of scientific assessment cannot surprise, but must appal, all those who watch the accumulation of profit and the neglect of knowledge.

DIETARY INTOLERANCE

The course of study of food intolerance as a cause of behavioural disturbance has not progressed smoothly. It has sometimes been trivialized and distorted by non-scientific pressures. The so-called Feingold hypothesis – that various types of food additive damage mental functioning – has had disproportionate emphasis. The predictable failure of the simple view that artificial dyes and preservatives are the main cause of behavioural disorder has led to some discrediting of the entire enterprise of studying links between diet and mental function. Several studies, however, point to the significance of dietary effects in individual cases of disorder – so it is important that the methodological problems should be overcome.

There is now a long history of speculation and study concerning links between behaviour disorders and food intolerance. Shannon (1922) argued that behaviour problems could be a primary allergic reaction; Schneider (1945) asserted that allergy was important in causing the 'syndrome' of childhood hyperkinesis. Speer (1954) described an 'allergic tension–fatigue syndrome' including behavioural changes in children. Kittler (1970) presented some case studies of children with 'minimal brain dysfunction' whose difficult behaviour had improved when dietary allergens (such as chocolate and milk) were excluded.

Objectors for a long time protested that the brain was so strongly protected against immune attack that allergy was highly implausible as an explanation. With time, however, this argument has lost some of its force. Allergic reactions to food have long been known to cause changes in the central nervous system (Kennedy, 1938). Even without accepting this mechanism, when allergic reactions take place elsewhere in the body the brain is affected. This may be as non-specific as a feeling of malaise after eating tartrazine (Neuman *et al.*, 1978) or as precise as alterations in noradrenaline turnover in rat brains (Besedovsky *et al.*, 1983). Non-allergic causes of intolerance have become increasingly recognized. The existence of plausible mechanisms is certainly no guarantee that effects exist, but they do make it impossible to dismiss clinicians' claims as absurd.

Trials of diets excluding additives

Empirical investigations were scanty until the 1970s, when a strong interest was shown by mass media in Feingold's (1975) hypothesis that artificial additives caused hyperactivity. This produced scientific trials and funding for research, which was all to the good.

To eliminate additives from the diet is quite difficult. The outcome is usually a wholesome diet. But to achieve it requires cooperation and firmness of purpose. One will therefore expect quite strong placebo effects.

For this reason there is little point in mentioning the early, open trials. They simply described families who started on the diet, knowing what they were doing, and who said their children got better. It is not in dispute that this will happen for many children in the short term.

An early controlled trial came from Conners' team, who compared a Feingold diet with another exclusion diet in 15 hyperactive children, and assessed outcome with rating scales (Conners *et al.*, 1976). They found a significant difference in favour of the Feingold diet. They qualified this heavily because there was an unexplained order effect (see below) and because just a few of the children accounted for the good outcome. One heavy reservation to add to theirs is that we have to doubt whether it was truly blind. Parents were running the diet, and even by that stage they could have been expected to know what the diet sheets meant and what they were in fact excluding. It was only parent ratings that changed; teachers saw no differences between diets. Placebo effects could therefore have been involved.

Harley and his numerous colleagues (1978) then did a better funded and more ambitious comparison. They had 30 hyperactive children and this time it was the researchers who organized the diets. They supplied and delivered all the family food week-by-week, and rotated foods so that it would have been very hard for anyone to guess when they were getting the additive-free diet and when the control diet. They even supplied food at the schools to minimize infractions. They also used a battery of measures, with ratings and observations and neuropsychological tests. They found no consistent diet effects. Parent ratings for the preschool children in the study suggested a significant diet effect in that group only, but direct observations did not, and it was in any case a rather *post hoc* sort of analysis.

Interestingly, the same order effect was present as in the Conners study. The Feingold diet was only superior when it followed the control. One explanation would be an enduring effect of the diet which persists even through a control diet if the control comes last. Another explanation would invoke placebo effects.

Any stimulus properties of the colourings could break the blind, and therefore lead to an amplification of the normal placebo effect. If a first treatment period has gone by, and no change has been experienced or seen, then parents and child must have an enhanced expectation of the second period. This would amplify any placebo action in the second period only. This only requires that there is some slight cue as to which diet is which. Such a cue could come from the child's sensations or the parents' uncertain suspicions about what he is eating. Future studies could therefore well include invitations to guess which treatment is which.

Challenges

The challenge studies followed logically on. If children improve with the exclusion of additives then of course they can be maintained on the diet and given either additives or placebo in a standard double-blind design. Harley *et al.* (1978) reported a negative study. Goyette *et al.* (1978) followed up the Conners *et al.* study and found no benefit on rating scales but a transient effect on a visual-motor tracking test that lasted for about an hour. They therefore followed it up by another study giving the questionnaires just 3 hours after the challenge – to catch short-lived effects. This time they obtained a significant worsening on parent ratings. Unfortunately they had no teacher ratings because there was a teachers' strike in progress. So they did the study all over again on a new set of children and this time got no positive results at all on any test (Conners, 1980). This group of investigations therefore argues only for evanescent actions of additives at most.

The Williams *et al.* (1978) study was a more complicated design because it tested both additives against placebo and also methylphenidate against placebo in 26 hyperactive children who had previously responded to stimulant drugs. The customary Conners Classroom Rating Scale showed a big effect of the drug treatment, as of course one would expect. The additives showed a small but significant effect – but this time not consistently on the parents' ratings, but only on teacher ratings. Levy *et al.* (1978) found no sign of differences between additives and placebo substances.

All these studies with small or absent effects have used only moderate doses, around 25 mg of additives or less. Maybe this is not enough. Swanson & Kinsbourne's (1980) work began with a similar absence of effects using standard doses. Then, however, they did what hindsight suggests should have been done from the start. They looked for a dose–response relationship. With a bigger dose of 100 mg they still found no behavioural effect. They did find an effect 1 to 2 hours after the high dose on a paired-associate learning test of short-term memory; and found it only in children who had previously responded to stimulant drugs.

Because of this, Mattes & Gittelman (1981) carried out a study using high doses on 11 children who were all definite responders to the diet according to their parents and had been identified through the Feingold Association. They found nothing. Rating scales did not worsen, and neither did distractibility. However, they did not use any cognitive test so findings are not directly comparable with that of Swanson & Kinsbourne (1980).

Another group study (Thorley, 1984) capitalized on a natural experiment. A voluntary residential school in Yorkshire decided to adopt the diet and requested evaluation. Thorley took the opportunity with a placebo-controlled challenge study after the children had been maintained on their diet. They were a group of 10 mildly retarded children with conduct problems including hyperactivity. It was a closed society, so the diet was certainly adhered to. After a fortnight on the diet, he began a daily challenge with a high-dose of colourings or a placebo. There were no significant differences between treatments. However, the non-significant trend on the Paired Associate Learning test might have become significant if he had used as many cases as did Swanson & Kinsbourne (1980).

The total of these challenge studies is rather slight. Only in the Williams *et al.* (1978) study is there any clear effect on behaviour – and that was small. But there are counterarguments to suggest that real effects could have been missed.

The first argument is one raised in Weiss's (1982) review. The negative results on behaviour may be because the very transient effects have not been caught in a questionnaire relating to a whole day at a time, let alone a whole week (as in Mattes & Gittelman, 1981). The trouble with this argument is that it is the exact opposite of the argument which saved the hypothesis from the comparison-diet studies. For them we had to suppose a long-lasting effect only. The two arguments cannot both be true. Yet both were deployed by the same reviewer in the interest of Feingold's story.

The second counterargument is that nobody ever said that *all* hyperactive children responded. This argument can be abused. For instance, a review by Mayron (1979) states that 'even if only 2 children out of 100 are helped by this diet, the problems of these 2 children have been solved'. He then runs through the studies, pointing out that 5/15 responded in the Conners study, 6/26 in the Williams, and so on. In the same way, reviewers point to the considerable fraction of children even in the negative studies who drop by 10% or 20% in their Conners' Classroom Rating Scale scores. The fallacy in this should be obvious. Chance alone will produce much the same subgroup effect. This is the kind of argument that keeps charlatans in business. Nevertheless, negative group results may well fail to record substantial changes in individuals. This must be addressed by single-case studies.

The third counterargument is considered in more detail below: the children may have reacted adversely to other substances besides the additives themselves – including the control foods to which the colourings were compared. Since the range of substances provoking reactions may vary from child to child, this objection can also be addressed by a single-case methodology.

Single cases

Single-case studies allow individualized hypotheses to be tested, and therefore escape the problems that I have just discussed. They do, of course, have problems of their own. One needs a reasonably large number of repeated observations to be able to make any kind of statistical inference. Without this, one is prey to falsely positive findings, especially as it is quite likely that only positive findings are publishable and a very large number of negative case studies can exist yet go unreported. This need for many data points tends to rule out the usual kinds of psychometric test, since they are likely to show practice effects. There are now a few cases published as persuasive evidence. Two of them were published by Rose in 1978. He searched a Florida community for hyperactive children who had responded well to the diet and been able to come off medication. He found just two; both of them were 8-year-old girls. Both of them went through a BABAB design with 1 mg tartrazine or no additives at all present in a daily cookie. Both children reacted to the tartrazine with a large and highly significant increase in off-task behaviour by comparison with the placebo cookie. The odd thing about this study is that both the girls were apparently responders to very low doses of the one dye that the investigator happened to pick. The coincidence is striking, but might result from some unstated selection factor.

The next single case was reported by Mattes & Gittelman-Klein (1978). A 10-year-old boy went through a design in which his daily cookies contained either wholesome ingredients or a dose of additives in a multiple reversal design. Formal questionnaire ratings gave no significant results. The significant finding was entirely based upon his mother's ability to guess which cookie he had taken – which just made the 0.05 level when they included the times she was not sure and made a forced guess.

A case reported by Weiss *et al.* (1980) showed a response that was clear, large, dramatic and significant at the 1 in 10 000 level. The design gave a daily soft drink on each of 77 days. On 8 of the days the drink contained artificial colourings. On those days the child's behaviour was much more disturbed than on others. The child (a girl, aged nearly 3 years) was the only clear responder in a group of 22 children, all identified as good responders to the diet, who went through exactly the same design.

She yields a solid piece of evidence, but is also a part of a negative trial. The conclusion seems to be that the diet often works, but not because of the hypothesis. It has a real, physical, idiosyncratic effect on the behaviour of an occasional child; and group studies make it possible that there is a relatively subtle effect upon cognition in a subgroup of children.

This is a positive, but quite a modest conclusion. It does not sustain the wild claims of Feingold or his imitators who have produced at least twelve books written for parents which tell them unequivocally that hyperactivity is due to artificial additives. I don't think it is unfair to say that there is an element here of exploitation.

Multiple food intolerance

Multiple food intolerance is not a parsimonious explanation, but seems to justify more study than it has received. Trites *et al.* (1980) conducted a series of studies suggesting that the hyperactive had more physical evidence of food allergies than normal controls. Removing the allergens from their diets produced a small but encouraging improvement in behaviour.

This raises another explanation for the mixed findings on Feingold diets. The elimination of additives may have led to the alteration of the diet in other ways, and to the unwitting avoidance of a quite different agent that was itself harmful. Chocolate, for instance, is usually withheld from children on Feingold diets because it is so frequently believed to contain additives. By the same token, the elimination of an allergen from the diet of an allergic individual may fail to alleviate symptoms because many other harmful substances are still present. Indeed, most controlled double-blind challenge studies have used, as placebo and excipient, either a cookie containing wheat flour or a chocolate drink. Wheat and chocolate are common instigators of immune responses in allergic children. They could therefore have been as harmful as the synthetic dyes to which they were compared. The Feingold hypothesis would still fail, but the more plausible hypothesis of a wide range of antigens would not be harmed by an apparent absence of effect for colourings in such a design.

Egger *et al.* (1985) described a controlled trial of a range of possible allergens, removed by a radical exclusion diet, reintroduced one at a time, and finally compared with placebo. The results were dramatically positive, and could have been inflated by the same interaction between treatment and order of administration that was noted in the work by Conners *et al.* (1976) and Harley *et al.* (1978). The effect size was also hard to interpret since significant results were largely confined to parental ratings. These ratings are the most likely of any to be sensitive to any failure of the maintenance of 'blind' status. Furthermore, the children in the trial could have been highly selected by referral bias. Replication will be important. Kaplan *et al.* (1989) have recently provided a brief report of the comparison between a multiple-exclusion and a control diet, that seems to add force to the possible value of this approach.

Caffeine is another, potentially harmful part of the normal diet. It is found in many soft drinks as well as in tea and coffee. It increases activity, and probably irritability, to a level that can cause problems (Elkins *et al.*, 1981).

The most promising lines of research now seem to be to try to confirm the suggestions in studies by Trites *et al.* (1980) and Egger *et al.* (1985) on multiple intolerance; to explore the cognitive effects in dose–response studies; and to combine single-case studies with testing for evidence of immune complex formation, mast cell instability, lymphocyte activity and other possible predictors of response. If we knew how to predict which children would respond, current clinical uncertainties would be resolved.

Future research should be more systematic in examining details determining response. Dose–response determination is important, but neglected because of the dominance of the original theories of idiosyncratic action. In the case of tartrazine, the effect of high doses has been investigated, with little evidence of a major effect (see above). However, other additives were never explored in this way. The effect of low doses also needs examination, in case they have a greater effect than higher ones through immune mechanisms. Many unanswered questions remain about action in spite of a considerable amount of research activity.

The lesson appears to be that, in the early stages of investigation, one should avoid the temptation of testing only one theoretical type of action of a substance. Rather, the substances to be tested should be examined systematically for the dose and time characteristics of response on a variety of measures prior to a full-scale trial.

The behavioural and learning effects should also be studied in their own right rather than assuming that they can all be subsumed into 'hyperactivity'. After all, children with brain damage display high rates of nearly all types of psychological upset, not just hyperactivity. Individual cases described in the literature as showing reactions to additives have not been confined to hyperactivity but include irritability, tempers and miserable affect as prominent symptoms. This could explain some apparent contradictions in the literature. Epidemiological surveys have not found that hyperactive children show the physical symptomatology that would be expected from a group with multiple allergies. On the contrary, Taylor *et al.* (1991) have found that physical symptoms of ill health are associated with emotional disorder rather than hyperactivity; and that the 8-year-old boys with pervasive, persistent hyperactivity in a community do not show elevated rates of atopic symptoms (in themselves or relatives) over a control group. The high rates of headaches, fits and other symptoms in the subjects of the Egger *et al.* (1985) and Kaplan *et al.* (1989) trials might therefore be pointers to a responsive subgroup.

Group results and decisions about individuals

The conclusion that seems to emerge is quite different from that of the lead studies. The small effect size associated with effects of additives is not a small action across individuals but a substantial effect upon a few individuals.

Until research gives grounds for diagnosing individuals, clinical practice has an element of detective work. Only a time-consuming and placebo-controlled single-case study will show definitely whether an individual responds. The judgement about who to submit to such a process needs to take into account the potential benefit to the individual (so that only handicapping levels of behaviour disturbance should qualify); the burden to the family (so that only those able to cope with the process should proceed); and the existence of other effective therapies – so that a concern with the chemical environment should not become exclusive nor a distortion of nutrition. At the same time, public concern is pressing. About 4% of parents in a nation-wide survey in the UK considered their children to be allergic to food and treated accordingly (Rona & Chinn, 1987). The demand for advice is great; the supply needs firmer research evidence.

The 1980s have seen the accumulation of evidence that a number of chemicals can adversely affect the behaviour and learning of children. This chapter has outlined the issues remaining for research in establishing the size and importance of these effects, the mechanisms of their pathogenesis and their effects upon development. In most of the examples chosen the conclusion has been that the effect is small in size and by comparison with the effects of the psychological environment. A small effect size can still be important – either because it can be removed readily, or because of the public health importance of clear knowledge, or because the effect is small only in group terms and has a large impact upon individual children. Methods have developed to the point of being able to detect small effects. The methods can now be applied to a wider range of supposed hazards.

REFERENCES

Barr, H. M., Streissguth, A. P., Darby, B. L. & Simpson, P. D. (1990) Prenatal exposure to alcohol, caffeine, tobacco, and aspirin: effects on fine and gross motor performance in 4-year-old children. *Developmental Psychology*, **26**, 339–48.

Bellinger, D., Leviton, A., Waternaux, C., Needleman, H. & Rabinowitz, M. (1987) Longitudinal analyses of prenatal and postnatal lead exposure and early cognitive development. *New England Journal of Medicine*, **316**, 1037–43.

Benton, D. (1988) Vitamin/mineral supplementation and non-verbal intelligence. *The Lancet*, **i**, 408–9 (letter).

Benton, D. & Roberts, G. (1988) Effect of vitamin and mineral supplementation on intelligence of a sample of schoolchildren. *The Lancet*, **i**, 140–3.

Besedovsky, H., del Rey, A., Sorkin, E., Da Prada, M., Burri, R. & Honegger, C. (1983) The immune response evokes change in brain noradrenergic neurones. *Science*, **221**. 564–6.

Bingham, S. (1987) *Nutrition Abstracts and Reviews*, **57**, 705–42.

Clarren, S. K. & Smith, D. W. (1978). The fetal alcohol syndrome. *New England Journal of Medicine*, **198**, 1063–7.

Cohen, J. (1988) *Statistical power analysis for the behavioral sciences*, 2nd edn. New York: Erlbaum.

Conners, C. K. (1980) *Food Additives and Hyperactive Children*. New York: Plenum.

Conners, C. K., Goyette, C. H., Southwick, D. A., Lees, J. M. & Andrulonis, P. (1976) Food additives and hyperkinesis. *Pediatrics*, **58**, 154–66.

David, O. J., Hoffman, S. P., Sverd, J., Clark, J. & Voeller, K. (1976). Lead and hyperactivity: behavioral response to chelation: a pilot study. *American Journal of Psychiatry*, **133**, 1155–8.

David, O. J., Hoffman, S. P., Sverd, J. & Clark, J. (1977) Lead and hyperactivity: lead levels among hyperactive children. *Journal of Abnormal Child Psychology*, **5**, 405–16.

Dietrich, K. N., Krafft, K. M., Bornschein, R. L., Hammond, P. B., Berger, O., Succop, P. A. & Bier, M. (1987) Effects of low-level fetal lead exposure on neurobehavioral development in early infancy. *Pediatrics*, **89**, 721–30.

Egger, J., Carter, C. M., Graham, P. J., Gumley, D. & Soothill, J. F. (1985) Controlled trial of oligoantigenic treatment in the hyperkinetic syndrome. *Lancet*, **i**, 540–5.

Elkins, R. N., Rapoport, J. L., Zahn, T. P. *et al.* (1981) Acute effects of caffeine in normal prepubertal boys. *American Journal of Psychiatry*, **138**, 178–83.

Ernhart, C. B., Morrow-Tlucak, M., Marler, M. R. & Wolf, A. W. (1987) Low level lead exposure in the prenatal and early preschool periods: early preschool development. *Neurotoxicology and Teratology*, **9**, 259–70.

Feingold, B. F. (1975) Hyperkinesis and learning disabilities linked to artificial food flavors and colors. *American Journal of Nursing*, **75**, 797–803.

Fergusson, D. M., Fergusson, J. E., Horwood, L. J. & Kinzett, N. G. (1988) A longitudinal study of dentine lead levels, intelligence, school performance and behaviour. *Journal of Child Psychology and Psychiatry*, **29**, 781–824.

Fulton, M., Raab, G., Thomson, G., Laxen, D., Hunter, R. & Hepburn, W. (1987) Influence of blood lead on the ability and attainment of children in Edinburgh. *Lancet*, **i**, 1221–6.

Goyette, C. H., Conners, C. K., Petti, T. A. & Curtis, L. E. (1978) Effects of artificial colors on hyperactive children: a double-blind challenge study. *Psychopharmacology Bulletin*, **14**, 39–40.

Graham, J. M., Jr, Hanson, J. W., Darby, B. L., Barr, H. M. & Streissguth, A. P. (1988) Independent dysmorphology evaluations at birth and 4 years of age for children exposed to varying amounts of alcohol in utero. *Pediatrics*, **81**, 772–8.

Hansen, O. N., Trillingsgaard, A., Beese, I., Lyngbye, T. & Grandjean, P. (1988) Neuropsychological profile of children in relation to dentine lead level and socioeconomic group. In Smith, M. A., Grant, L. D. & Sors, A. E. (eds). *Lead exposure and child development: an international assessment.* Dordrecht: Kluwer Academic Publishers.

Harley, J. P., Ray, R. S., Tomasi, L., Eichman, P. L., Matthews, C. G., Chun, R., Cleeland, C. S. & Traisman, E. (1978) Hyperkinesis and food additives: testing the Feingold hypothesis. *Pediatrics*, **61**, 818–28.

Harrell, R. F. (1946) Mental response to added thiamine. *Journal of Nutrition*, **31**, 283–98.

Harvey, P. G., Hamlin, M. W., Kumar, R. & Delves, H. T. (1984). Blood lead, behaviour and intelligence test performance in preschool children. *Science of the Total Environment*, **40**, 45–60.

Harvey, P. G., Hamlin, M. W., Kumar, R., Morgan, J., Spurgeon, A. & Delves, H. T. (1988) Relationships between blood lead, behaviour, psychometric and neuropsychological test performance in young children. *British Journal of Developmental Psychology*, **6**, 145–56.

Hatzakis, A., Kokkevi, A., Maravelias, C., Katsouyanni, K., Salaminios, F., Kalandidi, A., Koutselinis, A., Stefanis, C. & Trichopoulos, D. (1988) Psychometric intelligence deficits in lead-exposed children. In Smith, M. A., Grant, L. D. & Sors, A. E. (eds.) *Lead exposure and child development: an international assessment.* Dordrecht: Kluwer Academic Publishers.

Hawk, B. & Schroeder, S. R. (1983) Factors interactive with IQ and blood lead levels in children. Paper presented at the XVIth Annual Conference on mental retardation and developmental disabilities, Gatlinburz, TN, March.

Hawk, B. A., Schroeder, S. R., Robinson, G., Otto, D., Mushak, P., Kleinbaum, D. & Dawson, G. (1986) Relation of lead and social factors of IQ of low-SES children: a partial replication. *American Journal of Mental Deficiency*, **91**, 178–83.

Jones, K. S. & Smith, D. W. (1973) Recognition of the fetal alcohol syndrome in early infancy. *The Lancet*, **ii**, 999–1001.

Kaplan, B. J., McNicol, J., Conte, R. A. & Moghadam, H. K. (1989) Dietary placement in preschool-aged hyperactive boys. *Pediatrics*, **83**, 7–17.

Kennedy, F. (1938) Allergy and its effect on the central nervous system. *Archives of Neurological Psychiatry*, **39**, 1361–6.

Kittler, F. J. (1970) The effect of allergy on children with minimal brain damage. In Speer, F. (ed.) *Allergy of the Nervous System*. Springfield: Charles C. Thomas.

Kuzma, J. & Sokol, R. (1982) Maternal drinking behaviour and decreased intrauterine growth. *Alcoholism: Clinical and Experimental Research*, **6**, 396–402.

Landrigan, P. J., Whitworth, R. H., Baloh, R. W., Staehling, N. W., Barthel, W. F. & Rosenblum, B. T. (1975) Neuropsychological dysfunction in children with chronic low-level lead absorption. *The Lancet*, **i**, 708–12.

Lansdown, R., Yule, W., Urbanowicz, M.-A. & Hunter, J. (1986) The relationship between blood-lead concentrations, intelligence, attainment and behavior in a school population: the second London study. *International Archives of Occupational and Environmental Health*, **57**, 225–35.

Levy, F., Dumbrell, S., Hobbes, G., Ryan, M., Wilton, N. & Woodhill, J. M. (1978) Hyperkinesis and diet: a double-blind crossover trial with a tartrazine challenge. *Medical Journal of Australia*, **1**, 61–4.

Lucas, A., Morley, R. & Cole, T. J. (1988) Adverse neurodevelopmental outcome of moderate neonatal hypoglycaemia. *British Medical Journal*, **297**, 1304–8.

McBride, W. G., Black, B. P. & English, B. J. (1982) Blood lead levels and behavior of 400 preschool children. *Medical Journal of Australia*, **2**, 26–9.

McMichael, A. J., Vimpani, G. V., Robertson, E. F., Baghurst, P. A. & Clark, P. D. (1986) The Port Pirie cohort study: maternal blood lead and pregnancy outcome. *Journal of Epidemiology and Community Health*, **40**, 18–25.

McNeil, J. L. & Ptasnik, J. A. (1975) Evaluation of long-term effects of elevated blood lead concentrations in asymptomatic children. In *Recent advances in the assessment of the health effects of environmental pollution*. Vol. 2. Luxembourg: Commission of the European Communities, pp. 571–90.

Mattes, J. A. & Gittelman-Klein, R. (1978) A cross-over study of artificial food colorings in a hyperkinetic child. *American Journal of Psychiatry*, **135**, 987–8.

Mattes, J. A. & Gittelman, R. (1981) Effects of artificial food colorings in children with hyperactive symptoms. *Archives of General Psychiatry*, **38**, 714–8.

Mayron, L. W. (1979) Allergy, learning, and behavior problems. *Journal of Learning Disabilities*, **12**, 32–42.

Naismith, D. J., Nelson, M., Burley, V. J. & Gatenby, S. J. (1988) Can children's intelligence be increased by vitamin and mineral supplements? *The Lancet*, **ii,** 335.

Needleman, H. L. & Bellinger, D. C. (1988) Type II fallacies in the study of childhood exposure to lead at low dose: a critical and quantitative review. In Smith, M. A., Grant, L. D. & Sors, A. E. (eds.) *Lead exposure and child development: an international assessment.* Dordrecht: Kluwer Academic Publishers.

Needleman, H. L., Gunnoe, C., Leviton, A., Reed, R., Peresie, H., Maher, C. & Barratt, P. (1979) Deficits in psychologic and classroom performance of children with elevated dentine lead levels. *New England Journal of Medicine*, **300,** 689–95.

Neuman, I., Elian, R., Nahum, H., Shaked, P. & Creter, D. (1978). The danger of 'yellow dyes' (tartrazine) to allergic subjects. *Clinical Allergy*, **8,** 65–8.

Otto, D. A. (1988) Electrophysiological assessment of sensory and cognitive function in children exposed to lead: a review. In Smith, M. A., Grant, L. D. & Sors, A. E. (eds.) *Lead exposure and child development: an international assessment.* Dordrecht: Kluwer Academic Publishers.

Ouelette, E. M., Rosett, H. L., Rosman, N. P. & Weiner, L. (1977) Adverse effects on offspring of maternal alcohol abuse during pregnancy. *New England Journal of Medicine*, **297,** 528–30.

Plant, M. L. & Plant, M. A. (1987) Family alcohol problems among pregnant women: links with maternal substance use and birth abnormalities. *Drug and Alcohol Dependence*, **20,** 213–9.

Plant, M. L. & Plant, M. A. (1988) Maternal use of alcohol and other drugs during pregnancy and birth abnormalities: further results from a prospective study. *Alcohol and Alcoholism*, **23,** 229–33.

Pocock, S. J., Ashby, D. & Smith, M. A. (1987) Lead exposure and children's intellectual performance. *International Journal of Epidemiology*, **16,** 57–67.

Rapoport, J. & Quinn, P. O. (1975) Minor physical anomalies (stigmata) and early developmental deviation. *International Journal of Mental Health*, **4,** 29–44.

Ratcliffe, J. M. (1977) Developmental and behavioral functions in young children with elevated blood lead levels. *British Journal of Preventive and Social Medicine*, **31,** 258–64.

Rona, R. J. & Chinn, S. (1987) Parents' perceptions of food intolerance in primary school children. *British Medical Journal*, **294,** 863–6.

Rose, T. L. (1978) The functional relationship between artificial food colors and hyperactivity. *Journal of Applied Behavior Analysis*, **11,** 439–46.

Russell, M. & Skinner, J. B. (1988) Early measures of maternal alcohol misuse as predictors of adverse pregnancy outcomes. *Alcoholism*, **12,** 824–30.

Rutter, M. (1980) Raised lead levels and impaired cognitive/behavioral functioning. *Developmental Medicine and Child Neurology* (Suppl.), **42,** 1–26.

Schneider, W. F. (1945) Psychiatric evaluation of the hyperkinetic child. *Journal of Pediatrics*, **26,** 559–70.

Schroeder, S., Hawk, B., Otto, D., Mushak, P. & Hicks, R. (1985) Separating the effects of lead and social factors on IQ. *Environmental Research*, **38,** 144–54.

Shannon, W. R. (1922) Neuropathic manifestations in infants and children as a result of anaphylactic reactions to foods contained in their diet. *American Journal of Diseases of Children*, **24**, 89–94.

Silva, P. A., Hughes, P., Williams, S. & Faed, J. M. (1988) Blood lead, intelligence, reading attainment, and behavior in eleven year old children in Dunedin, New Zealand. *Journal of Child Psychology and Psychiatry*, **29**, 43–52.

Smith, M., Delves, T., Lansdown, R., Clayton, B. & Graham, P. (1983) The effects of lead exposure on urban children: the Institute of Child Health/Southampton study. *Developmental Medicine and Child Neurology* Suppl. 47, **25**(5).

Speer, F. (1954) The allergic tension–fatigue syndrome. *Pediatric Clinics of North America*, **1**, 1029–7.

Streissguth, A. P., Herman, S. C. & Smith, D. W. (1978) Intelligence behaviour and dysmorphogenesis in the fetal alcohol syndrome: a report on 20 patients. *Journal of Pediatrics*, **92**, 363–7.

Streissguth, A. P., Martin, D. C., Barr, H. M. & MacGregor Sandman, B. (1984) Intrauterine alcohol and nicotine exposure: attention and reaction time in 4 year old children. *Developmental Psychology*, **20**, 533–41.

Swanson, J. M. & Kinsbourne, M. (1980) Food dyes impair performance of hyperactive children on a laboratory learning test. *Science*, **207**, 1485–7.

Tarter, R. E., Jacob, T. & Bremer, D. A. (1989) Cognitive status of sons of alcoholic men. *Alcoholism: Clinical and Experimental Research*, **13**, 232–5.

Taylor, E. A. (1986) Causes and development of hyperactive behaviour. In Taylor, E. (ed.) *The overactive child.* Clinics in Developmental Medicine No. 97. London: Mac Keith Press. Oxford: Blackwell Scientific Publications, pp. 118–60.

Taylor, E. A., Sandberg, S. J., Thorley, G. & Giles, S. (1991) *The epidemiology of childhood hyperactivity.* Oxford: Oxford University Press/Maudsley Monographs.

Thomson, G. O. B., Raab, G. M., Hepburn, W. S., Hunter, R., Fulton, M. & Laxen, D. P. H. (1989) Blood-lead levels and children's behaviour – results from the Edinburgh Lead Study. *Journal of Child Psychology and Psychiatry*, **30**, 515–28.

Thorley, G. (1984) A pilot study to assess the behavioural and cognitive effects of food colours in a group of retarded children. *Developmental Medicine and Child Neurology*, **26**, 56–61.

Trites, R. L., Tryphonas, H. & Ferguson, H. B. (1980) Diet treatment for hyperactive children with food allergies. In Knight, R. M. & Bakker, D. (eds.) *Treatment of hyperactive and learning disordered children.* Baltimore: University Park Press, pp. 151–66.

Vivoli, G., Bergomi, M., Borella, P., Fantuzzi, G., Simoni, L., Catelli, D., Sturloni, N., Cavazzuti, G. B., Montorsi, R., Campagna, R., Tampien, A. & Tartoni, P. L. (1988) Evaluation of different biological indicators of lead exposure related to neuropsychological effects in children. In Smith, M. A., Grant, L. D. & Sors, A. E. (eds.) *Lead exposure and child development: an international assessment.* Dordrecht: Kluwer Academic Publishers.

Weiss, B. (1982) Food additives and environmental chemicals as sources of childhood behaviour disorders. *Journal of the American Academy of Child Psychiatry*, **21**, 144–52.

Weiss, B., Williams, J. H., Margen, S., Abrams, B., Caan, B., Citron, L., Cox, C., McKibben, J., Ogar, D. & Schultz, S. (1980) Behavioral response to artificial food colors. *Science*, **207**, 1487–9.

Werner, E. & Smith, R. (1977) *Kauai's children come of age.* Honolulu: University of Hawaii Press.

White, K. R. (1982) The relation between socioeconomic status and academic achievement. *Psychological Bulletin*, **91**, 461–81.

Williams, J. L., Cram, D. M., Tausig, F. T. & Webster, E. (1978) Relative effects of drugs and diet on hyperactive behaviours: an experimental study. *Pediatrics*, **61**, 811–7.

Winneke, G., Hrdina, K.-G. & Brockhaus, A. (1982) Neuropsychological studies in children with elevated tooth lead concentrations. Part I: pilot study. *International Archives of Occupational and Environmental Health*, **51**, 169–83.

Winneke, G., Kramer, U., Brockhaus, A., Ewers, U., Kujanek, G., Lechner, H. & Janke, W. (1983) Neuropsychological studies in children with elevated tooth-lead concentrations. Part II: extended study. *International Archives of Occupational and Environmental Health*, **51**, 231–52.

Yule, W., Lansdown, R., Millar, I. B. & Urbanowicz, M.-A. (1981) The relationship between blood lead concentrations, intelligence and attainment in a school population: a pilot study. *Developmental Medicine and Child Neurology*, **23**, 567–76.

Yule, W., Urbanowicz, M.-A., Lansdown, R. & Millar, I. B. (1984) Teachers' ratings of children's behaviour in relation to blood lead levels. *British Journal of Developmental Psychology*, **2**, 295–305.

9 The long-term psychosocial sequelae of specific developmental disorders of speech and language

MICHAEL RUTTER AND LYNN MAWHOOD

There are many reports that children with specific developmental speech and language disorders show a raised rate of educational retardation, behavioural difficulties and psychiatric problems. There is also increasing evidence that these sequelae may persist long after competence in spoken language has been acquired. In this chapter we review the empirical research findings on these associations in order to consider which features are associated with the greatest psychosocial risk, and to discuss the possible mechanisms involved.

Six main methodological problems bedevil this field of research. First, the groups studied have been quite heterogeneous in both type and severity of speech/language disorder (Bishop & Rosenbloom, 1987). Thus, the disorders investigated have ranged from uncomplicated abnormalities of articulation alone to pervasive disorders of receptive, expressive, and pragmatic language. Second, the investigations have varied widely in the level of detail on individual diagnosis and on the extent to which children with associated handicaps have been excluded. A major limitation in several of the epidemiological studies is that the sequelae of *specific* language deficits cannot be differentiated from those associated with *general* cognitive impairment which include language deficits as part of the overall problem. Accordingly, it is not always possible to determine whether the psychosocial sequelae were a function of associated mental retardation or some underlying medical condition rather than language impairment *per se*. A developmental origin (rather than a postnatally acquired illness or trauma) is usually implied (Benton, 1964), but the aetiology has been left unknown in most cases. Third, some studies concerned clinic samples with unknown referral biases whereas others were epidemiologically based (Stevenson, 1984). Fourth, investigations vary in the extent to which data on psychosocial sequelae have been both standardized and detailed. Fifth, studies differ in the degree to which longitudinal data have been available and statistically utilized in an effective manner. The consequence is that few studies separate the effects of *transient* language delay from those of *persistent* language impairment. Sixth, only some of the projects have used control groups or had general population data that allowed estimation of the degree to which the level of psychosocial disorder in the developmental language disorder was truly significantly raised. No one study adequately meets all the relevant research criteria but we have placed most reliance on those investigations that are methodologically most satisfactory.

The initial findings on associations between language delay and psychosocial disturbance stemmed from cross-sectional studies of clinic samples – either of children referred for speech or language difficulties (Cantwell *et al.*, 1979; Caulfield *et al.*, 1989; Crookes & Green, 1963; Fitzsimons, 1958; Lindholm & Touliatis, 1979; Mykelbust, 1954; Solomon, 1961; Trapp & Evan, 1960), or those seen for psychiatric problems (Chess & Rosenberg, 1974; Cohen *et al.*, 1989; Wing, 1969). These were followed by epidemiological studies which confirmed that the association was not simply a consequence of referral biases (Beitchman *et al.*, 1986, 1987; Drillien & Drummond, 1983; Fundudis *et al.*, 1979; Jenkins *et al.*, 1980; McGee *et al.*, 1984; Rutter *et al.*, 1970; Stevenson & Richman, 1978). Brief reference will be made to these findings but our main focus is on longitudinal studies.

Such studies face a host of methodological difficulties (Weiner, 1985) and no single investigation is free of constraints and limitations. Nevertheless, data are available from several well-planned prospective enquiries. The extent to which they meet a range of important methodological criteria is indicated in Table 9.1, which summarizes the characteristics of follow-up studies undertaken with samples of 15 or more, and which extend to age 7 years or older. The sample size restriction has meant the omission of the Ripley & Lea (1984) follow-up of 14 receptive aphasic children; however, most of these had acquired language disorders. It also leaves out several other informative follow-up studies of small samples (e.g. Petrie, 1975) where the numbers were too few for valid estimates of rates of psychological sequelae. More crucially, it leaves out the systematic longitudinal study undertaken by Tallal *et al.* (1989a), because the published follow-up data do not as yet extend into the school age period. However, because the study raises important issues, its findings are briefly discussed later in the chapter.

The findings in Table 9.1 bring out several important points. First, there are more studies of educational outcome than of emotional/social/behavioural sequelae. However, only a few of the investigations of the scholastic performance of children with a developmental language disorder used adequate controls or adjustment for general intellectual level. Second, most of the behavioural assessments relied on questionnaires or clinical impressions rather than detailed standardized interview measures. Accordingly, there are rather few data on the particular psychopathological problems associated with language

Table 9.1. *Criteria on methodology of longitudinal studies*

(Sample with 15 or more subjects and follow-up to age 7 years or older)

	Criteria								
Study	1	2	3	4	5	6	7	8	9
I. Epidemiological									
Fundudis *et al.* (1979)	+	−	−	+	+	+	+	+	+
Sheridan & Peckham (1975, 1978)	+	+	−	+	−	−	(Q)	+	−
Silva *et al.* (1983, 1984)	+	+	−	+	+	−	(Q)	+	+
Stevenson *et al.* (1985)	−	−	−	+	−	−	(Q)	−	−
II. Clinic studies									
Aram *et al.* (1984)	−	−	+	−	+	+	(Q)	+	+
Baker & Cantwell (1982, 1987 a, b)	−	−	−	−	+	+	+	+	+
Billard *et al.* (1989)	+	−	−	−	+	−	−	+	+
Bishop and colleagues (1987 a, b; 1989; 1990)	+	+	−	+	+	+	−	+	+
De Ajuriaguerra *et al.* (1976)	−	+	−	−	+	−	−	+	−
Debray-Ritzen *et al.* (1976)	+	−	−	−	+	+	−	+	+
Garvey & Gordon (1973)	−	−	−	−	±	−	−	−	+
Griffiths (1969)	+	−	−	−	+	+	−	+	+
Hall & Tomblin (1978)	−	−	+	+	+	−	−	+	+
Huntley *et al.* (1988)	−	−	−	−	+	−	−	+	−
King *et al.* (1982)	−	−	+	−	+	+	−	−	−
Levi *et al.* (1982)	?	−	−	−	+	+	−	+	?
Mason (1967)	−	−	−	+	−	−	−	+	?
Mawhood, L., Rutter, M. & Howlin, P. (unpublished data)	+	+	+	−	+	+	+	+	+
Paul & Cohen (1984)	−	−	+	−	+	+	(Q)	+	+
Stark *et al.* (1984)	+	−	−	±	+	−	−	+	+

Note: (Q) = questionnaire assessment only;
+ = definitely meets specified criterion;
− = does not meet specified criterion;
± = partially meets specified criterion;
? = not known.

Criteria

1 = At least 70% sample studied.
2 = Data from three or more time points.
3 = Follow-up into adult life.
4 = Normal control group.
5 = Detailed initial assessment of speech/language.
6 = Comparison of different types of language/speech disorder.
7 = Systematic standardized assessment of psychological abnormalities (at follow-up).
8 = Systematic standardized assessment of intellectual/educational level (at follow-up).
9 = Associated handicaps, including mental handicap, taken into account or excluded.

delay. Third, detailed initial assessments of speech and language were usually available in the studies of clinic samples but not in the epidemiological studies; conversely, few of the clinic studies used control groups. All the epidemiological studies had comparable follow-up data on children without an intial language delay but few sought to match the groups on other relevant variables. Fourth, most of the clinic studies had data missing on at least 30% of the group, with consequent uncertainties on the extent to which the findings may have been biased or unrepresentative. Fifth, very few studies have used data from three or more time points so that little is known on developmental course (as distinct from outcome). Finally, there is least information available on psychosocial functioning in adult life. It is because of this, that we discuss our own findings at greater length than might otherwise be warranted. With these methodological cautions in mind, the findings on different aspects of psychosocial outcome may be considered in more detail.

COURSE OF LANGUAGE DEVELOPMENT

The first issue necessarily concerns the extent to which early language deficits persist as children grow older. It may reasonably be assumed that some, perhaps many, instances of delay in acquiring spoken language represent no more than normal variations (in extreme cases the delay may be thought of as a 'maturational lag'). Just as normal children vary greatly in the age when teeth erupt or when puberty is reached, so children are likely to vary in the age when they first begin to speak. These differences in maturational timing may have important psychosocial consequences (they do, for example, in the case of puberty: Brooks-Gunn & Petersen, 1984; Clausen, 1975; Magnusson *et al.*, 1986), but the sequelae arise as a result of the sociocultural meaning of variations in timing rather than through biological risk stemming from some underlying neurodevelopmental disorder. At the other extreme, it is clear that some cases of marked language delay reflect pathology, in some cases due to a known medical condition such as a chromosomal abnormality (Walzer, 1985) and in other cases inferred rather than proven. Few would doubt that there are these two broad classes of language delay but their differentiation at an individual level has proved somewhat difficult (Bishop & Rosenbloom, 1987; Stark *et al.*, 1983).

The best data in early childhood are provided by Bishop & Edmundson (1987a, b) who undertook a prospective longitudinal study of 87 four-year-old children with a marked language impairment, together with a cross-sectional control group. All but 2 of the 87 children had a score on at least one language measure below the 3rd percentile with no more than one score (out of 9) above the 10th percentile;

thus, they comprised a group with a clinically significant severe delay. Nineteen of the 87 children had a non-verbal score on the Leiter more than two standard deviations below the mean; they were termed a 'general delay' group, with the remainder termed 'specific delay'. At follow-up at $5\frac{1}{2}$ years, 44% (30 out of 68) of the former and 11% (2 out of 19) of the latter no longer met the above criteria for severe language impairment. This relatively 'good outcome' group was closely similar to controls in language functioning at $5\frac{1}{2}$ years (although the mean scores tended to be marginally lower). Further follow-up at 8 years of age (Bishop & Adams, 1990) confirmed this separation of groups. The children with a 'good outcome' at $5\frac{1}{2}$ years continued to progress and at 8 years their language skills were only slightly below those of controls, with a mean standard score of 96.5 on the British Picture Vocabulary Scale (BPVS) and 91.7 on the Test for Reception of Grammar (TROG). By contrast, the 'poor outcome' group continued to show very substantial language impairment, their standard score on the BPVS being 83.6 and on TROG 81.1. Not surprisingly, the 'general delay' group showed even greater language impairment.

The highest proportion of 'good' outcomes (78%) was for the children with a pure phonological impairment and the lowest (0%) was for children with global language impairment associated with a non-verbal IQ below 70. Within the middle range, prognosis was best for children with a narrow range of language functions impaired and with a milder degree of impairment. Thus, a persistent language deficit is predicted by both the severity and the breadth of the language deficit at 4 years of age.

It has sometimes been thought that persistent language disorders should differ from transient ones in terms of their *patterns* of language, with the persistent group being more likely to show unusual or deviant patterns. That was not found in the Bishop & Edmundson study (1987a, b). In particular, a general language impairment tended to have a much worse prognosis than an impairment in just one or two aspects of language. Thus, deviance in terms of a specificity of impairment (i.e. one aspect of language 'out of step' with others) is *not* an indicator of a poor prognosis. On the other hand, qualitatively abnormal features of language or an association with social abnormalities or with neuro-developmental impairment (such as shown by perceptuo-motor difficulties) may indicate a more persistent disorder (Bishop & Edmundson, 1987b; Paul *et al.*, 1983; Stark *et al.*, 1984); the possibility remains to be tested systematically. Both Paul *et al.* (1983) and Griffiths (1969) reported that the small group of children with a severe impairment in receptive language did particularly badly. Silva *et al.* (1983) also showed in the Dunedin longitudinal study that a persistence of language delay is especially likely when the language deficit is associated with low intelligence.

Further follow-up data were provided by Baker & Cantwell (1987b) in their study of a (somewhat unrepresentative) subsample of children from a community speech and hearing clinic. Approximately a quarter showed no disorder of speech or language when seen some 3 years later at a mean age of 9 years (range 6 to 20 years) but the remainder exhibited continuing problems. Auditory processing and language usage defiicts were particularly prominent. Similarly, Stark *et al.* (1984), in their follow-up of language-impaired children of normal IQ from a mean age of 6½ to 10 years, found that about a quarter had caught up in language but the overall mean level of language was still over 2 years retarded.

Our own follow-up (L. Mawhood, M. Rutter & P. Howlin, unpublished data) into the adult life of boys of normal non-verbal intelligence with a severe developmental receptive language disorder, showed that their language complexity as perceived by their family was normal in two-thirds of cases, although only half were thought to have normal conversational skills in adult life. Half showed some abnormality in articulation. Also, half showed prosodic oddities in terms of limited variations in pitch or tone with speech that was somewhat flat, exaggerated, slow, fast, jerky or unusual in volume. Scores on the BPVS showed that all were performing below the ceiling (19 years 6 months) and half had an age equivalent of 12 years or less. Thus, although most children with a developmental language disorder eventually go on to acquire adequate spoken language, among those with initially severe language deficits most continue to show some form of language deficit in adult life which, although usually mild, is sufficient to be evident to others. Bishop & Edmundson (1987b) found that the rate of progress in language development in the preschool years did not clearly differentiate those with poor and good outcomes. However, the finding that many children with severe developmental language disorders never attain fully normal language clearly indicates that a 'maturational lag' explanation cannot apply to them (see above).

An indication of the presence of broader cognitive deficits in many children with a severe developmental language disorder is provided by the relatively high proportion who show cognitive impairment on language-related tasks as they grow older. Thus, in Aram *et al.*'s (1984) group of 16 with a Leiter IQ of 70+ when tested as preschoolers, 5 had a Wechsler full-scale IQ in adolescence at least 14 points below their initial IQ and none showed a rise as great as that. In part this may reflect a change in test content, but even so on the performance scale 4 out of 16 showed a drop of at least 14 points, with only 2 showing a rise of similar magnitude. Adult follow-up data from Hall & Tomblin (1978) indicated that even after language develops, verbal cognitive deficits often remain. In their language-impaired group the mean verbal scale IQ on the WAIS (Wechsler Adult Intelligence Scale) was 88 compared with a mean of 109 on the performance scale. This difference was not evident in those with articulation problems alone (110 vs 108). Stark *et al.*'s (1984) language-impaired group had a mean verbal IQ of 87 as compared with a mean performance IQ of 102 at the age of 10 years. Similarly, in our own follow-up of boys of normal non-verbal IQ with a developmental disorder of receptive language, the mean WISC (Wechsler Intelligence Scale for Children) performance IQ in middle childhood was 96 compared with a mean of 108 on Raven's Matrices when first tested in early childhood (Cantwell *et al.*, 1989). In adult life the mean WAIS verbal scale IQ was 75 and the mean performance scale 78 (L. Mawhood, M. Rutter & P. Howlin, unpublished data). Fundudis *et al.* (1979) found that their group of children with specific speech delay had a mean verbal IQ of 84 compared with a performance IQ of 99 on the WISC (their control group had scores of 93 and 101 respectively).

As their name implies, developmental disorders of language are usually conceptualized in terms of a 'pure' language deficit. However, Tallal and her colleagues have shown that the language problems tend to be associated with perceptual-motor impairments and especially with difficulties in temporal sequencing (see Tallal, 1985). Similarly, Bishop & Edmundson (1987b) noted close links between motor and language development, and Stark *et al.* (1983) found that the degree of perceptual-motor impairment predicted language outcome. Children with language disorders have been shown to have deficits in representational or symbolic thinking (Kahmi *et al.*, 1984; Morehead & Ingram, 1973), associative imagery and short-term memory (Eisenson, 1968; Graham, 1974; Masland & Case, 1968; Menyuk, 1969), auditory processing (Tallal, 1976; Tallal & Piercy, 1975) and sequencing (Efron, 1963; Poppen *et al.*, 1969). On this basis, Tallal has argued that temporal perceptual-motor dysfunction (rather than language problems *per se*) may account for the association with psychopathology (see below).

It might also be supposed that a strong family history of language delay could be relevant. There is evidence that developmental language disorders are associated with a familial loading for speech delay (Robinson, 1987; Tallal *et al.*, 1989b; Tomblin, 1989) and it has been thought that, at least in part, this represents genetic mediation. However, the genetic inference remains untested (there are difficulties in testing due to the much increased rate of language delay in twins compared with singletons – Rutter *et al.*, 1990) and it is not known whether the familial loading mainly applies to extreme normal variations in language development or to more pathological varieties of language delay. Bishop & Edmundson (1987b) found that a familial loading was somewhat more common in children with a worse outcome at $5\frac{1}{2}$ years but the difference fell short of statistical significance.

It is clear that much remains to be learned on the factors associated with the course of language development in children with developmental language disorders. Nevertheless, in considering psychosocial sequelae, it is apparent that it will be necessary to determine the effects of persistence of language impairment, the severity and breadth of the language deficit, associated low IQ and associated perceptual-motor and other neurodevelopmental problems.

READING AND OTHER SCHOLASTIC DIFFICULTIES

Numerous other studies have documented the findings that children with developmental language disorders have a substantially increased risk for later reading difficulties (Aram & Nation, 1980; Billard *et al.*, 1989; Debray-Ritzen *et al.*, 1976; Fundudis *et al.*, 1979; Garvey & Gordon, 1973; Griffiths, 1969; Ingram, 1963; Levi *et al.*, 1982; Mason, 1967; Shriberg & Kwiatkowski, 1988; Silva *et al.*, 1983; Stark *et al.*, 1984; Urwin *et al.*, 1988). Six main issues arise from this finding: (a) whether the scholastic risk is mainly a function of general intellectual impairment or a specific language deficit; (b) whether the risk is specifically for reading difficulties or more generally for a broad range of scholastic problems; (c) which types of speech/language deficit lead to the greatest scholastic risk; (d) whether the scholastic risk associated with a specific language disorder differs in degree or pattern from that associated with developmental disorders of non-language functions (such as motor or perceptual skills); (e) following the last point, whether the risk stems from the fact that language as such is impaired or from neurodevelopmental or cognitive deficits that may underlie the language disorder; and (f) whether the risk applies only when there is persistent language impairment or whether it applies also to transient language difficulties. These points are discussed more fully in this and the following sections.

Both epidemiological and clinical studies have shown that much of the scholastic risk stems from general intellectual impairment but, nevertheless, that reading difficulties arise with an increased frequency even when intellectual level has been taken into account. Thus, Silva *et al.* (1984), using data from the Dunedin epidemiological/longitudinal study, reported that the mean full-scale WISC IQ for children with a language score at or below the 5th percentile at age 3, 5 or 7 years (amounting to just less than 6% of children) was 93. Within this group, those with an IQ of 90 or greater still had a reading delay of about 4 months at 7 years of age. Aram *et al.* (1984) found that of 16 children with language delay and an IQ within the normal range, two-thirds had required special tutoring or had repeated one or more school grades by adolescence. Of the 11 with an initial IQ of at least 90, 5 were in the lowest decile for at least one subject out of reading, spelling and mathematics. It was notable, however, that the scholastic difficulties were as evident in mathematics as in reading or spelling. Stark *et al.* (1984), in their follow-up of language-impaired children attending a special class, found that at 10 years of age, 23 out of 29 had reading scores at least two grades below age level. Similarly, in Debray-Ritzen *et al.*'s (1976) sample of language-delayed children of normal intelligence, over two-thirds had reading difficulties. Billard *et al.* (1989), in their follow-up of 20 language-delayed children with a WISC performance IQ of at least 70, also found that the great majority had reading difficulties.

Fundudis *et al.* (1979), in their follow-up of a general population sample of children with a specific speech delay, found that they had a mean reading quotient of 83 compared with 94 for the control groups. This difference was maintained after controlling for differences in social background.

Richman *et al.* (1983), in their general population study, categorized language delayed at 3 years on the basis of an expressive language age on the Reynell scales at least 6 months below chronological age. At 8 years, half the language delay group had a spelling age below 80 months (compared with 23% of controls), and 41% had a reading accuracy age below 80 months (compared with 14% of controls). However, although only 2 out of 22 children had a full-scale IQ below 70, 36% had a full-scale IQ below 85 (compared with 4% of controls). Unfortunately, it was not determined whether language delay still predicted reading/spelling difficulties after IQ was taken into account.

Hall & Tomblin (1978), in their follow-up into adult life of 18 language-impaired and 18 articulation-impaired children with an IQ of 80 or more and from predominantly middle class families, found that the former group had a mean reading score half a standard deviation below the mean and a mean mathematics score approximately at the mean. The articulation group, by contrast, had scores for reading and mathematics well above the mean (plus a half to three quarters of a standard deviation). In our own follow-up into adult life of boys of initially normal IQ with a developmental disorder of receptive language, 8 out of 19 had a reading comprehension score with an age equivalent at or below 10 years, on oral reading 9 out of 19 were at or below this level, and on spelling it was 12 out of 19 (L. Mawhood, M. Rutter & P. Howlin, unpublished data). None had passed any national examinations at school, although 2 had later obtained City and Guild certificates in technical subjects. The assessment of performance in mathematics was less thorough. However, the arithmetic subtest score on the WAIS scale was one and a half standard deviations below the mean. This indicated a deficit in areas of scholastic achievement outside of reading and spelling, but the arithmetic performance was not markedly discrepant from that expected on the basis of the level of IQ in adult life. As already noted, this was well below that in early and middle childhood.

Crookes & Green (1963) found that reading difficulties were similarly affected in language-impaired children and in those with pure articulation problems but arithmetical difficulties were greater in the former group. However, Levi *et al.* (1982) found that reading difficulties at 7 years were more frequent in children with semantic–syntactic problems (unfortunately, it is not stated whether the groups differed in IQ). Huntley *et al.* (1988) in a follow-up of children who had been in a language intervention programme found mild scholastic deficits in relation to performance IQ but scores were not much below verbal IQ. Attainment was worse in reading and spelling than in mathematics. Debray-Ritzen *et al.* (1976) found that reading problems were most frequent in children with global language impairment and least frequent in those with isolated difficulties in articulation.

Much the most thorough analysis has been undertaken by Bishop & Adams (1990), with most informative findings. They compared the reading/spelling attainments at 8 years of children with 'resolved', or transient, specific language impairment (the children with a 'good outcome' at $5\frac{1}{2}$ – see above), those with 'persistent' specific language impairment (SLI), those with a general language delay and controls. All the first three groups had shown a clinically significant language deficit at age 4 years. In keeping with other investigations, 17 (20.7%) out of the 82 children with some form of initial language deficit showed specific reading retardation at 8 years (defined in terms of accuracy or comprehension more than 1.96 standard deviations below the level predicted on the basis of two subsets of the WISC IQ test); the comparable figure for controls was only 4.6%. However, a more detailed analysis brought out five important findings: (a) reading difficulties were evident in the persistent SLI but *not* in the resolved SLI group (a mean reading comprehension standard score of 84.0 versus 102.0; the mean score in the control group was 97.9 and in the general delay group it was 72.6); (b) the deficits applied as much to reading comprehension and spelling as to reading accuracy (mean standard scores of 84.0, 83.0 and 89.0 respectively in the persistent SLI group); (c) the persistent SLI group showed nonverbal as well as verbal deficits; thus, their mean standard scores on the two performance subtests of the WISC, block design and picture completion, were 91.5 and 94.1 respectively; (d) when intellectual level was taken into account, it was evident that the association between language impairment and reading skills was largely confined to reading comprehension; (e) phonological (articulation) impairment showed only a very weak association with reading/spelling difficulties. However, very few of the phonological problems persisted in the absence of a broader language impairment.

We may conclude that, even when there is normal non-verbal intelligence, severe developmental language disorders tend to be followed by substantial difficulties in reading comprehension and spelling. However, this risk is largely confined to the group of children with *persistent* language impairment, which frequently is associated with verbal cognitive defiicts. Scholastic progress can be expected to be normal in most instances when children have 'caught up' in their language development by the time they start school. Particularly in early childhood, but to some extent later too, there may also be poor performance in mathematics. However, on the whole, the deficits in reading and spelling tend to be both more severe and more persistent than those in mathematics. Research findings are consistent in showing that scholastic difficulties are much greater when the developmental disorder involves receptive or expressive language than when there is only an abnormality of articulation; however, findings are contradictory on whether there is any scholastic risk in the latter group once IQ and social background have been taken into account. We may tentatively conclude that the main scholastic risk occurs when phonological difficulties are associated with a broader language impairment; that there is little or no risk when articulation skills have largely resolved by the time of starting school; but that there may be some scholastic risk with very persistent phonological problems. We have been unable to find any investigations that have directly compared language disorders with perceptual-motor (or other non-language) developmental disorders. However, studies of clumsy children (Henderson & Hall, 1982) do not seem to show any marked increase in reading difficulties. Also, the Rourke & Strang (1983) studies of learning disabled children showed that those with reading difficulties tended to have verbal deficits whereas those with mathematical difficulties tended to have visuo-spatial deficits.

Although the data are too sparse and too unsystematic for firm conclusions, it appears that the scholastic risk associated with language delay is mainly (but not exclusively) for reading and spelling difficulties, and that this pattern probably also differs from that found with developmental disorders of non-language functions. Data that could separate the risks for language deficits *per se* from those associated with the postulated neurodevelopmental or cognitive impairment are lacking. Such a differentiation would in any case be difficult because marked language difficulties tend to be accompanied by deficits in verbal intelligence and by evidence of broader neurodevelopmental impairment. Nevertheless, the apparent difference in scholastic functioning between children with language disorders and those with perceptual-motor deficits suggests that the involvement of language, and of associated verbal cognitive deficits, is important in determining the pattern, and possibly the severity, of scholastic difficulties.

SOCIO-EMOTIONAL–BEHAVIOURAL DISORDERS IN CHILDHOOD

Numerous studies attest to the raised frequency of psychopathological problems in children with development disorders of speech and language (Baker & Cantwell, 1982; Beitchman *et al.*, 1986; Fundudis *et al.*, 1979; Jenkins *et al.*, 1980; Silva *et al.*, 1984; Stevenson *et al.*, 1985). Issues somewhat similar to those already discussed with respect to scholastic problems apply, but in addition there are a number of other considerations. Tallal *et al.*, (1989a) argued on the basis of their Achenbach Child Behavior Checklist findings at age 4 years that the raised scores in the language delayed group largely reflected neuro-developmental impairment rather than emotional disturbance. This was because items such as 'clumsy', 'confused', and 'can't concentrate' differentiated the groups. However, in males, 'cries too much' and 'clings to adults', and, in girls, 'withdrawn', 'secretive' and 'compulsions' also did so. The point raised is an important one but it is necessary to turn to findings on older age groups to test the hypothesis.

At age 5 years, in their community study using the Conners scale, Beitchman *et al.* (1986) found that speech/language impaired boys differed from controls on conduct disturbance and girls did so on 'anxious-passive' and 'day dreams'. Clinical diagnoses showed an excess of attention deficit disorders (although the Conners scores showed no significant difference on the hyperactivity factor) and of emotional disturbance. At 7 years, Fundudis *et al.* (1979) in the Newcastle epidemiological/longitudinal study found that children who had been speech retarded had only a non-significant increase on the teacher questionnaire measure of behavioural deviance and a trend towards increased introversion. On the other hand, in the Waltham Forest epidemiological/longitudinal study, Stevenson *et al.* (1985) found an *increase* in emotional/behavioural disturbance between 3 and 8 years in children with low language scores at 3 years. Of the children with a language delay at 3 years, 18% showed emotional disturbance as judged from parental questionnaire at age 8 years (versus 0% in controls); the comparable figures on the teacher questionnaire were 25% versus 15%. The language delay group showed no increase in conduct disturbance (Richman *et al.*, 1983). Silva *et al.* (1984), in the Dunedin epidemiological/longitudinal study, found a significantly raised rate of teacher-reported problems in their delayed-speech normal-IQ group but the increase on the parent scale fell short of significance.

There are considerable difficulties in resolving these differences in findings because studies have varied greatly in their definitions of developmental speech/language disorder and in their measures of psychopathology. That the latter is likely to influence results was evident in Caulfield *et al.*'s (1989) findings that observations revealed differences not evident on parental reports, and in the findings from the Beitchman *et al.* (1986) epidemiological study. On questionnaire designations of deviance the case:control ratio (pooling sexes) was about 1.5, whereas on clinical appraisal it was 4.1, with about half the speech/language children showing some form of psychiatric disorder. This proportion is almost exactly the same as that found in the Baker & Cantwell (1982 & 1987a, b) and Griffiths (1969) clinic studies (which lacked control groups). The clinic case–control studies of Fitzsimons (1958) and Solomon (1961), although not based on standardized measures, also showed higher rates of peer relationship difficulties and anxiety symptoms. Ingram (1959), too, reported that psychiatric problems mainly involved social difficulties or anxiety disorders. Thus, as judged by all available data, the main increase in psychopathology seems to be in the domains of anxiety, social relationships and attention-deficit problems rather than in conduct disturbance or antisocial behaviour.

The few follow-up data available suggest that psychopathological problems tend to increase, rather than diminish, as children grow older. Thus, Baker & Cantwell (1987b) in their follow-up of clinic children found that the proportion with psychiatric disorder rose from 44% to 60%. A quarter of the sample were without disorder at the time of initial appraisal but developed a disorder during the follow-up period, whereas only 8% of the sample had a disorder when young and became well when older. Of the 72 children who developed psychopathology during the follow-up, 38 showed an attention deficit disorder and 20 some type of anxiety disorder. In our own follow-up, 35% showed poor peer relations in early childhood but 50% did so in middle childhood (Cantwell *et al.*, 1989), and in adult life 70% showed impaired social functioning (L. Mawhood, M. Rutter & P. Howlin, unpublished data).

It may be concluded that it is extremely unlikely that the socio-emotional difficulties consistently found to be raised in individuals with speech/language impairment are simply reflecting *direct* manifestations of neurodevelopmental impairment, as suggested by Tallal *et al.* (1989a). The increase is not just in terms such as inattention or clumsiness, but also in anxiety and poor peer relations. Whether or not the socio-emotional difficulties stem specifically from speech/language impairment *per se* or more generally from neurodevelopmental or cognitive deficits that may underlie the language delay is another matter. Systematic comparisons with other types of specific developmental disorder are lacking and are much needed. Without them, it cannot be known whether the psychopathological risk with language delay differs in severity or type with that associated with, say, the clumsy child syndrome.

There are, however, some data showing the relative risk with different types of speech/language disorder. Baker & Cantwell (1987b), Beitchman *et al.* (1989a, b) and Silva *et al.* (1984), found that psychopathological problems were more frequent if language delay was accompanied by lower than average intelligence; similarly, Fundudis *et al.* (1979) reported that disturbance was greater when speech delay was associated with motor delay (implying a greater likelihood of intellectual or general developmental impairment). However, several studies have shown that emotional and social problems are common even in children with speech/language impairment whose IQ is in the normal range (Baker & Cantwell, 1982, 1987a, b; Beitchman *et al.*, 1986; Cantwell *et al.*, 1989; Griffiths, 1969; Ingram, 1959; L. Mawhood, M. Rutter & P. Howlin, unpublished data; Solomon, 1961). Within that group, the psychopathological risk tends to be greater when there is a deficit in language (especially involving comprehension) and not just an articulation problem, and when there is some impairment in cognitive functioning (Baker & Cantwell, 1987b; Beitchman *et al.*, 1989a, b). Findings are contradictory on whether the risk is substantially increased in children with a pure phonological (articulation) problem. However, it seems that this group is mainly at risk for emotional problems and 'immaturity' rather than attention deficit disorders. Unfortunately, the published studies do not include multivariate analyses that have separated the risks associated with the pattern of speech/language disability, those stemming from the severity of cognitive impairment, and those deriving from neurodevelopmental impairment outside language. This is particularly necessary as the three are intercorrelated.

So far as we know, there are no direct comparisons of language and non-language developmental disorders with respect to psychopathological sequelae. However, Rourke (1988) has compared verbal and visuo-spatial varieties of learning disability with the findings that socio-emotional disturbances involving anxiety and depression are more commonly associated with the latter type. The possibility that the psychopathological sequelae of specific developmental disorders vary according to whether language or visuo-spatial functions are involved warrants further study.

Most reports have focussed on common psychopathological problems but there is evidence that at least severe disorders of receptive language are also associated with risks for serious social abnormalities and for later psychoses. Paul *et al.* (1983; Paul & Cohen, 1984), in their study of a severely affected clinic sample (many of whom were also mentally retarded), noted that half showed autistic-like social abnormalities (although they did not meet the usual diagnostic criteria for autism). Our own follow-up into adult life of boys of normal non-verbal IQ with severe receptive language difficulties similarly showed that even by their mid-twenties only a quarter had developed normal friendships and over a third had never had a peer relationship involving selectivity and sharing (L. Mawhood, M. Rutter & P. Howlin, unpublished data). Similarly, half had never had a girlfriend (or a close homosexual relationship) and only 15% were married. These findings raise the question of whether it is helpful to consider the association with social difficulties in terms of risk for psychiatric disorder. In most instances in our samples, the affected individuals did not exhibit a behavioural pattern that fitted any accepted psychiatric diagnoses. It is not possible from other published papers (see above) to determine whether this also applied as the structured instruments that were used were designed specifically to make psychiatric diagnoses.

In addition, out of our sample of 20 boys with a severe developmental disorder of receptive language and 5 with a similar disorder involving some autistic features, 3 developed florid paranoid psychoses in late adolescence (2 from the former group and 1 from the latter). There were no cases of psychosis from the similarly studied autistic group (L. Mawhood, M. Rutter & P. Howlin, unpublished data). A large scale follow-up into adult life by S. Goode & M. Rutter (unpublished data) of over a hundred children with autism diagnosed according to Rutter's (1978) criterion has also revealed no instances of schizophrenic-type disorders. On the other hand, there are occasional reports in the literature of schizophrenia arising in individuals thought to show autism (Watkins *et al.*, 1988; Howells & Guirguis, 1984; Petty *et al.*, 1984). Our data suggest that this outcome is found only in individuals with *atypical* autistic syndromes and not in those with the characteristic autistic pattern as usually diagnosed. Also, of course, it is well recognized that some cases of schizophrenia are preceded by developmental problems, although typically not in language alone (Rutter & Garmezy, 1983). It is not known what differentiates this group from other cases of schizophrenia. Lewis & Mezey (1985) reported six cases in which a cavum septum pellucidum was found with the combination of early developmental abnormalities (usually including but confined to language) and the emergence of a paranoid psychosis in late adolescence or early adult life. The finding awaits replication.

There has been scarcely any research into the mechanisms underlying these psychopathological associations. Howlin & Rutter (1987) suggested that several needed consideration. First, it was possible that, in some cases, common antecedents might explain both the language delay and the associated psychopathology (Cantwell & Baker, 1977). Such antecedents include low IQ, temperamental difficulty, neurodevelopmental impairment and family disadvantage or psychosocial deprivation. Second, that speech/language disability may predispose to social or emotional problems because of the child's difficulties in communication or because language oddities increase the risk of social rejection. Third, the scholastic problems that frequently follow language delay may create their own risks as a result of the stresses associated with educational failure (Yule & Rutter, 1985). Fourth, the social impairments found in early childhood (Siegal *et al.*, 1985) may constitute an intrinsic part of the language disorder, with both the language delay and the social impairment stemming from some underlying specific cognitive deficit. Finally, the language delay and the later psychopathology may be different manifestations of the same constitutional liability. This may be the case, for example, in the links between early developmental delay and the emergence of schizophrenia in late adolescence or early adult life.

It is obvious that we lack adequate data to test these competing alternative explanations. However, it may be assumed that no one mechanism is likely to explain all the psychopathologial associations. Tentatively, it may be suggested that the link with schizophreniform psychoses may stem from a genetic liability that underlies both, perhaps with some risk added by prenatal/perinatal complications (Murray *et al.*, 1989). It is not as yet known what distinguishes those language disorders that are associated with schizophrenia. Our data indicate that it is exceedingly rare for them to fulfil the traditional diagnostic criteria for autism but equally our data, as well as those of others (Hanson *et al.*, 1976), suggest that the developmental disorders that lead onto schizophrenia are usually accompanied by substantial social difficulties. Usually, too, the developmental delay is not restricted to language.

As indicated above, the highly persistent social deficits that are seen with some severe disorders of receptive language probably constitute a basic part of the same communication disorder. In these cases, it is likely that both the language and the social deficits are associated with a broader pattern of cognitive impairment (in spite of a normal nonverbal IQ).

Perhaps some of the attention deficit disorders seen in language-impaired children stem from an underlying neurodevelopmental disorder rather than from language difficulties as such. If so, they should prove to be equally common in *non*-language developmental disorders.

Possibly, the anxiety disorders are those most likely to stem from the stressful social sequelae of language impairment, although it may well be that some constitute an element in the hypothesized basic social deficits noted above.

OUTCOME IN ADULT LIFE

Reference has been made already to some of the findings in adult life but some further points need to be made. Our findings showed that by their mid-twenties only a quarter were living independently away from parents; 13 out of 20 were still in the parental home and 2 lived in a sheltered (but semi-autonomous) apartment. Only 2 out of 20 had any type of vocational qualification (none received professional training) or tertiary academic education. Nevertheless, despite this, most were in some form of employment at follow-up (during a period when unemployment in the United Kingdom was exceptionally high). Out of the 20 subjects, 12 were in regular paid jobs (10 in unskilled or semiskilled jobs); 2 were in sheltered jobs or performing voluntary work; 2 attended adult training centres for the mentally handicapped; and 4 were out of work at the time (although all 4 had previously held jobs). At first sight, this work situation seems quite encouraging given the severity of the initial language disorder. However, closer examination of their work histories showed that difficulties were quite common. A third (35%) had been in continuous (or almost continuous) paid employment; a third (30%), despite having at least one period of employment lasting a year, had had long periods out of work or in temporary jobs; a quarter (25%) had only ever had brief temporary jobs and 10% had never had paid employment. The reasons given for the work difficulties varied; they included both social problems and an inability to cope satisfactorily with work demands.

As already noted, over half the group had substantial deficits in their social relationships, both in terms of same-sex friendships and love relationships (heterosexual or homosexual). Only a third showed normal functioning in both types of relationships and a third lacked any form of adequate relationship in either. It might be supposed that this lack reflected either lack of opportunity or shyness stemming from earlier communication problems, but this didn't seem to be so. Of the 7 men who had no friends of any type, 4 expressed no unhappiness about their situation and even the 3 who said they would like social contacts did not express this in terms of loneliness. Over half the group had experienced marked teasing when younger but it was currently a serious difficulty for only 2 men. Reports from parents (or other close relatives) indicated that about a third seemed to have difficulty appreciating other people's feelings. The pattern of these findings strongly suggested that, at least in many cases, the relationship difficulties stemmed from a basic social deficit rather than from shyness or social sensitivity. There was a trend for these social difficulties to be greater in those individuals whose language/communicative functioning was reported to be poorer in adult life but there was not a significant association with scores on the BPVS.

CHALLENGES FOR THE FUTURE: THE ROLE OF LONGITUDINAL STUDIES

It is clear that many key issues have yet to be resolved. There is no doubt that the presence of a specific delay in the development of speech and language is associated with a substantial increase in the risk for a range of psychosocial disorders, not only in early childhood at the time when language impairment is most evident but also in later childhood and adolescence and even adult life. What is much less well-understood is which mechanisms and processes are involved. It may be accepted that it is extremely unlikely that any single explanation will be found. Thus, we have to account for the continuities between language delay and later reading comprehension and spelling difficulties – a link that may well reflect shared underlying cognitive deficits. Then, there is the association with a range of non-specific emotional and behavioural problems – an association that may involve interconnected temperamental adversities and family disadvantage as well as the social sequelae of communication difficulties. However, the long-term limitations in social relationships that are still manifest in early adult life seem to require reference to more basic deficits that span language and socialization. This issue raises crucial questions about the classification of developmental language disorders. Are the persistent social sequelae, for example, explicable in terms of semantic–pragmatic deficits rather than syntactic or articulation difficulties? The extent to which semantic–pragmatic deficits constitute a distinctive syndrome remains uncertain but the inappropriate conversational features that create the impression of oddness (Bishop & Adams, 1989) could well have social implications. The possibility certainly warrants study (Bishop & Rosenbloom, 1987; Rapin & Allen, 1983, 1987). Or does the differentiation need to be in terms of medical or neuropathological or genetic distinctions? Finally, it appears that some forms of language delay carry an increased risk for the development of schizophrenia and schizophreniform conditions arising in late adolescence or early adult life. Does this reflect a risk stemming from early language delay or deviance *per se*, or from an underlying neurodevelopmental or genetic abnormality that just happens to involve language problems? Until recently, risk processes have generally been studied just in terms of the number and severity of risk variables. However, it has become apparent that with most risk factors there is huge individual variability in outcome. In recent times, there has been a growing awareness that some of this variability may reflect protective mechanisms as well as risk processes (Rutter, 1987, 1989). Which protective mechanisms operate to foster normal psychosocial development in children with language delay? We do not yet know the answers to these difficult, but fundamental, questions. In looking ahead to the future, we need to consider the particular role of longitudinal studies.

Obviously, there will continue to be a most important role for cross-sectional and retrospective research. Much remains to be done, for example, in sorting out the classification of developmental language disorders and, in particular, in taking further the study of possible connections between the types of language or speech abnormality as considered in a psycholinguistic framework and the types as considered from a medical or aetiological perspective (Bishop & Rosenbloom, 1987). Also, in charting the territory of associations between early language delay and later psychosocial sequelae, retrospective studies will continue to be highly informative. Nevertheless, for certain sorts of questions, longitudinal studies are absolutely essential. Weiner (1985) has pointed out the numerous methodological and practical difficulties inherent in the longitudinal study of uncommon disorders. These difficulties are real enough but they should not be exaggerated, as numerous investigators have shown that it is possible to accumulate sizeable samples of well studied subjects and to follow their development over periods of decades. Some of the particular strengths of longitudinal studies may be summarized as follows.

First, they are crucial for the investigation of time relationships. This is because, although people are quite good at remembering *whether* they have experienced major problems, they are much less good at recalling *when* these happened. The value of prospective data in this connection is illustrated by the Stevenson *et al.* (1985) finding that language-impaired children who did *not* show emotional/behavioural disturbance at 3 years of age, had a substantially increased risk of such disturbance at age 8 years.

Second, longitudinal data are essential for elucidation of the particular features of language delay that carry an increased risk for later psychosocial problems. Adolescents and young adults with disorders, as well as normal controls, are quite likely to remember that they were slow in gaining speech but ordinarily they will not be able to report the relative extent to which their language impairment involved syntactic, semantic, pragmatic and prosodic difficulties. Of course, reference to contemporaneous clinic records may provide what is needed but, usually, routine (non-research) records will prove to be too variable in quality and comparability for this to be a truly effective solution. The advantage of prospective designs is that discriminating, standardized, quantified measurement of different elements of speech and language is readily possible. The prospective longitudinal study undertaken by Bishop and her colleagues (Bishop & Edmundson 1987 a, b; Bishop & Adams, 1989) illustrates these advantages very well, as does the Baker & Cantwell (1982, 1987b) study and our own.

Third, prospective designs are needed for the assessment of postulated mediating variables such as temperamental difficulty, auditory processing, or metacognitive deficits that are most unlikely to have been assessed systematically in routine clinical care and cannot readily be recalled because the individuals will not have had adequate awareness of these aspects of their problems. The Tallal *et al.* (1989a) study exemplifies the potential of longitudinal data for this purpose, although follow-up into middle childhood has yet to take place.

Fourth, only longitudinal studies are likely to detect either unexpected outcomes or sequelae that do not readily fall into categories that coincide with recognized clinical syndromes. Thus, this applied to our finding that some subjects with developmental disorders of receptive language developed acute florid paranoid psychosis in late adolescence. It is pertinent that the psychiatrists who cared for these subjects during these psychoses did not link the psychotic disorders with the early language delay. The subjects had long since gained fair language competence and their early language difficulties seemed too far in the past to be relevant for the genesis of psychopathological disturbance in the late teenage period. Similarly, although the social difficulties that we found in early adult life were often quite severe and pervasive, they did not constitute any recognized psychiatric syndrome. Accordingly, it is unlikely that they would have been identified for retrospective study as having any coherence or significance.

Fifth, prospective studies are desirable to determine the rate of 'escape' from risk. It is important to find out what proportion of older individuals with some psychosocial disorder experienced the early risk factor, in this case, early language delay, and to assess the extent to which this percentage exceeds that in people free from disorder. However, it is equally necessary to find out the proportion of children with the specified early risk factor who do *not* go on to develop the psychopathological sequelae; continuities and discontinuities over time need to be examined looking forwards as well as looking backwards (Rutter *et al.*, 1983).

Sixth, if developmental processes are to be understood, it is necessary that risk relationships be investigated over *multiple* time points; it is not sufficient simply to relate the risk factor at time 1 to some outcome at time 2. There are many reasons why this is so. These range from the need to have at least three data points in order to separate real change from regression to the mean effects; to the power given to the testing of causal hypotheses when changes over time in one variable can be related to subsequent changes over time in some other variable. Within-individual change needs to be investigated and not just between-group differences if causal mechanisms are to be put to the test in adequate fashion (Farrington, 1988).

Finally, longitudinal data are needed in order to determine whether some hypothesized underlying mechanism is responsible for the connection between feature A at time 1 with feature B at time 2 in the same individual. For example, it might be postulated that the early language delay and the later social deficits both derive from the *same* genetic factor. In order to test that hypothesis it is necessary to use a genetic design that can span the interconnecting time period. For example, a longitudinal twin study could be used to find out whether patterns of concordance within MZ (monozygotic) and DZ (dizygotic) pairs link the early language delay with the later social deficits. There are, of course, special problems in employing twin research strategies with developmental language disorders because the rate of such disorders in twins is much higher than in singletons – with the implication that environmental factors are more important in the genesis of language disorders in twins than in singletons (Rutter *et al.*, 1990). That difference means that it is especially important to integrate different research designs, but the need to use them within a longitudinal framework remains.

In conclusion, it is well-established that developmental language disorders constitute a significant risk factor for a diverse range of later psychosocial disturbances. The mechanisms that mediate that risk remain ill-understood but they are susceptible to investigation and longitudinal studies will be particularly important in their elucidation.

ACKNOWLEDGEMENTS

We are most grateful to Thierry Deonna for helpful suggestions and comments.

REFERENCES

Aram, D., Ekelman, B. & Nation, J. (1984) Pre-schoolers with language disorders 10 years later. *Journal of Speech and Hearing Research*, **27**, 232–44.

Aram, D. & Nation, J. (1980) Pre-school language disorders and subsequent language and academic difficulties. *Journal of Communication Disorders*, **13**, 159–98.

Baker, L. & Cantwell, D. (1982) Psychiatric disorder in children with different types of communication disorders. *Journal of Communication Disorders*, **15**, 113–26.

Baker, L. & Cantwell, D. (1987a) Comparison of well, emotionally disordered and behaviorally disordered children with linguistic problems. *Journal of the American Academy of Child and Adolescent Psychiatry*, **26**, 193–6.

Baker, L. & Cantwell, D. (1987b) A prospective psychiatric follow-up of children with speech/language disorders. *Journal of the American Academy of Child and Adolescent Psychiatry*, **26**, 546–53.

Beitchman, J., Hood, J., Rochun, J., Peterson, M., Mantini, T. & Majumdar, S. (1989a) Empirical classification of speech/language impairment in children I. Identification of speech/language categories. *Journal of the American Academy of Child and Adolescent Psychiatry*, **28,** 112–7.

Beitchman, J., Hood, J., Rochun, J., Peterson, M. (1989b) Empirical classification of speech/language impairment in children II. Behavioral characteristics. *Journal of the American Academy of Child and Adolescent Psychiatry*, **28,** 118–23.

Beitchman, J., Peterson, M. & Clegg, M. (1987) Speech and language impairment and psychiatric disorder: the relevance of family demographic variables. *Child Psychiatry and Human Development*, **18,** 191–207.

Beitchman, J., Nair, R., Clegg, M., Ferguson, B. & Patel, P. (1986) Prevalence of psychiatric disorders in children with speech and language disorders. *Journal of the American Academy of Child Psychiatry*, **25,** 528–35.

Benton, A. (1964) Developmental aphasia and brain damage. *Cortex*, **1,** 40–52.

Billard, C., Dufour, M., Gillet, P. & Ballanger, M. (1989) Evolution du langage oral et du langage écrit dans une population de dysphasie de développement de forme expressive. *Approche Neuropsychologique des Apprentissages chez l'Enfant*, **1,** 16–22.

Bishop, D. & Adams, C. (1989) Conversational characteristics of children with semantic–pragmatic disorder. II. What features lead to a judgement of inappropriacy? *British Journal of Disorders of Communication*, **24,** 241–63.

Bishop, D. & Adams, C. (1990) A prospective study of the relationship between specific language impairment, phonological disorders and reading retardation. *Journal of Child Psychology and Psychiatry*, **31,** 1027–50.

Bishop, D. & Edmundson, A. (1987a) Language-impaired 4-year olds: distinguishing transient from persistent impairment. *Journal of Speech and Hearing Disorders*, **52,** 156–73.

Bishop, D. & Edmundson, A. (1987b) Specific language impairment as a maturational lag: evidence from longitudinal data on language and motor development. *Developmental Medicine and Child Neurology*, **29,** 442–59.

Bishop, D. & Rosenbloom, L. (1987) Childhood language disorders: classification and overview. In Yule, W. & Rutter, M. (eds.) *Language development and disorders*. London: MacKeith Press, pp. 16–41.

Brooks-Gunn, J. & Petersen, A. (1984) Problems in studying and defining pubertal events. *Journal of Youth and Adolescence*, **13,** 181–96.

Cantwell, D., Baker, L., Rutter, M. & Mawhood, L. (1989) Infantile autism and developmental receptive dysphasia: a comparative follow-up into middle childhood. *Journal of Autism and Developmental Disorders*, **19,** 1, 19–32.

Cantwell, D., Baker, L. & Mattison, R. (1979) The prevalence of psychiatric disorder in children with speech and language disorder. An epidemiologic study. *Journal of the American Academy of Child Psychiatry*, **18,** 450–61.

Cantwell, D. & Baker, L. (1977) Psychiatric disorder in children with speech and language retardation: a critical review. *Archives of General Psychiatry*, **34,** 583–91.

Caulfield, M. B., Fischel, J. E., De Baryshe, B. D. & Whitehurst, G. J. (1989) Behavioral correlates of developmental expressive language disorder. *Journal of Abnormal Child Psychology*, **17,** 187–201.

Chess, S. & Rosenberg, M. (1974) Clinical differentiation among children with initial language complaints. *Journal of Autism and Childhood Schizophrenia*, **4**, 99–109.

Clausen, J. (1975) The social meaning of differential physical and sexual maturation. In Dragastin, S. & Elder, G. (eds.) *Adolescence in the life cycle: psychological change and social content.* London: Halsted Press, pp. 25–48.

Cohen, N., Devine, M. & Meloche-Kelly, M. (1989) Prevalence of unsuspected language disorders in a child psychiatric population. *Journal of the American Academy of Child and Adolescent Psychiatry*, **28**, 112–7.

Crookes, T. & Green, M. (1963) Some characteristics of children with two types of speech disorder. *British Journal of Educational Psychology*, **33**, 31–7.

De Ajuriaguerra, J., Jaeggi, A., Gulgnard, F., Kocher, F., Maquard, M., Roth, S. & Schmid, E. (1976) The development and progress of dysphasia in children. In Morehead, D. & Morehead, A. (eds.) *Normal and deficient child language.* Baltimore: University Park Press, pp. 345–85.

Debray-Ritzen, P., Mattinger, M. & Chapuis, C. (1976) Etude statistique du devenir lexique des enfants présentant un retard de langage. *Revue Neurologique (Paris)*, **132**, 651–5.

Drillien, C. & Drummond, M. (1983) *Developmental screening and the child with special needs.* Clinics in Developmental Medicine, No. 86. London: S.I.M.P. with Heinemann.

Efron, R. (1963) Temporal perception, aphasia and *déjà vu*. *Brain*, **86**, 403–24.

Eisenson, J. (1968) Developmental aphasia (dyslogia). A postulation of a unitary concept in the disorder. *Cortex*, **4**, 184–200.

Farrington, D. (1988) Studying changes within individuals: the causes of offending. In Rutter, M. (ed.) *Studies of psychosocial risk: the power of longitudinal data.* Cambridge: Cambridge University Press, pp. 158–83.

Fitzsimons, R. (1958) Developmental, psychosocial and educational factors in children with nonorganic articulation problems. *Child Development*, **29**, 481–9.

Fundudis, T., Kolvin, I. & Garside, R. (eds.) (1979) *Speech retarded and deaf children: their psychological development.* London: Academic Press.

Garvey, M. & Gordon, N. (1973) A follow-up study of children with disorders of speech development. *British Journal of Disorders of Communication*, **8**, 17–28.

Graham, N. (1974) Response strategies in the partial comprehension of sentences. *Language and Speech*, **17**, 205–221.

Griffiths, C. (1969) A follow-up study of children with disorders of speech. *British Journal of Disorders of Communication*, **4**, 46–56.

Hall, P. & Tomblin, J. (1978) A follow-up study of children with articulation and language disorders. *Journal of Speech and Hearing Disorders*, **43**, 227–41.

Hanson, D., Gottesman, I. & Heston, L. (1976) Some possible childhood indicators of adult schizophrenia inferred from children of schizophrenics. *British Journal of Psychiatry*, **129**, 142–54.

Henderson, S. & Hall, D. (1982) Concomitants of clumsiness in young school children. *Developmental Medicine and Child Neurology*, **24**, 448–60.

Howells, J. & Guirguis, W. (1984) Childhood schizophrenia 20 years later. *Archives of General Psychiatry*, **41**, 123–8.

Howlin, P. & Rutter, M. (1987) The consequences of language delay for other aspects of development. In Yule, W. & Rutter, M. (eds.) *Language development and disorders.* Oxford: MacKeith Press, pp. 271–94.

Huntley, R., Holt, K., Butterfill, A. & Latham, C. (1988) A follow-up study of a language intervention programme. *British Journal of Disorders of Communication,* **23,** 127–40.

Ingram, T. (1963) Delayed development of speech with special reference to dyslexia. The association of speech retardation and educational difficulties. *Proceedings of the Royal Society of Medicine.* **56,** 199–203.

Ingram, T. (1959) Specific developmental disorders of speech in childhood. *Brain,* **82,** 450–67.

Jenkins, S., Bax, M. & Hart, H. (1980) Behavioural problems in pre-school children. *Journal of Child Psychology and Psychiatry,* **21,** 5–17.

Kahmi, A., Catts, H., Koenig, L. & Lewis, B. (1984) Hypothesis testing and non-linguistic symbolic abilities in language impaired children. *Journal of Speech and Hearing Disorders,* **49,** 169–76.

King, R., Jones, C. & Lasky, E. (1982) In retrospect: a fifteen year follow-up report of speech–language disordered children. *Language, Speech and Hearing Services in Schools,* **13,** 24–32, 69, 87–94.

Levi, G., Capozzi, F., Fabrizi, A. & Sechi, E. (1982) Language disorders and prognosis for reading disabilities in developmental age. *Perceptual and Motor Skills,* **54,** 1119–22.

Lewis, M. & Mezey, G. (1985) Clinical correlates of septum pellucidum cavities: an unusual association with psychosis. *Psychological Medicine,* **15,** 43–54.

Lindholm, B. & Touliatis, J. (1979) Behavior problems of children in regular classes and those diagnosed as requiring speech therapy. *Perceptual and Motor Skills,* **49,** 459–63.

Magnusson, D., Stattin, H. & Allen, V. (1986) Differential maturation amongst girls and its relation to social adjustment: a longitudinal perspective. In Featherman, D. & Lerner, R. (eds.) *Life span development, Vol. 7.* New York: Academic Press, pp. 135–72.

Masland, M. & Case, L. (1968) Limitation of auditory memory as a factor in delayed language development. *British Journal of Disorders of Communication,* **3,** 139–42.

Mason, A. (1967) Specific (developmental) dyslexia. *Developmental Medicine and Child Neurology,* **9,** 183–90.

McGee, R., Silva, P. & Williams, S. (1984) Perinatal, neurological environments and developmental characteristics of seven year old children with stable behavior problems. *Journal of Child Psychology and Psychiatry,* **25,** 573–86.

Menyuk, P. (1969) *Sentences children use*; *Research monograph no. 52*. Cambridge Mass; MIT Press.

Morehead, D. & Ingram, D. (1973) The development of base syntax in normal and linguistically deviant children. *Journal of Speech and Hearing Research,* **16,** 330–52.

Murray, R., Lewis, S., Owen, M. & Foerster, A. (1989) The neurodevelopment origins of dementia praecox. In McGuffin, P., Bebbington, P. (eds.) *Schizophrenia: the major issues.* London: Heinemann, pp. 90–107.

Mykelbust, H. (1954) *Auditory Disorders in Children.* New York: Grune & Stratton.

Paul, R. & Cohen, D. (1984) Outcomes of severe disorders of language acquistion. *Journal of Autism and Developmental Disorders,* **14,** 405–22.
Paul, R., Cohen, D. & Caparulo, B. (1983) A longitudinal study of patients with severe developmental disorders of language learning. *Journal of the American Academy of Child Psychiatry,* **22,** 525–34.
Petrie, I. (1975) Characteristics and progress of a group of language-disordered children with severe receptive difficulties. *British Journal of Disorders of Communication,* **10,** 123–33.
Petty, L., Ornitz, E., Michelman, J. & Zimmerman, E. (1984) Autistic children who became schizophrenic. *Archives of General Psychiatry,* **41,** 129–35.
Poppen, R., Stark, J., Eisenson, J., Forrest, T. & Wertheim, G. (1969) Visual sequencing performance of aphasic children. *Journal of Speech and Hearing Research,* **12,** 288–300.
Rapin, I. & Allen, D. A. (1987) Developmental dysphasia and autism in preschoold children: characteristics and subtypes. In *Proceedings of the first international symposium on specific speech and language disorders in children.* London: AFASIC, pp. 20–35.
Rapin, I. & Allen, D. (1983) Developmental language disorders: nosologic considerations. In Kirk, U. (ed.) *Neuropsychology of language, reading and spelling.* New York: Academic Press, pp. 155–84.
Richman, N., Stevenson, J. & Graham, P. (1983) The relationship between language, development, and behaviour. In Schmidt, M. & Remschmidt, H. (eds.) *Epidemiological approaches in child psychiatry II.* New York: Thieme-Stratton, pp. 57–70.
Ripley, K. & Lea, J. (1984) *A follow-up study of receptive aphasic ex-pupils.* Oxted, England: Moor House School, private publication.
Robinson, R. (1987) The causes of language disorder: introduction and overview. In *Proceedings of the first international symposium on specific speech and language disorders in children.* London: Association for All Speech Impaired Children, pp. 1–19.
Rourke, B. (1988) Socioemotional disturbances of learning disabled children. *Journal of Consulting and Clinical Psychology,* **56,** 801–10.
Rourke, B. P. & Strang, J. D. (1983) Subtypes of reading and arithmetical disabilities: a neurospsychological analysis. In Rutter, M. (ed.) *Developmental neuropsychiatry.* New York: Guilford Press, pp. 473–88.
Rutter, M. (1978) Diagnosis and definition. In Rutter, M. & Schopler, E. (eds.) *Autism: a reappraisal of concepts and treatment.* New York: Plenum.
Rutter, M. (1987) Psychosocial resilience and protective mechanisms. *American Journal of Orthopsychiatry,* **57,** 316–31.
Rutter, M. (1989) Pathways from childhood to adult life. *Journal of Child Psychology and Psychiatry,* **30,** 23–51.
Rutter, M., Tizard, J. & Whitmore, K. (eds.) (1970) *Education, health and behaviour.* London: Longmans. (Reprinted, 1981, Melbourne, FA: Krieger).
Rutter, M., Quinton, D. & Liddle, C. (1983) Parenting in two generations: looking backwards and looking forwards. In Madge, N. (ed.) *Families at risk.* London: Heinemann Educational. pp. 60–98.
Rutter, M. & Garmezy, N. (1983) Developmental psychopathology. In Hetherington, E. (ed.) *Socialization, personality and social development.* Vol. 4, *Mussen's handbook of child psychology,* 4th edn. New York: John Wiley, pp. 775–911.

Rutter, M., Bolton, P., Harrington, R., Le Couteur, A., MacDonald, H. & Simonoff, E. (1990) Genetic factors in child psychiatric disorders. I. A review of research strategies. *Journal of Child Psychology and Psychiatry*, **31**, 3–37.

Sheridan, M. & Peckham, C. (1975) Follow-up at 11 years of children who had marked speech defects at 7 years. *Child: Care, Health and Development*, **1**, 157–66.

Sheridan, M. & Peckham, C. (1978) Follow-up to 16 years of school children who had marked speech defects at 7 years. *Child: Care, Health and Development*, **4**, 145–57.

Shriberg, L. & Kwiatkowski, J. (1988) A follow-up study of children with phonologic disorders of unknown origin. *Journal of Speech and Hearing Disorders*, **53**, 144–55.

Siegel, L., Cunningham, C. & van der Spuy, H. (1985) Interactions of language-delayed and normal preschool boys with their peers. *Journal of Child Psychology and Psychiatry*, **26**, 77–83.

Silva, P., Justin, C., McGee, R. & Williams, S. (1984) Some developmental and behavioural characteristics of seven-year old children with delayed speech development. *British Journal of Disorders of Communication*, **19**, 107–54.

Silva, P., McGee, R. & Williams, S. (1983) Developmental language delay from 3 to 7 years and its significance for low intelligence and reading difficulties at age seven. *Developmental Medicine and Child Neurology*, **25**, 783–93.

Solomon, A. (1961) Personality and behavior patterns of children with functional defects of articulation. *Child Development*, **32**, 731–7.

Stark, R., Bernstein, L., Cordino, R., Bender, M., Talla, P. & Catts, H. (1984) Four-year follow-up study of language impaired children. *Annals of Dyslexia*, **34**, 49–68.

Stark, R., Mellits, E. & Tallal, P. (1983) Behavioral attributes of speech and language disorders. In Ludlow, C. & Cooper, J. (eds.) *Genetic aspects of speech and language disorders.* New York and London: Academic Press, pp. 37–52.

Stevenson, J. (1984) Predictive value of speech and language screening. *Developmental Medicine and Child Neurology*, **26**, 528–38.

Stevenson, J. & Richman, N. (1978) Behaviour, language and development in three-year-old children. *Journal of Autism and Childhood Schizophrenia*, **8**, 299–313.

Stevenson, J., Richman, N. & Graham, P. (1985) Behaviour problems and language abilities at 3 years and behavioural deviance at 8 years. *Journal of Child Psychology and Psychiatry*, **26**, 215–30.

Tallal, P. (1985) Neuropsychological foundations of specific developmental disorders of speech and language: implications for theories of hemispheric specialisation. In Cavenar, J. Jr (Ed.) *Psychiatry: Volume 3*. Philadelphia: Lippincott, pp. 1–15.

Tallal, P. (1976) Rapid auditory processing in normal and disordered language development. *Journal of Speech and Hearing Research*, **19**, 561–71.

Tallal, P. & Piercy, M. (1975) Developmental aphasia: the perception of brief vowels and extended stop consonants. *Neuropsychologica*, **12**, 83–93.

Tallal, P., Dukette, D. & Curtiss, S. (1989a) Behavioral/emotional profiles of preschool language-impaired children. *Development and Psychopathology*, **1**, 51–67.

Tallal, P., Ross, R. & Curtiss, S. (1989b) Familial aggregation in specific language impairment. *Journal of Speech and Hearing Disorders*, **54**, 167–73.

Tomblin, B. (1989) Familial concentration of developmental language impairment. *Journal of Speech and Hearing Disorders*, **54**, 287–95.

Trapp, E. & Evan, J. (1960) Functional articulatory defect and performance on a non-verbal task. *Journal of Speech and Hearing Disorders*, **25**, 176–80.

Urwin, S., Cooke, J. & Kelly, K. (1988) Preschool language intervention: a follow-up study. *Child: Care, Health and Development*, **14**, 127–46.

Walzer, S. (1985) X chromosome abnormalities and cognitive development: implications for understanding normal human development. *Journal of Child Psychology and Psychiatry*, **26**, 177–84.

Watkins, J., Asarnow, R. & Tanguay, P. (1988) Symptom development in childhood onset schizophrenia. *Journal of Child Psychology and Psychiatry*, **29**, 865–78.

Weiner, P. (1985) The value of follow-up studies. *Topics in Language Disorders*, **6**, 78–92.

Wing, L. (1969) The handicaps of autistic children: a comparative study. *Journal of Child Psychology and Psychiatry*, **10**, 1–40.

Yule, W. & Rutter, M. (1985) Reading and other learning difficulties. In Rutter, M. & Hersov, L. (eds.) *Child and adolescent psychiatry*, 2nd edn. Oxford: Blackwell, pp. 444–64.

10 Reproductive hormones

JOHN BANCROFT

INTRODUCTION

Reproductive development is unique in its time course. There is the initial, and fundamental, process of sexual differentiation into male or female during fetal development. After birth there is a phase of developmental quiescence until puberty, or shortly before. Once reproductive maturity is attained it persists in men, with variable degrees and speeds of decline in late life, whilst in women it clearly terminates with the process of ovarian ageing that leads to the menopause. Women have a more complex, and potentially more problematic, reproductive development as they have to cope with a transition from the 'prereproductive to reproductive' in adolescence and from the 'reproductive to postreproductive' at the perimenopause. In addition they have to contend with three quintessentially female phenomena: the menstrual cycle, pregnancy and lactation.

The process of sexual differentiation is most elegant in its biological simplicity. In most respects the capacity for development along both male and female lines exists in each fetus from conception. The process of selecting one or other line of development then depends on one genetically controlled factor: the hormonal production of the gonad. If the primitive gonad develops as a testis, (and the genetic factor determining this probably resides in the first segment of the Y chromosome (Josso, 1989)) then the Mullerian Inhibiting Factor produced by the primitive Sertoli cells will inhibit female development (e.g. in the Mullerian duct), and the testosterone produced by the differentiated Leydig cells will stimulate development of incipient male structures.

Beyond this process of sexual differentiation, however, hormonal control of reproduction is highly complex, involving interacting systems which are as yet only partially understood. In addition to the gonadal steroid hormones, principally oestrogens, progesterone and androgens, there is an ever growing number of neuropeptides recognized to play a part, in the pituitary control of the gonads (i.e. luteinizing hormone

(LH) and follicle-stimulating hormone (FSH)), the hypothalamic control of the pituitary (i.e. luteinizing hormone releasing hormone (LHRH)), and the various functions in the brain mediating between steroid feedback or other central influences and the hypothalamo–pituitary complex (e.g. prolactin, β-endorphin). This chapter focuses on the steroids.

Steroid hormones have two distinct types of effect on reproductive development: (a) *organizing* and (b) *activating.*

Organizing effects are involved in sexual differentiation, leading *prenatally* to anatomical differentiation and some differentiation of brain function, and *at puberty,* to development of secondary sexual characteristics. Organizing effects in the brain, for the most part, can be seen as *structural,* and hence immutable, but with important exceptions, particularly in the primate and human domain. Organization is usually viewed as structural in the sense that specific neural tissues and neurocellular connections become established. This has been clearly demonstrated in lower mammals, such as rodents. But organization can also be seen in more functional terms, e.g. certain types of reproductive function may depend on the continued presence of a certain hormonal milieu. An example of this in the human context is given below.

Activating effects are functional and depend on the activation of hormone-sensitive target organ receptors. The number and distribution of such receptors are in part a consequence of earlier hormonal organization. Three broadly different approaches to the study of activating effects will be considered. One involves the measurement of specific hormones or neurotransmitters in the circulation or urine, relating their levels to measures of behaviour. The second approach recognizes the complexity of hormonal mediation and the cascade of neuromodulating effects that mediate between a hormonal effect and a behavioural consequence; it therefore measures a number of such potential factors at the same time, using multivariate methods of analysis. The third approach views neuroendocrine mechanisms as systems, and tests the functioning of such systems by challenging them and measuring the response (e.g. pituitary function tests; neuroendocrine challenge tests).

The univariate measurement of gonadal steroids remains a valid approach where sexuality is involved. Although a variety of neuromodulators and neurotransmitters may be involved in the mediation of such steroid effects, our knowledge of steroid receptors in the brain indicates the specific effects that such steroids have in relation to reproductive behaviour. When we consider the possible effects of reproductive hormones on mood and well-being the picture is very different. Here we are not considering specific hormonal effects, but rather the modulation of highly complex self-regulating systems the natures of which are not understood. In such circumstances, univariate methodology has been extensively used (e.g. in an attempt to explain the 'premenstrual syndrome') and has been consistently unhelpful. Alternative approaches are required and these will be discussed later in the chapter.

ORGANIZING EFFECTS OF HORMONES

The organizing effects of relevance to this chapter are those involving brain function. The reproductive hormone most clearly involved is testosterone, although it is possible that its organizing effects result from its aromatization intracellularly to oestradiol 17-β. The male fetal brain is normally exposed to testosterone, the female brain is not. There are, however, high levels of oestrogens extracellularly, and some form of protective mechanism (e.g. alphafetoprotein) prevents the oestrogens from entering the cells and producing the same effects as androgens. Such effects have been clearly identified in non-primate research, and can be summarized under two headings: (a) *masculinization* and (b) *defeminization*.

Masculinization is manifested in male-type behaviour: sexual behaviour expressed as mounting, and non-sexual, as rough-and-tumble, aggressive type play. The first is of uncertain relevance to the human, because there is no clear gender dimorphism of human sexual behaviour as there is in rodents. The second is of potential importance and will be considered further.

Defeminization is manifested behaviourally, by the suppression of the female lordosis response; and neuroendocrinologically, by suppression of development of the positive-feedback response of the hypothalamo-pituitary–gonadal axis which is central to the female reproductive cycle. In primates (including humans) there is no behavioural counterpart of lordosis. The presence or absence of positive feedback remains a sexually dimorphic characteristic, but whereas in the rodent it results from early 'structural' organization of the hypothalamus, in primates and humans it appears to be dependent on the prevailing hormonal milieu. This has crucial implications for extrapolating from rodent to human.

The distinction between masculinization and defeminization confronts us with an important issue: masculinity and femininity are biologically independent dimensions. Whilst there is general agreement on this point, there is some debate on the extent of this independence, whether the two dimensions are in effect 'orthogonal' or 'oblique' (Reinisch & Sanders, 1987).

Relevant evidence from both lower and higher mammals is now substantial, much of it derived from experimental manipulations of developmental processes. Such experimentation is not possible with humans, and as a consequence our human evidence is much more limited and less conclusive. Whilst some developmental phenomena are sufficiently universal to allow us to assume that they exist in humans also, we must nevertheless be wary with our extrapolations.

When we consider the limited human evidence, the importance of longitudinal studies is obvious. The principal evidence available to us comes from three types of 'natural experiment': (a) inborn errors of metabolism, resulting in abnormal levels of reproductive hormones during fetal development, (b) exposure to drugs during fetal development, and (c) sex chromosome abnormalities. This evidence has been extensively reviewed elsewhere (e.g. Money & Ehrhardt, 1972; Reinisch & Sanders, 1987; Bancroft, 1989) and will be summarized here only briefly. The effects that have been studied include gender-related behaviours, cognitive function and sexual orientation or preference.

Inborn errors of metabolism

There are three principal conditions in this category.

Adrenogenital syndrome

This results from an autosomal recessive gene defect in cortisol synthesis, usually due to a deficiency in the 21-hydroxylase enzyme. In most cases adequate cortisol production is maintained by means of excessive adrenocorticotrophic hormone (ACTH) stimulation, but at the expense of adrenal cortical hyperplasia and an associated excess of androgenic steroids.

In the male this causes precocious puberty. In girls it leads to virilization with varying degrees of masculinization of the external genitalia. Usually the anomaly is diagnosed soon after birth, and since the availability of corticosteroids, has been treatable. Prior to such treatment, affected girls would be exposed to excess androgens both postnatally as well as prenatally. Whether treated or not, females with this condition have shown evidence of greater 'tomboyish' behaviour during childhood together with some 'male stereotype' preferences during adulthood, e.g. preference for male clothes, and putting career before marriage. Women who were not treated, and hence were exposed to high androgen levels during childhood, were more likely to report homosexual or bisexual fantasies, though clear Lesbian identities did not occur (Money & Ehrhardt, 1972; Lev Ran, 1977). This apparent effect on sexual preferences may have been secondary to gender-role effects.

The precocious puberty in boys with this syndrome is associated with an early onset of sexual interest, although accompanying sexual imagery is consistent with the boy's social and emotional age (Money & Alexander, 1969).

The main limitations of this source of evidence are that: (a) the condition is rare; (b) appropriate controls for comparison are not easily chosen, given the small number of cases involved; and (c) the varying degrees of genital virilization are likely to produce confounding effects on how such children are raised, making the attribution of developmental differences to hormonal effects less certain.

Androgen insensitivity syndrome

The basic defect in this condition is a reduced affinity of cellular receptors for androgens. This results in a failure of androgenic effects at the cellular level, probably in all tissues where androgen receptors are involved. The syndrome is transmitted either as an X-linked recessive trait or a male-limited dominant trait, so that only genetic males are affected.

This condition demonstrates clearly the role of Mullerian Inhibiting Factor, because this functions normally, resulting in the suppression of Mullerian duct development (i.e. absence of Fallopian tubes, uterus and upper third of the vagina). But because of the absence of androgenic stimulation, there is no male development. The result is external genitalia of female type, and a short, blind vagina (the lower two thirds of the vagina develop with the external genitalia, the upper third from the Mullerian duct). Affected individuals with the complete syndrome are reared as girls and their psychosexual development appears to be normally female.

As this condition is most often diagnosed following the failure to menstruate, there is an absence of the confounding effect of the diagnosis on childhood development. However, by the same token, it is only possible to assess the prediagnosis childhood development of these individuals retrospectively. There are a number of unanswered questions about this condition. Why, for example, do these women have apparently normal levels of sexual desire in spite of their androgen insensitivity; why do they not show normally female 'positive feedback' in their hypothalamo-pituitary responsiveness? (This may result from an unidentified 'testicular factor' inhibiting positive feedback; see below.) The condition is also very rare and the problem of obtaining suitable controls again arises.

5-alpha reductase deficiency

5-alpha reductase is necessary for the conversion of testosterone to dihydrotestosterone (DHT). DHT is necessary for male development of the urogenital sinus into normal male external genitalia. The rare inborn deficiency of 5-alpha reductase results in inadequate masculinization of the external genitalia, although at puberty, for reasons that are not well understood, there is sometimes growth of the previously undeveloped penis.

This rare condition was brought to prominence by Imperato-McGinley *et al.* (1974) who found a number of such cases in a few neighbouring villages in the Dominican Republic. Their reports of how such individuals often developed male gender identities after puberty led these workers to conclude that gender identity was hormonally determined and not a consequence of social learning. However, their evidence of the early gender identity of these children was inadequate, and the fact that they were usually given a particular name (i.e. guavedoces or 'penis at 12') suggested that they grew up with ambiguous rather than unequivocal female gender identities (Imperato-McGinley *et al.*, 1979). If so the change of identity at puberty tells us little about the determinants of normal gender identity.

More recently Herdt & Davidson (1988) have reported a small series of such cases in a community in Papua New Guinea. The importance of this report is that it is based on an extensive ethnographic study of the society involved (something missing in the Dominican study), so that attitudes to child-rearing and the reactions to these particular individuals during childhood were much better documented. This society also contrasts with the Dominican rural culture in having a very segregated gender structure. Most of the individuals affected with the 5-alpha reductase deficiency were recognized as pseudohermaphrodites at birth and reared as such, usually with considerable associated stigma. A few were brought up as girls only to be discovered for what they were by their husbands at marriage, who rejected them traumatically. This account certainly does not support the earlier conclusion that pubertal increases in testosterone reorganized gender identity along male lines. Whilst of considerable interest, this condition does not tell us much about the role of hormones in the development of gender identity.

The administration during pregnancy of drugs which influence steroid mechanisms. (For review see Reinisch & Sanders, 1987)

Progestagenic steroids

The administration of progestagens during pregnancy to prevent spontaneous abortion has been used for some time. Early progestagens used for this purpose were subsequently found to possess androgenic properties. When given early enough during pregnancy this led to some degree of virilization of the external genitalia. A few studies have examined the effects of such administration, usually given later than required to affect anatomical differentiation, on behavioural development. Some masculinizing effects have been observed, including activity level, play patterns, mental abilities and aggression/assertion (e.g. Reinisch & Karow, 1977; Beral & Colwell, 1981; Reinisch, 1981). However, not all the evidence has been consistent, with some studies suggesting enhanced femininity in females taking progestagen (Ehrhardt *et al.*, 1977; Meyer-Bahlburg *et al.*, 1977).

Oestrogens

Comparable inconsistency arises with the evidence from the administration of oestrogens during pregnancy, in particular diethylstilboestrol (DES); some studies have shown a masculinizing effect (Kester *et al.*, 1980; Hines & Shipley, 1984), others feminization (Yalom *et al.*, 1973; Reinisch, 1977).

Barbiturates

There is substantial evidence from the animal literature of the disruptive effects that barbiturates have on fetal development. Much of this appears to be due to a direct action on neural tissues. However, an additional mechanism involves the alteration of hepatic metabolism of steroids that results from the induction of enzymes by the barbiturates. The animal evidence certainly suggests that an 'antiandrogenic' influence on sexual differentiation can result (Reinisch & Sanders, 1982). As yet there is little evidence of such steroid-mediated effects on sexual differentiation in humans, although longitudinal studies are in progress.

There are formidable methodological problems in interpreting evidence in this category. The timing and dosage of drug administration varies enormously. In many respects, when synthetic steroids with varied hormonal effects are involved, it is difficult to predict the developmental consequences. The use of steroid preparations during pregnancy is now much more limited and cautious. The potential effects of barbiturates, however, remain a matter of considerable potential importance. In the 1950s and 1960s as many as 25% of pregnant women were likely to have taken barbiturates at some stage during pregnancy. Their prescription is now much reduced, but they remain sufficiently often used for conditions such as hypertension or nausea, as well as drugs of abuse, to be of importance (Reinisch & Sanders, 1982).

Sex chromosome abnormalities

These conditions, whilst of considerable interest and not particularly uncommon (approximately 1 in 700 births), do not help us much in understanding the effects of reproductive hormones on behaviour. In the XXX syndrome there is no obvious hormonal abnormality, although it is not unusual for menarche to be delayed. In the XYY syndrome hormonal abnormalities are very subtle. The XXY syndrome is of most interest endocrinologically. Whereas degeneration of seminiferous tubules is inevitable, leading to infertility, Leydig cell function is often relatively normal. But in any case many of the abnormalities of this condition, both behavioural and somatic, arise before hypogonadism is established. Endocrine factors in the causation of Klinefelter's syndrome remain very uncertain. Turner's syndrome or 45 XO is associated with specific cognitive deficits which will be considered further below.

Longitudinal studies of sex chromosome abnormalities have, however, confronted us with a crucial ethical issue for developmental research. Screening of neonates allows the early recognition of these abnormalities. It is clearly possible that some of the stigmata associated with such conditions could result from knowledge of the chromosomal condition and hence expectation of negative developmental consequences. It is therefore necessary, to avoid the confounding effects of such environmental influences, to carry out longitudinal studies on children whose parents and health care providers are unaware of the chromosomal status. Attempts to carry out such research in the United States have led to considerable opposition, on the grounds of human rights. Such longitudinal studies are in progress elsewhere (e.g. Edinburgh), but these ethical problems should not be underestimated.

Other types of evidence

Longitudinal studies of the relationship between perinatal hormone levels and later behavioural development

If variations in the level of androgens (or oestrogens) during fetal development are reflected in variations in Central Nervous System (CNS) organization as it relates to gender–role behaviour, then it should be possible to demonstrate such effects in longitudinal studies in which perinatal androgen levels are correlated with subsequent behaviours.

The main obstacle to such research is the inaccessibility of steroid hormone levels in the fetus in normal circumstances. There is a brief window in time when perinatal blood is readily available and its collection poses no ethical problems, viz. the collection of cord blood at birth.

One group has measured levels of steroid hormones in the cord blood of male and female infants and related them to levels of timidity (measured as response to a novel toy) at ages 6 to 18 months. For the boys, timidity was negatively correlated with testosterone and progesterone and positively correlated with oestradiol. For the girls, no significant correlations were found (Jacklin *et al.*, 1983). The relationship of these hormone levels to subsequent mood was also assessed. Androstenedione, oestrogen and progesterone were positively correlated with 'happy/excited' mood and negatively correlated with time spent in 'calm/quiet' mood in boys. Hormone–mood relationships in girls, whilst not significant, were all in the opposite direction. These authors concluded that 'if hormones do have an organizational effect, the nature of this effect is different for the two sexes' (Marcus *et al.*, 1985).

The reliance on cord blood does pose problems of interpretation. First it involves sampling at one point in time, and possibly a time when blood levels are already falling, or at least temporarily variable. It is also a very specialized time. At birth the male infant has circulating levels of testosterone that are approximately half those of the normal adult, whereas in female infants, levels are similar to those in the adult. In both sexes there is a dramatic drop within the first few days, presumably due to the withdrawal of human chorionic gonadotrophin (HCG). Clearly these findings of the Jacklin group, whilst of considerable interest, require replication.

A further opportunity presents itself in the immediate postnatal period. In the male, circulating testosterone starts to rise in the second or third week postnatally, reaching a maximum similar to levels in the cord blood between the 30th and 60th day, and then gradually declining to low prepubertal levels. There is no such postnatal androgen surge in the female (Forest *et al.*, 1976). This androgen rise in boys is not as impressive as it looks because it is accompanied by a substantial increase in sex hormone binding globulin (SHBG) and consequently only a modest rise in free T (testosterone). Salivary T, which is thought to be highly correlated to plasma free T does not show this surge. The function of this postnatal surge is not known. However, it is conceivable that it plays a role in masculinization and defeminization of the brain. The main problem in studying this phenomenon is that, once again, there are ethical objections to collecting blood samples from infants for purely research purposes. As yet no studies have been reported where the level of this postnatal surge is related to behavioural development or sexual orientation.

Cross-sectional studies of 'organizing' effects in adults; the determinants of sexual orientation

Attempts to relate 'organizing' effects of prenatal hormones to adult sexual orientation have provided telling examples of how 'cross-sectional' studies can mislead. Dorner and his colleagues (Dorner, 1980) found that, in rats, exposure to inadequate amounts of androgens during male fetal development resulted in inadequate masculinization, as shown by a reduced tendency to mount, and inadequate defeminization, in the form of partial hypothalamo-pituitary 'positive feedback' to oestrogen. They therefore proceeded with human studies on the basis that the presence in the male of positive feedback in response to oestrogen provocation would indicate inadequate defeminization *and* masculinization of the fetal brain. If such incomplete defeminization was present in homosexual men this would suggest that their homosexuality was based on inadequate prenatal masculinization of their brains. They proceeded to test the pituitary response to oestrogen provocation in homosexual and heterosexual men and heterosexual women. They found an LH response in the homosexual men that was midway between the normal female (positive feedback) and normal male ('negative feedback' patterns). They took this as evidence of incomplete brain masculinization. These findings were replicated by Gladue *et al.* (1984).

The first flaw in this line of reasoning was to equate the opposite-sex mounting of the male rodent with human male heterosexuality, and conversely lack of opposite sex mounting with human homosexuality. As mentioned earlier, there is no dimorphism of sexual behaviour in humans, and the tendency of the male rat to mount and the female to be mounted is best conceptualized in terms of 'complementarity' of behaviour rather than the expression of a sexual preference (Beach, 1979). The second flaw was to assume that the positive feedback response in the human is 'organized' at the prenatal stage as a structural development normally blocked by exposure to testosterone. There is now substantial evidence, in both primates and humans, that a positive feedback response can be elicited from otherwise normal males after they have been castrated (see Gooren, 1988a, for review). It now seems likely that there is a testicular factor present (as yet unidentified) which inhibits positive feedback in the male. The differences between homosexual and heterosexual men reported by Dorner (1980) and Gladue *et al.* (1984) (but not found in all comparable studies; see Gooren, 1988a) probably reflect differences in current testicular function and not in early brain organization. The reason for such differences in testicular function has not been identified, but there are a number of possibilities including life style, recreational drugs, infections, which need to be considered.

In general, attempts to account for adult sexual orientation in terms of early hormonal organization are unlikely to be successful. The evidence of increased homophilic interest or fantasy, reported in some of the studies of endocrine abnormalities reviewed above, may reflect other aetiological mechanisms, e.g. the psychosocial consequences of having an anomalous anatomical differentiation or a direct effect of hormones on gender role behaviour, which in turn influences the process of sexual learning (Bancroft, 1989).

Sex differences in cognitive function

One of the most robust findings in the field of cognitive sex differences is a relative male superiority in visuo-spatial skills (Maccoby & Jacklin, 1974). This difference becomes apparent only from puberty onwards. In addition there is now substantial evidence that boys are more likely to be mathematically gifted than girls. Once again the difference becomes apparent only around puberty, although this could reflect a lack of suitable tests for younger ages. The difference in visuo-spatial skills probably contributes to the difference in mathematical ability but is unlikely to be a sufficient explanation.

This evidence has recently been reviewed by Benbow (1988) who herself has extensively studied gifted children. Her review is accompanied by critiques from 42 other specialists, providing together a rich if varied appraisal of the field. Whilst there was consensus that the sex difference in mathematical ability had been established, there was considerable disagreement about the likely explanation for this difference. Amongst the explanations considered was an effect of reproductive hormones. One version of this is that the superiority of the male is due to the effects of testosterone or the testosterone–oestradiol ratio. The relevant evidence is mostly restricted to visuo-spatial ability, is limited and confusing. Broverman *et al.* (1964), for example, found that high androgen levels were associated with low spatial scores in male and high spatial scores in females, suggesting that there might be an optimal level. Nyborg (1983), with a different version, has proposed that oestradiol is the key hormone. He points to the gross visuo-spatial deficits in females with Turner's syndrome who are deficient in oestrogens, and the fact that after one year of cyclical oestrogen–progestogen replacement such women show normal female levels of performance on visuo-spatial tasks. Normal females, he proposes, have too much oestrogen, and in the male, the higher the testosterone the less likely there are to be optimal levels of oestradiol. This is a complex theoretical model designed to fit the confusing evidence that is available and which awaits appropriate experimental validation. The Turner's female shows her deficit from early childhood, whereas the usual sex difference visuo-spatially develops later. Whilst Nyborg strove to make his model accommodate this fact, his explanation lacks conviction and alternative genetically mediated mechanisms also deserve consideration. As yet the role of reproductive hormones in cognitive development remains an interesting possibility which awaits supportive evidence.

ACTIVATING EFFECTS OF REPRODUCTIVE HORMONES

In considering the 'activating' effects of reproductive hormones we can consider three phases of the life cycle: (a) *puberty and adolescence*, (b) *adulthood*, (c) *late adulthood and reproductive decline.*

Puberty and adolescence

Puberty is a major developmental stage of the life cycle when the child, after a period of relative stability in the late childhood role, undergoes the process of sexual maturation, with the development of secondary sexual characteristics, the unfolding of sexuality and the long-term process of adjusting to the adult role.

In addition to the increase in sexual interest and responsiveness that occurs during adolescence, there are other changes in emotional status, manifested ordinarily as a phase of relative emotional perturbation and reactivity, and in terms of morbidity, as a changing pattern of behavioural disorder and psychiatric illness (Rutter, 1990).

Whereas the increase in gonadal hormones that accompanies puberty is clearly responsible for the development of secondary sexual characteristics, the role of these hormones in the changing behavioural and affective state is less clear cut and remains somewhat controversial. Obviously there are various psychosocial processes that are likely to influence this developmental phase, leading some authorities to minimize or reject any effects of hormones on behaviour, other than the indirect consequences of their effects on physical maturation and the psychosocial reaction to this. Certainly any sensible attempt to evaluate the role of hormones at this stage of development will need to take into account how such biological mechanisms might interact with psychosocial mechanisms.

Attempts to study hormone–behaviour relationships during adolescence have so far been few, and mainly cross-sectional rather than longitudinal, reflecting the difficulties in carrying out research with this age group when sensitive issues such as sexuality are being assessed.

Hormones and adolescent behavioural problems

Nottelmann *et al.* (1987, 1990) reported a study of 56 normal boys and 52 normal girls aged 9 to 14 years. Whilst this was a longitudinal study, in that each child was assessed three times at six-month intervals, so far only evidence from the first assessment has been reported. Psychosocial adjustment was assessed by self-ratings of various aspects of self-image, and by parental ratings of adolescent behavioural problems. Pubertal status, in terms of Tanner stages, was determined, and hormonal assessment involved assay of plasma levels of gonadal steroids (testosterone and oestradiol), gonadotrophins, and adrenal androgens (androstenedione, dehydro-epiandrosterone (DHEA) and DHEA sulphate (DHEAS)).

The results as reported are complex and difficult to interpret and evaluate, partly because of the large number of correlations computed. In summary they observed correlations that suggested two types of hormone–behaviour relationship, one relating to the stage of pubertal development, the other to stress. In general, such relationships were more striking amongst the boys; their adjustment problems were associated with a multivariate hormone profile possibly indicative of late pubertal maturation, with relatively low gonadal steroids, relatively high adrenal androgens and often associated with high chronological age. Amongst the girls, hormone–behaviour relationships observed were more univariate; adjustment problems were associated with relatively high gonadrotrophins, low DHEAS and high androstenedione.

This study illustrates well the complexity of this type of research. The interaction between pubertal development and stress could work in two directions: late pubertal development could cause psychosocial stress, manifested as behavioural maladjustment and a characteristic hormonal profile; on the other hand, the endocrine consequences of stress could inhibit pubertal development. These interactions will not easily be disentangled, but are more likely to be so in longitudinal studies in which the timing of onset of stress and of pubertal development can be more accurately assessed. Rubin (1990), in commenting on the Nottelmann *et al.* studies, advocated the measurement of adrenal corticosteroids as well as androgens as a better way to monitor stress. Obviously there are many methodological problems and uncertainties to be resolved in this type of longitudinal study, and the efforts of Nottelman and her colleagues can be seen as a first pioneering step into this difficult area.

Hormones and adolescent aggression

Whereas the relationship between androgens and aggression is unequivocal in some species, as exemplified in ungulates such as the bull or stallion where castration effectively reduces aggressive behaviour, this relationship in primates and humans remains unclear. Part of the problem stems from the conceptual confusion over the term 'aggression'. There are a number of behavioural patterns, potentially independent of each other, which tend to be subsumed under the heading 'aggressive behaviour'. Examples include rough-and-tumble play of the immature male primate or human, assertiveness and the expression of dominance in interpersonal relationships, the preparedness to retaliate if attacked, the tendency to defend one's territory, the expression of dominance or physically assaultive behaviour during sexual interactions, reaction to frustration with hostile behaviour, preparedness to engage in physical contact sports such as rugby football or ice hockey and reacting to interpersonal conflict with hostile behaviour. Androgens may influence some of these behaviours and not others, and it is probable that their effects interact with psychosocial influences and the consequences of social learning. Much of the confusion in the evidence probably stems from the use of 'self-ratings' of aggressive tendencies; those studies that have shown a more convincing relationship between androgens and aggression have used some relatively objective concept of aggression, such as criminal behaviour, or observed aggressive interactions.

In the primate and human there is some evidence, discussed earlier, for an *organizing* role for androgens increasing the likelihood of certain types of 'aggressive', characteristically male behaviours such as rough-and-tumble play, and various forms of assertiveness. What is less clear is the extent to which androgens have an *activating* role in maintaining these behaviours. Such activating effects of androgens could be mediated in several ways: by stimulating physical development that endows the individual with a size and strength that might encourage the use of aggressive behaviour; by effects on energy levels increasing the likelihood of an 'active' rather than a 'passive' response; by effects on sexuality which might in turn release learnt aggressive responses, both in the subject and in others who might compete with him sexually; and by a direct effect on brain mechanisms underlying aggressive behaviour. The picture is further complicated by hormonal changes that occur *in response* to behaviour. Thus male primates may show a fall in testosterone levels if their position in the dominance hierarchy is lowered. There is now evidence of a similar pattern in human males, who may show a fall in testosterone in situations, such as officer selection, where they fare badly and their self-esteem suffers (Kreuz *et al.*, 1972), or increase in testosterone after some form of interpersonal victory, such as winning at tennis (Mazur & Lamb, 1980).

When we consider the primate evidence we find a link between androgens and aggression via the androgenic effects on sexuality. Once the young male enters puberty he becomes recognized as a sexual competitor by other males and hence the potential recipient of attack. He will then require his own aggressive behaviour to defend himself if he is not to fall lower in the dominance hierarchy and effectively lose his opportunities for sexual interaction. Whatever it is about his postpubertal condition that attracts this hostility is not dependent on androgens for its maintenance, as this pattern of response from other males continues even after the postpubertal male is castrated. Also castration, whilst it has an unequivocally adverse effect on the male's sexual behaviour, has much less effect on his pattern of aggressive behaviour, apart from the fact that he is less likely to get into sexual conflict with other males. Thus we see 'organizing' effects of androgens, in part manifestated as sexual maturity, and indirect 'activating' effects of androgens on aggression as a consequence of their sexual motivating effects, but no clear evidence that androgens stimulate aggressive behaviour *per se*.

The human studies of androgens and male aggression have been of four types: correlational studies of testosterone and self-ratings of aggressive behaviour in normal adult males, largely negative or with unreplicated effects (Persky *et al.*, 1971; Meyer-Bahlburg *et al.*, 1974); correlational studies in criminals, in which there has been some consistency in evidence showing that violent offenders are likely to have higher testosterone than non-violent offenders (Kreuz & Rose, 1972; Rada *et al.* 1976); studies of sportsmen, which have shown some correlation between testosterone and observer ratings of 'aggressive' physical contact during sports such as ice hockey (Scaramella & Brown, 1978); and studies of adolescents, which are of most relevance to us here. Olweus (1975) developed his 'multi-faceted aggression inventory for boys', pointing out that aggressive behaviours are probably more easily elicited and assessed in adolescent boys than in adult men. In a study of 58 boys aged 16, testosterone levels were related to measures of aggression from this inventory, measures based on ratings by peers, and assessment of the stage of pubertal development and body shape (Olweus *et al.*, 1980). Significant correlations were found between testosterone and physical and verbal aggression ($r = 0.36$ and 0.38 respectively). The individual items contributing to these correlations were those covering situations of provocation. Generally speaking they found little evidence that aggression could be accounted for by testosterone induced physical strength or size. The relationships between testosterone and pubertal development were, however, complex and the authors commented that to investigate the contributions of physical development to testosterone related aggression would require longitudinal studies. Comparable findings were found by this group in a further study of institutionalized young male delinquents (Mattsson *et al.*, 1980).

Although the evidence is far from adequate and open to various interpretations, there is one pattern beginning to emerge that deserves consideration. During adolescence the direct effects of androgens on certain types of aggression (i.e. response to provocation) may be further enhanced by the effects of testosterone on physical growth and sexuality. Beyond adolescence, however, these androgen effects become obscured by other consequences of social learning which allow the male to maintain his self-esteem, his sexual confidence and his sense of dominance with behaviours which are more socially acceptable and hence more effective without being androgen dependent. We see exceptions to this learning process in the form of poorly adapted individuals whose continuing 'androgen driven' behaviour is likely to lead them into criminal or otherwise antisocial behaviour. At the present time there is very little that can be said about hormones and female aggression.

Hormones and adolescent sexuality

There is now unequivocal evidence of the role of androgens in the activation and maintenance of adult male sexual desire and arousability (Bancroft, 1988). Hormonal control of female sexuality remains much less clear, though it would appear that at least for some women, or at some stages in the life cycle of women, androgen enhances female sexuality also (Bancroft, 1989).

Puberty is accompanied by a marked increase in sexual interest in both sexes. In boys spontaneous erections, whilst occurring prepubertally, increase in frequency as puberty is approached and there is a substantial increase in the frequency and duration of spontaneous erections during sleep (nocturnal penile tumescence) which reach a peak in adolescence and decline gradually thereafter. Whilst some boys are capable of orgasm prepubertally, seminal emission as well as spermatogenesis only become possible at puberty. It has been widely assumed that, at least in boys, this postpubertal surge of sexual interest and responsiveness is at least in part a consequence of the surge in testosterone at that stage. As mentioned earlier, however, this causal relationship is disputed by some (e.g. Gagnon & Simon, 1973) who see biological influences as largely confined to the psychosocial impact of physical maturation.

An unusual study of the relationship between hormones and sexuality around puberty has been reported by Udry *et al.* (1985) for boys and Udry *et al.* (1986) for girls. This was again a cross-sectional study in which school children between the ages of 9 and 14 were assessed hormonally, and by means of questionnaire, in terms of sexual interest, sexual activity and peer group relationships. The striking results of this study suggested that, in the case of boys, the level of free testosterone in the plasma was the best predictor of the extent of the boy's sexual interest and sexual activity, more so than his stage of pubertal development, or any of the psychosocial factors measured. In the case of girls, the picture was different; whereas there was some correlation between free T and measures of sexual interest, the likelihood of a girl being sexually active with a partner was much more strongly related to her pattern of peer group relationships, and especially to whether her female friends had also engaged in sexual activity. Here we have a strong suggestion of a sex difference in the role of hormones in influencing sexual behaviour, with male sexuality being pre-eminently determined by hormones (androgens) and female sexuality, at least of an interactional kind, by social mechanisms. Does this mean that female sexual learning is more susceptible to social pressures than male, or that female sexuality is less responsive to hormonal influence or both? These remarkable findings of Udry's group need replication. It would obviously be preferable to study such relationships using longitudinal methodology that allows assessment of a child's sexuality and peer group relationships before puberty and then observation of how these two aspects develop through early adolescence. The difficulties of such research should not be underestimated, however. Moral objections of the adult (parental) community may be the most serious obstacle.

We have already heard that the timing of the 'pubertal' surge in androgens may influence their effect on behavioural development. Thus boys with precocious puberty, whilst motivated sexually to some extent, nevertheless show an interest in sex that is in keeping with their stage of cognitive development. Boys whose puberty is delayed may be stressed and suffer adverse consequences to their psychoneuroendocrine system. Is there an optimal time in sexual development for hormonal effects and social learning to interact? One way of tackling this question is to study the effects of androgen replacement in states of hypogonadism with different ages of onset. Do males who have already experienced normal adolescent sexual development and who became hypogonadal in adult life react differently to androgen replacement, compared with males of similar age who have not gone through puberty? Gooren (1988b) recently reported a study in which he compared the treatment of two types of hypogonadism: hypergonadotrophic (i.e. secondary to testicular failure) and hypogonadotrophic (secondary to pituitary or hypothalamic failure) in boys around the age of 15. He found that the first group responded better and more quickly and comprehensively to androgen replacement than the second group. Given the similar chronological age of the two groups, this difference raises the possibility that the cause of the hypopophyseal-pituitary failure in the hypogonadotrophic group may have had adverse direct effects on psychosocial development other than via the gonadal route.

A recent study of young female university students (average age $21\frac{1}{2}$ years) has emphasized the need for longitudinal studies in assessing hormonal effects on the behaviour of women. In this study two groups were assessed, one using oral contraception the other not. Oral contraceptives lower circulating androgen levels quite substantially, mainly as a result of an increase in SHBG. Hence this offered a model for examining androgen–behaviour relationships in young women. Behavioural assessment was carried out by questionnaire (Bancroft *et al.*, 1991b, c), and in a sub-group, by daily ratings (Alexander *et al.* 1990). Four-weekly blood samples were taken to assess androgen levels (principally free T). Amongst the women in sexual relationships, those using oral contraceptives in spite of having substantially lower levels of free T, reported higher levels of sexual interaction with their partners than did the non-oral-contraceptive women. (This difference between groups did not apply to masturbation frequency.) Correlations between free T and some aspects of sexual behaviour were found, but only in the oral-contraceptive-using group. The pill using women also reported more satisfaction with their sexual partners.

It became obvious in this study that knowledge about the women's sexuality (and testosterone levels) and capacity for maintaining sexual relationships *before* they started on oral contraceptives was needed for interpreting these data. What are the psychosocial factors that influence a young woman's choice of contraceptive, and how would these influence her reaction to the hormonal effects of the oral contraceptive? It is a remarkable fact that there are virtually no prospective, longitudinal data of this kind relevant to oral contraceptive use (Bancroft & Sartorius, 1990). It also has to be borne in mind that the psychosocial factors obscuring hormone–behaviour relationships in women of this age group might be different from those affecting girls in early adolescence, and different again from those affecting women in the midst of their child-rearing, or around the menopause.

Adulthood

When we consider the relevance of reproductive biology to psychosocial disorders of adulthood we are immediately confronted by a striking sex difference. For men, reproductive function carries a low profile. They reproduce because they engage in sexual behaviour, which more often than not they enjoy, and in the majority of cases any reproductive consequences are unplanned. Decline in testicular function may be a biological risk factor for older men, though as yet the evidence for this is far from conclusive. For women, reproductive biology features large at least until middle age. An inescapable impact is from the menstrual cycle. Embedded in the life cycle of each woman is the reproductive phase which begins with the establishment of ovarian and menstrual cyclicity in early adolescence and ends with the decline of ovarian function around the menopause. For 35 to 40 years of each woman's life she experiences a cyclical pattern. At the beginning of this phase the transition from the neuroendocrine stability of childhood to this cyclicity requires adjustment. At the menopause she has to adjust back again to the postmenopausal non-cyclical state. In between these important transitional phases she is likely to experience pregnancy and lactation. In recent years there is also a good chance that she will have taken steroidal contraceptives for prolonged periods of time.

There are striking differences in the prevalence of psychiatric disorders in men and women (Weissman & Klerman, 1977; Nolen-Hoeksema, 1987). Women are much more prone to experience affective disorders (particularly unipolar depression, dysthymia and anxiety states) and men to have alcohol and drug related problems (Robins *et al.*, 1984; Regier *et al.*, 1988; Weissman *et al.* 1988). This sex difference first becomes apparent at puberty (Rutter, 1990); before puberty affective disorders are generally less common but are more likely in boys than girls. After puberty the sex ratio is reversed. The greatest difference between male and female rates occurs during the age period covering women's reproductive span. Whilst in some studies the sex difference persists in older age groups, others have reported minimal or no sex difference in the elderly (Nolen-Hoeksema, 1987).

This chapter focuses particularly on affective disorders and considers whether the fundamental differences in the reproductive biology of men and women contribute to this sex difference in morbidity. Whereas pregnancy, lactation and the use of steroidal contraceptives are part of women's reproductive history, detailed discussion is confined to the possible relevance of the menstrual cycle and its cessation at the menopause. Clearly it is unlikely that reproductive biology is a sufficient explanation for this sex difference, and if it is of relevance at all, it probably interacts with other factors. Before considering the possible role of reproductive/endocrine factors, the alternative explanations that have been put forward to account for the sex difference in affective disorders will be briefly summarized.

Non-biological explanations for the sex difference in affective disorders

Artefacts of reporting. There are some exceptions in the literature to the general finding of a female preponderance, e.g. the Amish, some student studies and some studies of the elderly, in which the usual sex ratio has not been apparent (Nolen-Hoeksema, 1987). It is possible that some of the reported sex difference results from males, particularly those susceptible, being less accessible to the researcher (e.g. in prison). Angst & Dobler-Mikola (1984) reported that men are less likely than women to recall depressive episodes that occurred more than a few weeks ago, so the sex difference is greater the longer the time interval being assessed. They attributed this to some form of selective forgetting that is more likely to occur in men. Weissman *et al.* (1984) by contrast found that the prevalence rates continued to show a similar sex ratio whether one month or one year periods were assessed. Also, psychiatric hospital admission rates predictably show the sex difference. On balance it appears that in spite of such possible artefacts the findings are sufficiently robust to justify the assumption that the sex difference is a real phenomenon requiring explanation.

Differential access to helping agencies. Women with symptoms of anxiety or depression are twice as likely to consult their GP as men with such symptoms. This may be because their symptoms tend to be more severe (Ingham & Miller, 1982). But it has also often been suggested that women in their role as mothers, have greater contact with health professionals and hence opportunities to present their own problems. However, Goldberg (1988) has recently shown that *en route* through the helping agencies to reach psychiatric care, women, particularly those with children, take longer to reach the psychiatrist, as if professionals accepted depression in such women as 'to be expected'. Similarly, McGuffin *et al.* (1988) found evidence that there was a lower threshold of symptoms for men to be referred for psychiatric help. It therefore appears likely that the reactions of helping agencies is a relevant issue. However, such effects appear likely to reduce rather than increase the sex difference in depression, at least in terms of its clinical presentation.

Sex differences in reactions to adversity. Whereas evidence for the importance of life events in predicting depression is now substantial, most studies have either been confined to women or have failed to examine gender differences. However, there have been some findings, tending to show that women are more susceptible to adversity. Miller & Ingham (1979) demonstrated that, while overall levels of anxiety and depression were significantly higher in women, these levels rose in nearly parallel fashion for both sexes as the number of major stressors increased – results in line with Byrne's (1979) finding that women showed higher levels of state anxiety than men following myocardial infarction. There is some evidence that life events may be more common in women in community samples (Surtees *et al.*, 1981; Blazer *et al.*, 1987) and perhaps among patients (Benjaminsen, 1981). In addition, Surtees *et al.* (1981) tentatively concluded that women might take longer than men to adapt to events that have similar magnitudes of threat. Regarding onsets of psychiatric disorder following life events no sex differences have been found in depression following bereavement (Bornstein *et al.*, 1973; McHorney & Mor, 1988). However, natural disaster (Shore *et al.*, 1986) seems to be associated with greater disorder among women. Finally a study by Hobbs *et al.* (1985) suggested that different types of adversity may be important for the two sexes. For women, being divorced or separated, having a poor relationship with either parent, or having three or more children and, for men, being unemployed, were most significantly associated with psychological disturbance.

Learned helplessness and other aspects of coping behaviour. One of the more researched models of the psychology of depression has been 'learned helplessness' as described first by Seligman (1975) and modified by Abramson *et al.* (1978). According to this model, depression results from expectations that outcomes are uncontrollable – that nothing one can do will improve the situation.

Nolen-Hoeksema (1987) showed that men when depressed tended to engage in activities designed to distract them from their mood. Women on the other hand tended to ruminate more about the possible causes of their mood. Folkman & Lazarus (1980) found that, in some circumstances, men used more 'problem focused coping' than women.

The large volume of work on social support is also likely to be relevant. As yet there is little comparative evidence of the use of social support by men and women. However, Miller & Ingham (1979), studying a general population sample, found that women without a good confidante were significantly more anxious and depressed than those with at least one. These differences were less marked and failed to reach significance for the men. Women with few casual friends were more depressed than other women in the sample, whilst men with few casual friends were more anxious than other men. Furthermore in a Camberwell project (Brugha, 1988) there was some evidence that women experiencing depression attached more importance to their social support than did men.

Social role explanations. It has been postulated that problems in the perception and enactment of social roles are relevant to the sex difference in rates of affective disorders and parasuicide. Several dimensions of role analysis are of particular salience in this context. Thus women may be more likely to suffer from role overload (too many duties associated with major social positions, e.g. parent, home-maker, worker), role conflict (where behaviour patterns in one role are incompatible with those of another role, requiring inconsistent behaviour or attitudes), and role strain (feelings of worry and guilt about performance in role). This complex area has not been systematically investigated in relation to the sex differences in question, and an adequate model of the processes linking role problems with these outcomes is not yet available.

All these explanations deserve consideration and all may be contributing in some instances. If reproductive biology is also contributing, it may do so by interacting with one or more of these non-biological mechanisms. Let us now consider the possible role of the menstrual cycle in this respect.

The menstrual cycle and related mood changes

Mood change in the form of irritability, tiredness and depression is commonly experienced by many women around the time of menstruation, with well-being at its best typically in the late follicular phase of the cycle (Sanders *et al.*, 1983). In a prevalence study of Swedish women, 34% reported premenstrual irritability and 9% premenstrual sadness of moderate or severe degree (Andersch *et al.*, 1986). Premenstrual changes of a physical kind, such as breast tenderness and bloating, are extremely common and occasionally are sufficiently severe to be a problem. The association of such cyclical physical changes with mood change is commonly called the 'premenstrual syndrome' (PMS).

Several studies have shown an association between this premenstrual mood change and depressive illness in women (e.g. Coppen, 1965; Kashiwaga *et al.*, 1976; Endicott *et al.*, 1981; Halbreich & Endicott, 1985; Mackenzie *et al.*, 1986). Rubinow *et al.* (1986) suggested that in susceptible women (i.e. women with a predisposition to depressive illness) the repeated challenge to their affective state, month after month, by something analogous to a 'kindling' phenomenon, increases the likelihood of more chronic depression developing. This monthly challenge could depend on either neuroendocrine mechanisms, psychological (i.e. cognitive) mechanisms or an interaction between the two.

What is the nature of this association between PMS and depressive illness? There are four fundamental questions requiring an answer.

(1) Are women with PMS more prone to develop depressive illness? If this is the case, the occurrence of PMS would act as a valuable indicator of those at risk for depression. This would not only have preventative implications, but also provide opportunities for studying the natural history of depressive illness.

(2) Is the mood change experienced perimenstrually comparable in quality and severity to the mood change of depressive illness and, if so, are the underlying mechanisms of mood change

similar? If this is the case, this would not only have implications for the management of PMS, but would provide rich opportunities for studying the aetiological mechanisms in women whose mood changes predictably and recurrently from depressed to normal.

(3) Does this recurrent mood change have a basic link to the menstrual cycle or is it an example of what Angst & Dobler-Mikola (1985) call 'recurrent brief depression' which is experienced by some men and women and is perhaps inappropriately attributed to the menstrual cycle by a proportion of such women?

(4) If there is a basic link between this recurrent mood change and the menstrual cycle, is there a neuroendocrine or other biological explanation for the link?

Methodological issues

The field of menstrual cycle related mood change is beset with methodological problems. As these problems are of crucial importance to the design and implementation of longitudinal research, some of these methodological issues will be considered in closer detail.

Retrospective versus prospective assessment. Many studies of PMS have relied on retrospective assessments, either of what usually happens or what happened around the last menstruation. A number of studies have found that when women report themselves as having PMS in this way and then proceed to keep daily ratings of how they feel (i.e. prospective assessment) symptom severity is generally lower than originally reported (Endicott & Halbreich, 1982; Rubinow *et al.*, 1984; McMillan & Pihl, 1987). There is now a widely held view that retrospective methods cannot be relied upon for research purposes, owing to the extent of exaggeration and attribution involved. To reject retrospective ratings, however, would be to reject any large-scale survey of PMS; the large numbers necessary for such a survey would preclude prospective assessment, with its sustained subject co-operation. It is also important to remember that the overwhelming majority of assessments on which our understanding of psychosocial health and well-being is based are retrospective in nature and no less subject to sources of retrospective distortion. How justified is this rejection of retrospective assessment of PMS?

There is little doubt that discrepancies between the retrospective and prospective methods arise. However, the reasons for them need careful consideration; we should not just assume that one is valid and the other is not. Hart *et al.* (1987) found that recall of a cycle accounted for 72%

of the variance in that cycle's prospective scores, whereas prospective scores for one cycle predicted only 14% of the variance in prospective scores from the next cycle. In other words there is a considerable amount of intercycle variability. When this is combined with an apparent tendency for many women to experience a reduction in symptom severity when they start to keep daily records (Endicott & Halbreich, 1988), and the use of arbitrary criteria of cyclicity, the observed discrepancies are not so surprising. Any method of assessment has its sources of distortion and it seems sensible to regard both retrospective and prospective (i.e. daily) ratings of menstrual cycle changes as problematic but necessary for different purposes. Having said that, it is also worth emphasizing the potential for improvement for both types of assessment that will come from careful methodological studies.

The definition of the Premenstrual Syndrome. The field of PMS has been plagued by two fundamental and related problems: (a) the assumption that PMS is a distinct, homogeneous entity and (b) the use of varying methods of defining it. The second problem only arises in the presence of the first. Given the first assumption, there have been understandable and to some extent justified attempts to achieve consistency of definition, particularly for research purposes. Thus there is beginning to be a consensus for the use of criteria such as a 30% (or, 2 points on a 0 to a 5 rating scale) difference between premenstrual and postmenstrual scores (NIMH, 1983). But such consistency still leaves much room for confusion. First, we are applying an arbitrary cut-off point to what is, in reality, a continuum. Which symptoms should be involved in this way, given the large number of symptoms that are experienced by women on a cyclical basis? Should some composite score across different symptoms be used? Should physical symptoms (e.g. breast tenderness, bloating) and emotional symptoms (e.g. irritability, depression) be regarded separately?

I believe a justifiable conclusion at the present time is that what we usually regard as 'PMS' is a heterogeneous collection of cyclical phenomena that have in common some temporal relationship to the menstrual cycle and which are 'aggregated' both in women's and scientists' minds as a result of the shared concept of PMS. If so, it is premature and possibly counterproductive to be seeking a single definition of PMS. We should at least be distinguishing between symptom types and making no assumptions about their interrelationships. We can then apply sensible though arbitrary criteria, such as the 30% change, to each symptom.

Another potential problem stems from the preoccupation with the premenstrual phase of the cycle. Most definitions involve the cessation or rapid reduction of symptoms either at or soon after the onset of menstrual bleeding. Women whose symptoms persist through menstruation are likely to be excluded from the category 'PMS sufferer' (e.g. Steiner & Haskett, 1987). In our experience, both with clinical and research populations, symptoms, especially depression or negative mood, may start during the premenstruum but persist through much of the menstrual phase. It is not unusual for them to be maximal during menstruation. Whilst is is necessary to identify women whose problems are clearly menstrual (e.g. dysmenorrhoea), there seems to be no justification for excluding women from consideration because their premenstrual symptoms persist during menstruation, as if this was a different type of phenomenon with presumably different aetiology. There may be interesting differences between those with 'premenstrual only' and those with more prolonged symptoms which would help us to understand more about the nature of these menstrual cycle related problems. But we will not recognize these differences if we look only at one of the groups.

Investigating the association between PMS and depressive illness. The most substantial evidence of a link between PMS and a previous history of a depressive disorder comes from studies where established diagnostic schedules have been used to estimate the lifetime prevalence of various psychiatric diagnoses, based on Diagnostic and Statistical Manual III (DSM III) or Research Diagnostic Criteria (RDC). Thus Endicott *et al.* (1981), using the Schedule of Affective Disorders and Schizophrenia (SADS), found a link between PMS and lifetime occurrence of major depressive disorder. Stout *et al.* (1986) used the National Institute of Mental Health (NIMH) Diagnostic Interview Schedule (DIS), basically similar to the SADS but designed for non-clinical interviewers and large-scale epidemiological surveys. They applied this to first-time attenders of a PMS clinic and compared the rates with those from the local community (Piedmont, North Carolina) that had been one of the centres in the Epidemiological Catchment Area (ECA) study of psychiatric epidemiology (Weissman *et al.*, 1988). They found substantially higher rates amongst the PMS clinic attenders of dysthymia ('neurotic' depression), phobic anxiety and drug and alcohol related problems. In striking contrast to Endicott *et al.* (1981) they found a significantly *lower* rate for major depressive disorder amongst the PMS clinic attenders. They also stressed the amount of overlap there was between the symptoms of PMS and those of several other psychiatric diagnoses. It is possibly relevant that Endicott *et al.*'s (1981) findings were not based on PMS clinic attenders but women participating in a study of depression. Clearly, the setting in which a woman describes her 'lifetime history' could well influence the type of picture that emerges.

An important general issue for any of these studies is the validity of 'lifetime' prevalence rates, particularly in women with a history of PMS. To what extent does questioning about a woman's affective state many years before, and applying fairly concrete, inflexible diagnostic criteria, allow one to distinguish between major depressive disorder or dysthymia and long-standing perimenstrual mood change? Relevant to this is a further report from the Duke, North Carolina group (Blazer *et al.*, 1988). They exploited the fact that the DIS generates a list of symptoms that are relatively free of aetiological assumptions. They took such data from women in the ECA study and subjected them to a multivariate classification technique to see what 'symptom clusters' this type of analysis would generate. They found one grouping basically similar to the DSM III category of Major Depressive Disorder. But they also found a grouping they described as premenstrual dysphoria. They suggested that the occurrence of this type of experience amongst women in the community would tend to inflate the rates for other DSM III depressive disorders in such community-based studies. Generally, therefore, in assessing the relationship between PMS and depressive illness we have the confounding effect of this type of overlap to take into consideration.

With these methodological issues in mind let us consider to what extent we can answer the four questions posed earlier.

Are women with PMS more prone to develop depressive illness? In a large-scale retrospective survey of women's menstrual health (Warner & Bancroft, 1990) we found evidence of two groups of women, one reporting negative mood confined to the premenstrual week, the other, with negative mood, persisting into the menstrual phase. These two groups differed in their relation to age and parity. The first, 'premenstrual only', group showed an association with age; this particular pattern was more often reported by women in the older age groups. The other group, 'premenstrual and menstrual', showed no association with age but were more likely to be parous. This led us to postulate that these two groups were aetiologically distinct, and that it was the second group, with the more prolonged mood change, that would show the association with depressive illness. We set out to test this hypothesis in a recent study (Warner *et al.*, 1991). In 144 women perimenstrual mood was assessed retrospectively and, in 87 of these women, also prospectively. In each case the presence or absence of a previous history of depression treated with antidepressants was established. With both the retrospective and prospective data we found support for our hypothesis. Of those women showing depressive mood both premenstrually and menstrually on prospective ratings, 32% gave a history of treated depression. Of those whose perimenstrual depression was confined to the premenstrual week, none gave this history.

A further impression from this study was of a changing temporal pattern of perimenstrual mood over time. A proportion reported more prolonged mood change at the end of this two year period compared with their initial ratings. Is it possible that their premenstrual depression was gradually becoming more chronic and merging into a depressive illness? This is not an uncommon clinical impression in the PMS clinic. Given these uncertainties about assessment of past depressive episodes, the possibility of changing temporal patterns over time, and the likelihood that the association will be best demonstrated by the occurrence of depressive illness *after* a period of recurrent perimenstrual mood change, we will probably be unable to answer our first question with any confidence until we have carried out longitudinal studies in which women with different patterns of perimenstrual mood change are followed over a period of time, the stability of their patterns examined and their likelihood of developing a depressive illness assessed. As yet we have virtually no evidence of this kind. Only two studies have used the occurrence of PMS to *predict* depressive illness (Shuckit *et al.*, 1975; Wetzel *et al.*, 1975). They were limited studies, involving female undergraduates, at an age when neither PMS nor depressive illness is common in most women. In spite of such limitations, they did find some support for the association, strengthening the need for more substantial longitudinal studies in more appropriate populations.

Is the mood change associated with menstruation qualitatively and quantitatively similar to that occurring during depressive illness? Few studies have directly attempted to compare the severity of depression perimenstrually with that occurring during depressive illness. The measure that provides the most information in this respect is the Beck Depression Inventory (BDI) (Beck *et al.*, 1979) which has been widely used and compared with other measures of depressive severity (Beck *et al.*, 1988). In our recent study described above (Warner *et al.*, 1991) we asked 144 women to rate their degree of depression for a premenstrual and postmenstrual week, using the Beck Depression Inventory (BDI). Studies of PMS complainers have reported average premenstrual BDI scores of around 16 (Stout & Steege, 1985; Maddocks *et al.*, 1986; Graham, 1989). In our study of perimenstrual mood change we selected women on the basis of their perimenstrual *depression* ratings, rather than more generally because of 'premenstrual syndrome'. We found average BDI scores of 20 in women whose mood change was confined to the premenstruum, with 24% having BDI scores in the 'moderate to severe' range of clinical depression and 8% in the severe range. For those with mood change both premenstrually and menstrually, the mean premenstrual BDI score was 25, with 35% in the moderate to severe, and 31% in the severe ranges. On this basis a substantial proportion of women with perimenstrual mood change are experiencing mood of a severity comparable with clinical depression. However, this conclusion needs qualification. The BDI scores in our study did not relate well to the daily ratings of depression, and although the BDI and daily ratings were from different cycles, the possibility remains that the BDI used in these circumstances is measuring more than 'depression', perhaps reflecting more generally the negative effects of menstrual-related somatic symptoms. More work is required to establish satisfactory methods of quantifying depressive mood in relation to the menstrual cycle.

A few attempts have been made to apply qualitative criteria of depression to perimenstrual mood change. Halbreich *et al.* (1982) developed the Premenstrual Assessment Form (PAF) partly to identify specific types of depressive syndrome. They found that approximately 50% of PMS sufferers met their criteria of a 'major depressive syndrome', although rarely meeting the criteria of 'endogenous' subtype, and being most commonly 'atypical'. Whilst an interesting attempt by this group, they have not clearly related their PAF to DSM III or RDC diagnostic methods. Haskett *et al.* (1980) studied a group of 'severe PMS' sufferers, and in attempting to apply RDC criteria, concluded that these women were not suffering from a major depressive disorder, and that the premenstrual syndrome was characterized more by irritability, tension and lability of mood. However, they applied the usual 2 week duration criterion and they also defined PMS strictly so that women whose depressive mood persisted during menstruation would have been excluded.

In our study (Warner *et al.*, 1991) we devised a self-report questionnaire to cover the various qualitative features of major depressive disorder as defined for RDC, though we modified the duration criterion from 2 weeks to 1 week. On this basis we found that 49% of our 'premenstrual only' and 61% of the 'premenstrual and menstrual' groups met the criteria for major depressive disorder during their premenstrual phase. The numbers meeting the criteria for 'endogenous subtype' in the two groups were 11% and 15% respectively. Thus we have some evidence of depression qualitatively similar to depressive illness in women with PMS, particularly those whose depressive mood persists through the menstrual phase. Further research is required on this issue. It seems inherently likely that the cognitive features of perimenstrual depression would be different from those of chronic depression, with perhaps more emphasis on 'loss of control' and less on 'hopelessness'. Remarkably little attention has been paid to this aspect, and yet women with such cyclical depression offer a rich opportunity for investigating cognitive aspects of depression.

Does this recurrent mood change have a basic link to the menstrual cycle? Angst & Dobler-Mikola (1985) have introduced a new concept into the psychiatry of affective disorders – recurrent and non-recurrent brief depression. They pointed to the varieties of depressed state that were covered by diagnostic categories such as dysthymia, and defined a particular form characterized by its short duration – 'brief depressive episodes', lasting less than 2 weeks (usually 1 to 3 days), dividing this into two subtypes 'recurrent' and 'non-recurrent' brief depression. The recurrent variety occurred monthly over the preceding year, and was twice as common in women as in men (13.9% and 7.5% 3-month prevalence rates respectively). They showed that in terms of symptomatology the recurrent brief depression did not differ from chronic depressive illness, except that anxiety and *premenstrual and menstrual* symptoms were more likely in the recurrent form. Remarkably, nowhere in this paper is any possible relationship considered between this recurrent mood change and the menstrual cycle. If such mood changes are not related to menstruation, and obviously in men they will not be unless it is the menstruation of their female partners, then is it possible that some women are experiencing this pattern and incorrectly attributing it to the menstrual cycle? Alternatively, given that it occurs in both men and women, is it possible that in women it becomes entrained to the menstrual cycle after a period of time? This would be consistent with our own data showing a more variable temporal relationship between mood and menstruation than between cyclical physical changes such as breast tenderness (Bancroft *et al.*, 1988). It is more common to fail to meet the arbitrary criteria for cyclicity with mood changes than with physical symptoms.

Once again we are left with an intriguing and possibly important question that can only be answered by longitudinal studies in which women (and possibly men) are monitored for recurrent mood change over a period of time.

If there is a basic link between this recurrent mood change and the menstrual cycle, is there a neuroendocrine or other biological explanation for the link? At this stage of our knowledge we should keep an open mind about the extent to which the menstrual cycle determines cyclical mood change in women. Given that such a possibility has to be taken seriously, can we explain the relationship in biological terms or should it be attributed to the effects of social learning, expectation and attribution?

Much effort has been expended looking for a biological explanation for the premenstrual syndrome. In general, this large body of research has been unhelpful (Bancroft & Backstrom, 1985). There may be two principal reasons for this. First, the previously mentioned tendency to treat PMS as a homogeneous entity; it is for example, distinctly possible that certain cyclical phenomena, such as breast tenderness, may be direct consequences of the ovarian cycle and its varying levels of ovarian steroids affecting the target organs. Other phenomena, such as cyclical mood change, may have a different type of relationship to the ovarian cycle, reflecting more the temporal entrainment of a recurrent cycle and its 'biological clock' effects on the mood regulating mechanisms in the brain, rather than a direct effect of varying levels of oestrogen and progesterone on the brain (Bancroft & Backstrom, 1985). Secondly, almost all research to date has been 'cross-sectional', usually involving a comparison of the ovarian cycles of women with and without PMS. The methodological issues in studying hormone–behaviour relationships, briefly mentioned at the beginning of the chapter, are of particular relevance at this point. The typical and conventional approach has been to compare women with and without PMS for some hormonal or biochemical variable circulating in the blood. Earlier studies have focused on ovarian steroids such as oestradiol or progesterone or oestradiol/progesterone ratios, more recent studies on other hormones such as prolactin or β-endorphin. Such positive findings that have been reported have usually not been replicated, making such evidence of uncertain relevance. Should we pursue this line of research or is it in any case doomed to failure? A preferable alternative is to test the functioning of this highly complex system in some standardized empirical fashion. Examples of neuroendocrine challenge tests used in this way will be considered below.

A further, alternative, and as yet untried, approach would be to explore whether the development of PMS accompanies a subtle change in some characteristic of the ovarian cycle over time. For this we need parallel evidence of the natural history of PMS and of the menstrual cycle. In our large retrospective study (Warner & Bancroft, 1990) we found strong evidence that the likelihood of a woman describing herself as a PMS sufferer was related to the duration of her natural ovarian cycles, i.e. the length of time since menarche, pregnancy or the use of steroidal contraception, whichever was most recent. The peak time for reporting PMS was after 3 to 6 years of natural cycles, and it was at this stage in particular that stress-related factors seemed relatively unimportant as correlates of PMS reporting. Is it possible that after a certain number of years of repeated uninterrupted natural cycles there is some alteration to the system, or alternatively, is it a matter of an accumulated 'kindling' effect, as described earlier? This possibility can only be answered by longitudinal studies in which women are followed up over years of natural cycles to see whether any change in the neuroendocrine features of the cycle is related to change in cyclical symptomatology. There is also the important and related need to follow women through to the perimenopausal stage, which will be discussed later. To what extent are these changes in the cycle part of the process of decline of the ageing ovary?

As far as perimenstrual mood change is concerned, are there any biological features associated with this form of cyclical depression which are comparable to those found in depressive illness?

The search for biological markers of depressive illness of a neuroendocrine or biochemical kind is at an early but interesting stage of development. Both 'state' and 'trait' markers are being sought. Three broad areas of research have evolved.

The pituitary–adrenocortical axis. It is well established that depressed people have increased levels of circulating cortisol as a state characteristic (Sachar, 1967). This is most clearly evident as increased secretion of cortisol in the second half of the day.

As yet, little attention has been paid to cortisol production in women with PMS. Haskett *et al.* (1984) studied 42 women by means of Dexamethasone Suppression Test (DST) and 24 hour urinary cortisol production on two occasions during the cycle (follicular phase and premenstrually). No consistent differences, either in DST response or cortisol production were found between the two occasions. This makes it unlikely that women with perimenstrual mood change show the *increased* cortisol production characteristic of depressive illness.

Neurotransmitter receptors. Neurotransmitter receptors on blood platelets offer an indirect way of estimating receptor numbers within the brain. Thus, adrenergic, serotonergic and imipramine binding sites have been measured in states of depression and recovery. The results so far have been inconsistent and apart from the doubtful assumption of parallel changes in receptor numbers in both the platelets and the brain, there are formidable methodological problems with the receptor assays involved (Porter *et al.*, 1987). There have, however, been reports of abnormal levels of 5-hydroxytryptamine (5HT) platelet receptors in women with PMS (Taylor *et al.*, 1984; Rapkin *et al.*, 1987).

Neuroendocrine challenge tests. The administration of a L-tryptophan load by intravenous infusion produces, in normal subjects, a transient increase in both prolactin and growth hormone. This is believed to result from an increase in the turnover or availability of 5HT following the infusion. The administration of clonidine, an alpha2 adrenoreceptor agonist, produces changes in growth hormone (GH). In depressed subjects both types of response are blunted (Checkley *et al.*, 1981; Heninger *et al.*, 1984). At present it is not yet clear to what extent either of these neuroendocrine tests measure state or trait characteristics, a fundamental issue which needs to be resolved. However, they are examples of methods for 'testing the system' referred to above.

We have recently completed a study involving the neuroendocrine challenge of an infusion of tryptophan. We compared 13 women with demonstrable perimenstrual depression and 13 women with no perimenstrual mood change, carrying out the challenge test twice in each subject: just before menstruation and during the mid-to-late follicular phase (Bancroft *et al.*, 1991a). The results were striking and potentially of considerable importance. We found two types of effect. One characterized the phase of the cycle; we observed a blunted prolactin response to the challenge during the premenstrual phase in both groups of women. This suggests that there is typically some biochemical change premenstrually, which when combined with other vulnerability factors accounts for why depressive mood tends to occur at that phase of the cycle. The other type of effect distinguished women with and without premenstrual mood change; such an effect was observed with both GH and cortisol response to the infusion. The women with premenstrual depression did show a blunting of their GH response premenstrually, but the most striking effect was that their GH response was substantially less than that of the women with no mood change *at both phases of the cycle.* A cortisol response to tryptophan occurred both premenstrually and postmenstrually in the no mood change group, but did not occur *at either phase* in the mood change group.

Thus we have evidence that women with a propensity for perimenstrual depression show some abnormal neuroendocrine responses both premenstrually and postmenstrually. This possibly persisting abnormality may then combine with the changes that normally occur premenstrually to make such women vulnerable to depression *at that phase of the cycle.*

This is a radically new way of formulating the biological basis of perimenstrual mood change and opens up a number of exciting possibilities for further research. As yet we do not know whether the GH and cortisol abnormalities are *state* or *trait* phenomena, though this will be a researchable question within a longitudinal study of such women.

The unexpected cortisol findings are of particular interest. As mentioned above, people with chronic depression typically show raised cortisol production. The significance of this alteration, whether it is an epiphenomenon or is causally related to the mood change, has never been established. Nor do we know at what point in the development of a depressive illness this cortisol hypersecretion becomes established. Here we have evidence from a study of depressive mood of very recent onset, albeit recurrent. Is it possible that a normal woman's cortisol response to tryptophan premenstrually reflects an adaptive mechanism that protects her from depressive mood at that time? And is one of the characteristics of the woman prone to perimenstrual depression an inability to show this adaptive cortisol response? Does this characteristic make such women more at risk for depressive illness also?

If we can identify markers that would indicate women at risk they could play an important role in selecting women for longitudinal studies. So far we have only looked at this one neuroendocrine challenge test. Other studies of this kind, involving the adrenergic and dopaminergic systems may also be informative.

Later adulthood and reproductive decline

In women, later adulthood and reproductive decline involves the menopause; what are the psychosocial consequences of the menopause that may be hormonally determined?

In men, there is no direct counterpart of the menopause. There is a variable degree of ageing of the hypothalamo-pituitary-testicular axis which may have psychosocial consequences. But as yet we have little evidence showing a causal relationship between this hormonal decline and the common declines in sexual interest, energy and other aspects of well-being in men as they get older (for review see Bancroft 1989; Schiavi, 1990). This aspect will not be dealt with further in this chapter.

The menopause

The decline in ovarian function associated with the menopause reflects an ageing process in which primordial follicles become increasingly resistant to stimulation by FSH. In contrast to the testis, in which hormone production is independent of gametogenesis, the main hormone production of the ovary depends on follicular development. Once this ceases, ovarian production of oestradiol almost ceases and progesterone remains at 'early follicular' levels. The postmenopausal ovary continues to produce a certain amount of androgen (androstenedione and testosterone) which provides a source of oestrogen by its aromatization in the peripheral fatty tissues.

This process of ovarian decline is gradual, starting with an alteration and often reduced regularity of the menstrual cycle, an increased likelihood of anovular cycles and gradually rising levels of plasma FSH, and to a lesser extent, LH. The cessation of menses is one feature of this process, reflecting decline in the cyclical rise and fall of oestrogen to the point where endometrial hypertrophy and shedding no longer occurs. The process of ovarian decline and the adjustment to a postmenopausal stable state may continue for some time after the cessation of menses. This period of transition varies considerably in duration, although for the majority of women it is between 4 and 6 years (Treloar, 1981).

We can thus see that this process results in two relatively distinguishable stages in a woman's reproductive history: (a) the *transitional* stage, when a woman is adapting to a shift from a pattern of regular neuroendocrine cycles to a relatively steady neuroendocrine state, and

(b) a *postmenopausal* stage, when she experiences states of relative hormonal deficiency. The transitional stage can be seen as the counterpart of the transitional stage of adolescence, when the adolescent girl has to adjust from a state of neuroendocrine stability to one of cyclicity. At the menopausal end of the woman's reproductive phase, problems may occur in one or both stages. The classical symptom of the transitional stage is the vasomotor instability experienced as a 'hot flush' or 'cold sweat'. As we shall see there may be other complaints associated with this phase. The most convincing consequences of postmenopausal oestrogen deficiency are vaginal dryness and, as a gradual process, osteoporosis. A woman may find the transitional stage troublesome, but produce enough oestrogen postmenopausally to avoid the problems of oestrogen deficiency. Another woman may pass through the transitional stage with a minimum of difficulty but have problems with vaginal dryness or, later, osteoporosis. Some women suffer in both, probably the majority in neither respect. In this paper, the term 'perimenopausal' will be used to describe the transitional phase.

Methodological issues. In attempting to understand the impact of these stages on women's health we are again confronted with some fundamental methodological problems.

Definition. As should by now be clear, the term 'menopause' is unhelpful. It is in fact a discrete non-event which is recognizable as a biological marker, but only in retrospect. Furthermore, it is not a useful temporal marker of the stages that concern us. The transitional phase may stretch for 3 or 4 years either side of this marker. Greene (1984) has discussed the variable approaches to definition and in particular has distinguished two approaches used by McKinlay *et al.* (1972) and Jaszmann *et al.* (1969). The 'McKinlay' method defines 'premenopausal' status as 'having menstruated within the last 3 months'; 'perimenopausal' as 'having last menstruated between 3 and 12 months ago'; 'postmenopausal' as 'having last menstruated more than 12 months ago'. This system is therefore simply based on the date of the last period. The 'Jaszmann' method aims to judge whether the *pattern* of menstruation has changed. 'Premenopausal' means normal menses during the preceding year; 'perimenopausal' indicates an altered pattern of menstruation (shorter, longer or irregular cycles) during the preceding year; 'postmenopausal' means no menstruation for the past year. Most of the surveys of menopausal symptoms have used one or other of these definitions, or slight modifications of them (Greene, 1984).

Studies using the Jaszmann method have been consistent in finding evidence of increased psychosomatic morbidity in the perimenopausal stage, when a woman is still menstruating but with altered cycles (e.g.

Jaszmann *et al.*, 1969; Ballinger, 1975). Those using the McKinlay method have found an increase in hot flushes and night sweats as women move from 'premenopausal to postmenopausal' but no difference in other types of symptoms (Thomson *et al.*, 1973). Lock (1986) studied the menopause in Japanese women, in the usual age group of 45 to 55, and categorized them using a modification of the McKinlay method. Interestingly, vasomotor symptoms were unusual in this study, and in other symptoms there were no differences between the premenstrual, perimenstrual and postmenstrual groups. McKinlay & Jefferys (1974) used, in effect, both types of definition. Using the McKinlay method, they also found only vasomotor symptoms to be associated with menopausal status. When, however, they applied a modification comparable to Jaszmann's, and introduced a transitional group who were menstruating but with altered cycles, they found an increase in a number of symptoms such as dizziness, palpitations, depression, sleeplessness in the transitional group compared with the 'normal' premenopausal group.

A further method relies on age and our knowledge of the average age of menopause. Thus Bungay *et al.* (1980) divided their women into age groups and compared the 45 to 50 age group, who were assumed to be predominantly in the transitional perimenopausal stage, with the 50 to 55 age group, who were assumed to be predominantly postmenopausal. Whilst crude, this method produced results consistent with the Jaszmann method, showing an increase in vasomotor symptoms most marked in the 50+ age group, and an increase in psychosomatic and minor complaints in the assumed transitional 45 to 50 age group.

Socio-cultural attitudes to menopause. Given the complex and long-term nature of the perimenopausal transitional period, it is to be expected that its subjective manifestations will reflect socio-economically and culturally derived influences and attitudes. Greene (1984) has reviewed the relevant but limited evidence. He concluded that negative attitudes to the menopause are not as widespread or marked as is often assumed. They are more likely in women of lower socio-economic status and also in younger women rather than women of perimenopausal age. There is some evidence of cultural variation in the social significance of postmenopausal or postreproductive status, with women in some societies viewing the menopause as an entry point to a social role of much higher status. The evidence also suggests that women in such societies are less likely to complain of 'menopausal' symptoms.

However, Greene (1984) also found little support for the notion that menopausal complaints are manifestations of modern industrialized societies. The form in which such complaints are expressed are likely to be subject to social influences and vary cross-culturally. Thus Lock (1986), in her Japanese study, reported the predominance of complaints such as 'shoulder stiffness', a common complaint amongst the Japanese which has connotations of 'stress'.

In general the limited evidence suggests that vasomotor symptoms are not culture-sensitive and are found as clear manifestations of the menopausal state whenever studied (e.g. Sharma & Saxena, 1981). An interesting exception is Lock's (1986) study of Japanese women of whom a much smaller proportion reported 'hot flushes' compared with a Canadian study using a similar methodology (Kaufert, 1984). Ethnic differences of this kind could reflect genetic differences in responsiveness of the vasomotor system as much as different cultural stereotypes.

Co-existing problems. In assessing the role of endocrine change on the well-being and health of women at this stage in their life cycle, it is important to take into consideration the variety of life stresses that are likely to arise at this time. The 'empty nest' and parental death are two adverse influences that are likely to affect women in the 45 to 55 age range (Greene, 1983). As discussed above, negative connotations of this transitional phase will vary with socio-economic and cultural factors. The relationship between adverse life events and other types of health problem such as depression, is complex and detailed methods of assessment that allow for the 'matching' of event with the prior susceptibilities of the individual are necessary to demonstrate a causal relationship. As yet this type of investigation aimed specifically at women in the perimenopausal stage of development has been limited (e.g. Cooke & Greene, 1981; Greene, 1982). The results suggest that, with the exception of certain types of life event such as bereavement, there is no noticeable increase in adverse life events at this life stage. However, there does appear to be a reduced ability to cope with such ordinary adversity compared with younger women (Greene, 1984).

Competing tendencies. The transitional stage of the perimenopause is further complicated by the possibility that it is at a time when earlier adverse influences, related to regular menstruation, recede in importance, resulting in a reduction in morbidity, whilst other factors, such as oestrogen deficiency, increase in importance. This possibility will be considered more closely in relation to depressive illness.

The evidence. With these methodological issues in mind, let us briefly consider the evidence of a relationship between the perimenopause and the postmenopausal status on the health of women under three headings: (a) *general health and well-being,* (b) *depressive illness and* (c) *sexual function.*

General health and well-being. The weight of evidence from community-based studies is that, whereas both vasomotor symptoms and a variety of psychosomatic and minor affective problems are more prevalent in the 45 to 55 age group, their relationship to menopause is somewhat different. In particular, vasomotor symptoms, whilst often in evidence in the years before cessation of menses, tend to be most severe after menses have stopped. The other 'psychosomatic' type changes are most likely to peak in the few years before cessation of menses and reduce in frequency a year or so after the menopause. Vasomotor symptoms are also relatively specific to the menopause, although they are experienced by a proportion of younger women perimenstrually. The other symptoms, such as dizziness, minor depression, weight gain and sleeplessness, are common at any age and one is seeing an *increase* rather than an *onset* at this perimenopausal stage. Ballinger (1975) has also shown that the more psychiatric of these symptoms are more likely to occur in women with a previous history of psychiatric problems. In other words, whilst the perimenopause may be associated specifically with certain types of phenomena such as the hot flush, there are also changes during the perimenopause which make the woman more susceptible to other sources of stress and other types of emotional reactions of a non-specific nature.

So far only one longitudinal study of women passing through the menopause has been reported. McKinlay & McKinlay (1989) studied a cohort of 2300 premenopausal women over a $4\frac{1}{2}$ year period. Each woman was interviewed *by telephone* at nine-month intervals. During the study 55% of the women experienced the transition through natural or surgical menopause. They assessed whether women's menstrual status changed from 'regular' to 'irregular' to 'ceased'. Their reported results so far are confined to the first three follow-up assessments. Their principal conclusion was that *cessation of menses*, at least that associated with a natural menopause, had virtually no bearing on the women's well-being or physical health, which was more dependent on the presence of physical symptoms and other stresses present *before* cessation of menstruation. The main exception was in the group experiencing surgical menopause. But in these women there was a high level of morbidity both before and after their surgery. It is not entirely clear from this report whether the change from regular to irregular cycles was associated with any change in well-being or symptoms, and further analyses and reports are awaited from this important study. The limitations imposed by the use of telephone interviews should be borne in mind.

Depressive illness. The idea that the menopause or perimenopause is associated with depressive illness in women originated in the early nineteenth century leading to the concept of involutional melancholia with its distinct phenomenology (Hallstrom, 1973). Rosenthal (1968) in critically reviewing the earlier literature was largely responsible for laying the concept of involutional melancholia to rest; there is little sustainable evidence that depressive illness at the perimenopause is phenomenologically distinct. Also there has been a growing opinion that depressive illness is not more likely at the perimenopause although the evidence for this assumption has been somewhat indirect. One early and influential study by Winokur (1973) directly addressed the issue. He assessed 71 consecutive cases of depressive illness in women admitted to hospital and worked out the likelihood of such illness occurring during the menopause, which he defined as the 3 years after the reported date of cessation of menses. He assessed the number of previous episodes of depression reported by these women, but for some reason which he did not explain he used a different criterion for a depressive illness during the menopause (i.e. admission to hospital) from other times (when social disability but not hospital admission was required). He concluded on these somewhat doubtful grounds that there was no increased likelihood of depression during the menopause. Weissman & Klerman (1977), in their review of the sex difference in depression, dismissed the menopause as a contributory factor in the greater prevalence amongst women, citing Winokur's (1973) study, and commenting that 'similar findings have been noted by others'; to support this they cited a number of studies that did not address the menopause issue directly but rather gave rates of depressive illness by age group. One of the studies cited (Juel-Nielsen & Strömgren, 1965) actually reported rates showing a peak in the 45 to 55 age group. Generally speaking, more recent epidemiological studies, such as the American Epidemiological Catchment Area (ECA) study, have reported rates of depression highest in the 30 to 45 age group and declining somewhat in older women. Interestingly, this was the picture reported by Weissman *et al.* (1988) for major depressive disorder, although for dysthymia, a less severe and more prolonged form of depressive disorder, one month prevalence rates were slightly higher in the 45 to 64 age group than the 25 to 44 age group (Regier *et al.*, 1988). Certainly, there is no suggestion of a peak of major depression in the 45 to 55 age group. Against this are the various sources of evidence, cited above, of increased prevalence of minor affective disturbances in the perimenopausal phase, and also the common clinical experience of some women becoming depressed around the menopause and not recovering fully until oestrogen replacement is given.

The most substantial study to investigate depressive illness in relation to the climacteric was that of Hallström (1973) in Sweden. He studied representative samples of women in the community at the following ages: 38, 46, 50, 54 and 60. His definition of menopausal stages was comparable to Jaszmann's, although his 'perimenopausal' stage was defined as having had 'one or more periods of amenorrhoea lasting less than 12 months'. This would indicate a later stage of the transitional period than Jaszmann's definition. In line with other studies already mentioned, Hallström found that his perimenopausal women had increased likelihood of psychological morbidity, but this group did not differ in terms of depressive illness. He concluded that the most likely explanation was that the menopausal process was not relevant to the causation of depressive illness. However, he made one important qualification to this conclusion. 'This interpretation presupposes that other causative factors for mental illness are present in equal degree in the different climacteric phases. If this is not the case, then any possible causal relation between a climacteric phase and a change in the incidence rate might be obscured'. He went on to test the possibility that certain types of pathogenic factors might be associated with earlier or later menopause, and found no support for this possibility. There are, however, further possibilities along these lines which have not been considered previously. In particular, it is possible that there are factors associated with menstruation and the premenopausal status of women, which increase the likelihood of depression in susceptible women, and which therefore would cease to act *after* the menopause, leading to a reduction in the incidence of depression. At the same time, there may be other factors increasing the likelihood of depression in women with other susceptibilities which become active with the postmenopausal decline in oestrogen. In other words are there tendencies working in opposite directions around the menopause which would conceal a menopause-linked increase in depression occurring in a proportion of women?

Gater *et al.* (1989) have recently reported an epidemiological study of first-admission rates for affective psychosis. This showed the usual preponderance of women, but demonstrated that the excess in women could largely be attributed to parity. In fact non-parous women had a lower relative risk of admission than men. This effect of parity was evident up to the age of 54; thereafter parous and non-parous women had similar rates. This effect was not due to postpartum depression, and appeared to continue once women had experienced pregnancy. Bebbington (1988) examined the Camberwell data for less severe depressive episodes and found some support for the above findings, with the effect of parity being present until the age of 50. Kendell *et al.* (1987) also showed an increase in the incidence of depressive illness with parity which was not apparently dependent on the number of pregnancies. The implication of these interesting data is that pregnancy renders a woman more susceptible to depression, for reasons not yet identified, until she gets to the age around the menopause. Here we have one mechanism by which the rates of depression might fall when women get to the menopause.

The possibility remains that in some specifically vulnerable women, decline in oestrogen levels renders them susceptible to depression, which would respond to hormone replacement. If this is the case, the proportion of such women is not likely to be large but may nevertheless represent a clinically important group. Longitudinal studies should explore the possibility of such competing trends and aim to identify women at risk for these different types of effect. Once effective longitudinal studies of premenopausal women are carried out, it may become possible to identify those women whose vulnerability to depression may *lessen* once they are postmenopausal.

Sexual function. One unequivocal effect of postmenopausal decline in oestrogen levels, is vaginal dryness leading, when severe, to atrophic vaginitis. This is one of the few menopausal symptoms to show a correlation with circulating levels of oestradiol in the plasma (Chakravarti *et al.*, 1979). This can cause dyspareunia, and secondarily lead to loss of interest in sex. It is important to note that this vaginal effect is noticeable in only 8% to 10% of postmenopausal women, so that presumably most women produce enough oestradiol to avoid this problem. Leiblum *et al.* (1983) investigated the degree of vaginal atrophy and its relationship to sexual activity in postmenopausal women. They found the more sexually active women to have less vaginal atrophy. Either sexual activity protects the vagina, or women who do not have significant vaginal dryness are more likely to be sexually active.

A more difficult question is whether the hormonal changes accompanying the menopause contribute directly to the decline in women's sexual desire and enjoyment of sex that commonly occur, or whether such changes are related to other aspects of ageing. Hallström's (1973) epidemiological study suggested that the menopause is relevant. By holding age constant in his analysis, he found sexual decline more marked in postmenopausal than premenopausal women. Further evidence of this kind comes from Pfeiffer *et al.* (1972) and Bottiglioni & De Aloysio (1982).

The nature of this association between menopause and sexual decline, apart from the issue of oestrogen-dependent vaginal response, remains unclear. McCoy & Davidson (1985), for example, in a longitudinal study of postmenopausal women found no correlation between declining sexuality and declining oestrogen levels.

More clear-cut evidence comes from studies of hormone replacement following surgical menopause (i.e. removal of the ovaries). This procedure of course produces a more dramatic change in gonadal steroid levels as the normal postmenopausal ovarian production is also eliminated. This is particularly important in relation to androgens, the main product of the postmenopausal ovary.

The most convincing studies of hormone replacement in oophorectomized women come from Sherwin *et al.* (1985) and Sherwin & Gelfand (1987). They showed that by giving hormone replacement immediately following surgery in women who were previously normal sexually, sexual interest and enjoyment was maintained or enhanced by testosterone replacement but not by oestradiol. This is consistent with a fundamental role for testosterone in the sexuality of women, though as we have seen earlier this relationship has appeared complex or obscured in other studies. It should also be said that other studies of post-oophorectomized women have not always been consistent with those of Sherwin and her colleagues. Dennerstein *et al.* (1980) demonstrated a beneficial effect of oestrogen on sexual desire, though they did not compare it with testosterone. Dow *et al.* (1983) compared oestradiol with an oestradiol/testosterone combination and found that both regimes improved sexual function. A possibly important difference in this case was that, in contrast to Sherwin *et al.* (1985) subjects, the women in this study had already developed sexual problems when they entered the trial. The presence of interpersonal sexual difficulties does appear to obscure subtle hormone–behaviour relationships in women. It should also be pointed out that the beneficial effects of androgens reported by Sherwin *et al.* (1985) involve injections that raised the plasma testosterone to sustained levels well above the physiological.

Male–female differences

Male issues have not been dealt with in any depth in this chapter. In relation to hormones and male sexuality, the evidence has been reviewed elsewhere (Bancroft, 1988, 1989). What we have encountered at several points in this review, however, is evidence that hormones play a more direct role in influencing male behaviour, whereas with females hormonal effects are either obscured by psychosocial factors or appear to be inconsistent across women. In contrast to women, the evidence from men, at least as far as sexuality is concerned, is surprisingly consistent. A number of possible explanations for this apparent sex difference have been proposed (Bancroft, 1989), including the following:

(1) Females are more susceptible than males to social learning in their sexual development, so that hormone–behaviour effects are more likely to be obscured.

(2) Females are more variable than men in their behavioural responsiveness to reproductive hormones. This would be con-

sistent with the role that such effects play in fertility in the human species. It is more crucial for the male, if he is to reproduce himself, that he responds appropriately to his reproductive hormones. If he does not, he is less likely to get into a sexual relationship. In so far as such responsiveness is genetically determined, the genes of such men are less likely to be maintained in 'the genetic pool'. For women, their likelihood of being in a fertile relationship is less dependent on their hormone-driven behaviour. The pattern of sexual behaviour for human pairs typically involves a frequency of coitus, male initiated, which is sufficient for optimal fertility. Hence, greater genetic variability in hormone–behaviour sensitivity is possible for women.

If either of these explanations is valid, they serve to underline the importance of individual differences in hormone–behaviour interactions in women, and the need to identify 'types' of women in terms of their behavioural responsiveness to reproductive hormones. Such a view does offer some hope of explaining why a proportion of women are vulnerable to PMS, postnatal depression, adverse reactions to steroidal contraceptives, and difficulties through the perimenopause. Such variability clearly has to be taken into account in planning longitudinal studies in women, as a crucial consideration is the need to identify 'markers' which might allow us to select women for groups with different patterns of reactivity. This is particularly important when a certain 'response pattern' is likely to be present in a small but clinically relevant proportion of women.

CONCLUSIONS ABOUT LONGITUDINAL RESEARCH

The limitations of cross-sectional studies in explaining the relationship between reproductive hormones and behaviour of women through the life cycle should now be obvious, and the need for longitudinal studies incontrovertible. However, longitudinal research in this area is exceptionally difficult, particularly when studies of development are involved. 'Natural experiments' are extremely rare and in any case difficult to interpret. Exposure to drugs during pregnancy remains an important issue, and the longitudinal studies of the effects of barbiturates, underway with June Reinisch and her colleagues, should soon be bearing fruit. To make those studies feasible, however, an extremely ambitious research programme had to be funded and initiated in Denmark.

Studies of adolescent development are of considerable interest and those cited here whet our appetite for what is possible. Yet the practical and ethical problems of continuous or repeated assessment in this age group are considerable.

In the adult the potential for longitudinal studies in the areas covered by this review are real, particularly in relation to the menstrual cycle. There are already outstanding examples of longitudinal studies of the menstrual cycle, involving hundreds of women, thousands of cycles over many years (Treloar *et al.*, 1967; Vollman 1977). These serve to show just what many women are prepared to do in documenting their cycles. What is now needed are comparable studies of cohorts of women, representing different patterns of cycle-related changes, to see how stable these patterns are over time, how they relate to changes in ovarian function, whether they change after pregnancy and to what extent they are related to subsequent depressive illness. There are a number of fundamental methodological issues that need to be resolved before such studies will be feasible, some of them alluded to in this review. But the possibility is there.

REFERENCES

Abramson, L. Y., Seligman, M. E. P. & Teasdale, J. D. (1978) Learned helplessness in humans: a critique and reformulation. *Journal of Abnormal Psychology*, **87**, 49–74.

Alexander, G. M., Sherwin, B. B., Bancroft, J. & Davidson, D. W. (1990) Testosterone and sexual behavior in oral contraceptive users and non-users: a prospective study. *Hormones and Behavior*, **24**, 435–41.

Andersch, B., Wendestam, C., Hahn, L. & Olman, R. (1986) Perimenstrual complaints. I. Prevalence of premenstrual symptoms in a Swedish urban population. *Journal of Psychosomatic Obstetrics and Gynaecology*, **5**, 39–49.

Angst, J. & Dobler-Mikola, A. (1984) Do the diagnostic criteria determine the sex ratio in depression? *Journal of Affective Disorders*, **7**, 189–98.

Angst, J. & Dobler-Mikola, A. (1985) The Zurich study – a prospective epidemiological study of depressive, neurotic and psychosomatic syndromes. IV Recurrent and nonrecurrent brief depression. *European Archives of Psychiatry and Neurological Sciences*, **234**, 408–16.

Ballinger, C. B. (1975) Psychiatric morbidity and the menopause: screening of a general population sample. *British Medical Journal*, **3**, 344–6.

Bancroft, J. (1988) Reproductive hormones and male sexual function. In Sitsen, J. M. A. (ed.) *Handbook of sexology* Vol 6: *The pharmacology and endocrinology of sexual function.* Amsterdam: Elsevier, pp. 297–315.

Bancroft, J. (1989) *Human sexuality and its problems*, 2nd edn. Edinburgh: Churchill Livingstone.

Bancroft, J. & Backstrom, T. (1985) Premenstrual syndrome. *Clinical Endocrinology*, **22:** 313–36.

Bancroft, J., Cook, A. & Williamson, L. (1988) Food craving, mood and the menstrual cycle. *Psychological Medicine*, **18**, 855–60.

Bancroft, J. & Sartorius, N. (1990) The effects of oral contraceptives on well being and sexuality: a review. *Oxford Reviews of Reproductive Biology*, pp. 57–92.

Bancroft, J., Cook, A., Davidson, D. W., Bennie, J. & Goodwin, G. (1991a) Blunting of the neuroendocrine response to infusion of L-tryptophan in women with perimenstrual mood change. *Psychological Medicine*, in press.

Bancroft, J., Sherwin, B. B., Alexander, G. M., Davidson, D. W. & Walker, A. (1991b) Aspects of sexuality in oral contraceptive users and non-users. I. Sexual experience, sexual attitudes and gender role. *Archives of Sexual Behavior*, in press.

Bancroft, J., Sherwin, B. B., Alexander, G. M., Davidson, D. W. & Walker, A. (1991c) Aspects of sexuality in oral contraceptive users and non-users. II. The role of androgens. *Archives of Sexual Behaviour*, in press.

Beach, F. A. (1979) Animal models for human sexuality. In Ciba Foundation Symposium, Vol. 62 (New Series). *Sex, Hormones and Behaviour.* Amsterdam: Excerpta Medica, pp. 113–132.

Bebbington, P. (1988) Gender and parity in a community survey of psychiatric disorder. Paper at Annual Meeting, Royal College of Psychiatry, Brighton.

Beck, A. T., Rush, A. J., Shaw, B. F. & Emery, G. (1979) *Cognitive therapy of depression.* New York: Guilford.

Beck, A. T., Steer, R. A. & Garbin, M. G. (1988) Psychometric properties of the Beck Depression Inventory: twenty-five years of evaluation. *Clinical Psychology Review*, **8**, 77–100.

Benbow, C. P. (1988) Sex differences in mathematical reasoning ability in intellectually talented pre-adolescents; their nature, effects and possible causes. *Behavioural and Brain Sciences*, **11**, 169–232.

Benjaminsen, S. (1981) Stressful life events preceding the onset of neurotic depression. *Psychological Medicine*, **11**, 369–78.

Beral, V. & Colwell, I. (1981) Randomised trial of high doses of stilboestrol and ethisterone therapy in pregnancy: long term follow up of the children. *Journal of Epidemiology and Community Health*, **39**; 155–60.

Blazer, M. D., Hughes, D. & George, L. K. (1987) Stressful life events and the onset of a generalized anxiety syndrome. *American Journal of Psychiatry*, **144**, 1178–83.

Blazer, D., Swartz, M., Woodbury, M., Manton, K. G., Hughes, D. & George, L. K. (1988) Depressive symptoms and depressive diagnoses in a community population. Use of a new procedure for analysis of psychiatric classification. *Archives of General Psychiatry*, **45**, 1078–84.

Bornstein, P. E., Clayton, P. J., Halikas, J. A., Maurice, L. M. & Robins, E. (1973) The depression of widowhood after thirteen months. *British Journal of Psychiatry*, **122**, 561–6.

Bottiglioni, F. & De Aloysio, D. (1982) Female sexual activity as a function of climacteric condition and age. *Maturitas*, **4**, 27–31.

Broverman, D. M., Broverman, I. K., Vogel, W., Palmer, R. D. & Klaiber, E. L. (1964) The automization of cognitive style and physical development. *Child Development*, **35**, 1343–59.

Brugha, T. S. (1988) Gender differences in mental illness. Paper at Annual Meeting, Royal College of Psychiatry, Brighton.

Bungay, G., Vessey, M. & McPherson, C. (1980) Study of symptoms in middle life, with special reference to the menopause. *British Medical Journal*, **281**, 181–3.

Byrne, D. G. (1979) Anxiety as state and trait following survived myocardial infarction. *British Journal of Social and Clinical Psychology*, **18**, 417–23.

Chakravarti, S., Collins, W., Thom, M. & Studd, J. (1979) The relation between plasma hormone profiles, symptoms and response to oestrogen treatment of women approaching the menopause. *British Medical Journal*, **281**, 181–3.

Checkley, S. A., Slade, A. P. & Shur, E. (1981) Growth hormone and other responses to clonidine in patients with endogenous depression. *British Journal of Psychiatry*, **138**, 51–5.

Cooke, D. J. & Greene, J. G. (1981) Types of life events in relation to symptoms at the climacteric. *Journal of Psychosomatic Research*, **25**, 5–11.

Coppen, A. (1965) The prevalence of menstrual disorders in psychiatric patients. *British Journal of Psychiatry*, **111**, 155–67.

Dennerstein, L., Burrows, G. D., Wood, C. & Hyman, G. (1980) Hormones and sexuality: effect of estrogen and progestogen. *Obstetrics and Gynecology*, **56**, 316–22.

Dorner, G. (1980) Sexual differentiation of the brain. *Vitamins and Hormones*, **38**, 325–81.

Dow, M. G. T., Hart, D. M. & Forrest, C. S. A. (1983) Hormonal treatment of sexual unresponsiveness in post-menopausal women: a comparative study. *British Journal of Obstetrics and Gynaecology*, **90**, 361–6.

Ehrhardt, A. A., Grisanti, G. L. & Meyer-Bahlburg, H. F. L. (1977) Prenatal exposure to medroxyprogesterone acetate (MPA) in girls. *Psychoneuroendocrinology*, **2**, 391–8.

Endicott, J. & Halbreich, U. (1982) Retrospective report of premenstrual depressive changes: factors affecting confirmation by daily ratings. *Psychopharmacology Bulletin*, **18**, 109–12.

Endicott, J. & Halbreich, U. (1988) Practical problems in evaluation. In Gise, L. H., (ed.) *Contemporary issues in Obstetrics & Gynecology* Vol. 2. *The premenstrual syndrome.* Edinburgh: Churchill Livingstone, pp. 35–46.

Endicott, J., Halbreich, U., Schacht, S. & Nee, J. (1981) Premenstrual changes and affective disorders. *Psychomatic Medicine*, **43**, 519–29.

Folkman, S. & Lazarus, R. S. (1980) An analysis of coping in a middle-aged community sample. *Journal of Health and Social Behavior*, **21**, 219–39.

Forest, H. G., Deperetti, E. & Bertrand, J. (1976) Hypothalamic-pituitary-gonadal relationships from birth to puberty. *Clinical Endocrinology*, **5**, 551–69.

Gagnon, J. H. & Simon, W. (1973) *Sexual conduct: the social sources of human sexuality.* Chicago: Aldine.

Gater, R. A., Dean, C. & Morris, J. (1989) The contribution of childbearing to the sex difference in first admission rates for affective psychosis. *Psychological Medicine*, **19**, 719–24.

Gladue, B. A., Green, R. & Hellman, R. E. (1984) Neuroendocrine response to estrogen and sexual orientation. *Science*, **225**, 1496–9.

Goldberg, D. (1988) Sex differences in access to psychiatric care. Paper at Annual Meeting, Royal College of Psychiatry, Brighton.

Gooren, L. J. G. (1988a) An appraisal of endocrine theories of homosexuality and gender dysphoria. In Sitsen, J. M. A. (ed.) *Handbook of sexology* Vol 6: *The pharmacology and endocrinology of sexual function.* Amsterdam: Elsevier, pp. 410–24.

Gooren, L. J. G. (1988b) Hypogonadotropic hypogonadal men respond less well to androgen substitution treatment than hypergonadotropic hypogonadal men. *Archives of Sexual Behavior,* **17,** 265–70.

Graham, C. A. (1989) Treatment of premenstrual syndrome with a triphasic oral contraceptive: a double-blind placebo-controlled trial. Unpublished PhD thesis, McGill University, Montreal.

Greene, J. G. (1982) Psychosocial factors in women during the climacteric: a community study. In Main, C. J. (ed.) *Clinical psychology and medicine; a behavioural perspective.* New York: Plenum.

Greene, J. G. (1983) Bereavement and social support at the climacteric. *Maturitas,* **5,** 115–24.

Greene, J. G. (1984) *The social and psychological origins of the climacteric syndrome.* Aldershot: Gower.

Halbreich, U. & Endicott, J. (1985) The relationship of dysphoric premenstrual changes to depressive disorder. *Acta Psychiatrica Scandinavica,* **71,** 331–8.

Halbreich, U., Endicott, J., Schacht, S. & Nee, J. (1982) The diversity of premenstrual changes as reflected in the Premenstrual Assessment Form. *Acta Psychiatrica Scandinavica,* **65,** 46–65.

Hallström, T. (1973) *Mental disorder and sexuality in the climacteric.* Stockholm: Scandinavian University Books.

Hart, W. G., Coleman, G. J. & Russell, J. W. (1987) Assessment of premenstrual symptomatology: a re-evaluation of the predictive validity of self-report. *Journal of Psychosomatic Research,* **31,** 185–90.

Haskett, R. F., Steiner, M. & Carroll, B. (1984) A psychoendocrine study of premenstrual tension syndrome: model for endogenous depression? *Journal of Affective Disorders,* **6,** 191–9.

Haskett, R. F., Steiner, M., Osmun, J. N. & Carroll, B. J. (1980) Severe premenstrual tension; delineation of the syndrome. *Biological Psychiatry,* **15,** 121–39.

Heninger, G. R., Charney, D. S. & Sternberg, D. E. (1984) Serotonergic function in depression. *Archives of General Psychiatry,* **41,** 398–402.

Herdt, G. H. & Davidson, J. (1988) The Sambia 'Turnim-man': sociocultural and clinical aspects of gender formation in male pseudohermaphrodites with 5-alpha reductase deficiency in Papua New Guinea. *Archives of Sexual Behavior,* **17,** 33–57.

Hines, M. & Shipley, C. (1984) Prenatal exposure to diethylstilboestrol (DES) and the development of sexually dimorphic cognitive abilities and cerebral lateralisation. *Developmental Psychology,* **20,** 81–94.

Hobbs, P. R., Ballinger, C. B., McClure, A., Martin, B. & Greenwood, C. (1985) Factors associated with psychiatric morbidity in men – a general practice survey. *Acta Psychiatrica Scandinavica,* **71,** 281–6.

Imperato-McGinley, T., Petersen, R. E., Gautier, T. & Sturla, E. (1974) Steroid 5-alpha reductase deficiency in man; an inherited form of male pseudohermaphroditism. *Science,* **186,** 1213–43.

Imperato-McGinley, T., Guerrero, L., Gautier, T. & Petersen, R. E. (1979)

Androgens and the evolution of male gender identify among male pseudohermaphrodites with 5-alpha-reductase deficiency. *New England Journal of Medicine*, **300**, 1233–7.

Ingham, J. G. & Miller, P. McC. (1982) Consulting with mild symptoms in General Practice. *Social Psychiatry*, **17**, 77–88.

Jacklin, C. N., Maccoby, E. E. & Doering, C. H. (1983) Neonatal sex-steroid hormones and timidity in 6 to 18-month old boys and girls. *Developmental Psychobiology*, **16**, 163–8.

Jaszmann, L., Van Lith, N. & Zaat, J. (1969) The perimenopausal symptoms: the statistical analysis of a survey. *Medical Gynaecology and Sociology*, **4**, 268–77.

Josso, N. (1989) Fetal sex differentiation. In M. Serio (ed.) *Perspectives in Andrology*. Serono Symposium Publication Vol. 53. New York: Raven, pp. 1–9.

Juel-Nielsen, N. & Strömgren, E. (1965) A five year survey of a psychiatric service in a geographically delimited rural population given easy access to this service. *Comprehensive Psychiatry*, **6**, 139–65.

Kashiwaga, T., McClure, J. N. & Wetzel, R. D. (1976) Premenstrual affective syndrome and psychiatric disorder. *Diseases of the Nervous System*, **37**, 116–9.

Kaufert, P. (1984) Research note. Women and their health in the middle years: a Manitoba project. *Social Science and Medicine*, **18**, 279–81.

Kendell, R. E., Chalmers, J. C. & Platz, C. (1987) Epidemiology of puerperal psychosis. *British Journal of Psychiatry*, **150**, 662–73.

Kester, P. A., Green, R., Finch, S. J. & Williams, K. (1980) Prenatal 'female hormone' administration and psychosexual development in human males. *Psychoneuroendocrinology*, **5**, 269–85.

Kreuz, L. E. & Rose, L. M. (1972) Assessment of aggressive behavior and plasma testosterone in a young criminal population. *Psychosomatic Medicine*, **34**, 321–32.

Kreuz, L. E., Rose, R. M. & Jennings, J. R. (1972) Suppression of plasma testosterone levels and psychological stress: a longitudinal study of young men in officer candidate school. *Archives of General Psychiatry*, **26**, 479–82.

Leiblum, S., Bachman, G., Kemmann, E., Colburn, D. & Swatzman, L. (1983) Vaginal atrophy in the post-menopausal woman. The importance of sexual activity and hormones. *Journal of the American Medical Association*, **249**, 2195–8.

Lev Ran, A. (1977) Sex reversal as related to clinical syndromes in human beings. In Money, J. & Musaph H. (eds.) *Handbook of Sexology*. Amsterdam: Excerpta Medica, pp. 157–73.

Lock, M. (1986) Ambiguities of aging: Japanese experience and perceptions of menopause. *Culture, Medicine and Psychiatry*, **10**, 23–46.

Maccoby, E. E. & Jacklin, C. N. (1974) *The psychology of sex differences.* Stanford University Press.

Mackenzie, T. B., Wilcox, K. & Baron, H. (1986) Lifetime prevalence of psychiatric disorders in women with perimenstrual difficulties. *Journal of Affective Disorders*, **10**, 15–19.

Maddocks, S., Hahn, P., Moller, F. & Reid, R. L. (1986) A double-blind placebo-controlled trial of progesterone vaginal suppositories in the treatment of premenstrual syndrome. *American Journal of Obstetrics and Gynecology,* **154,** 573–81.

Marcus, J., Maccoby, E. E., Jacklin, C. N. & Doering, C. H. (1985) Individual differences in mood in early childhood: their relation to gender and neonatal sex steroids. *Developmental Psychobiology,* **18,** 327–40.

Mattsson, A., Schalling, D., Olweus, D., Low, H. & Svenson, J. (1980) Plasma testosterone, aggressive behavior and personality dimensions in young male delinquents. *Journal of the American Academy of Child Psychiatry,* **14,** 476–90.

Mazur, A. & Lamb, T. A. (1980) Testosterone, status and mood in human males. *Hormones and Behavior,* **14,** 236–46.

McCoy, N. & Davidson, J. M. (1985) A longitudinal study of the effects of the menopause on sexuality. *Maturitas,* **7,** 203–10.

McGuffin, P., Katz, R., Adrich, T. & Bebbington, P. (1988) The Camberwell Collaborative Depression Study. II. Investigation of family members. *British Journal of Psychiatry,* **152,** 766–74.

McHorney, C. A. & Mor, V. M. (1988) Predictors of bereavement depression and its health service consequences. *Medical Care,* **26,** 882–93.

McKinlay, S. & Jefferys, M. (1974) The menopausal syndrome. *British Journal of Preventative and Social Medicine,* **28,** 108–15.

McKinlay, S., Jefferys, M. & Thompson, B. (1972) An investigation of the age of menopause. *British Journal of Preventative and Social Medicine,* **28,** 108–15.

McKinlay, S. & McKinlay, J. B. (1989) The impact of menopause and social factors on health. In Hammond, C. B., Haseltime, F. P. & Schiff I. (eds.) *Menopause: evaluation, treatment and health concerns.* New York: Alan Liss, pp. 137–61.

McMillan, M. & Pihl, R. O. (1987) Premenstrual depression; a distinct entity. *Journal of Abnormal Psychology,* **96,** 149–54.

Meyer-Bahlburg, H. F. L., Boon, D. A., Sharma, M. & Edwards, J. A. (1974) Aggressiveness and testosterone measures in man. *Psychosomatic Medicine,* **36,** 269–74.

Meyer-Bahlburg, H. F. L., Grisanti, G. L. & Ehrhardt, A. A. (1977) Prenatal effects of sex hormones on human male behavior: medroxyprogesterone acetate (MPA). *Psychoneuroendocrinology,* **2,** 383–90.

Miller, P. McC. & Ingham, J. G. (1979) Reflections on the life-event-to-illness link with some preliminary findings. In Sarason, I. G. & Spielberger, C. D. (eds.) *Stress and Anxiety,* Vol. 6. Washington: Hemisphere.

Money, J. & Alexander, D. (1969) Psychosexual development and absence of homosexuality in boys with precocious puberty; a review of 18 cases. *Journal of Nervous and Mental Diseases,* **148,** 111–23.

Money, J. & Ehrhardt, A. A. (1972) *Man and woman, boy and girl; differentiation and dimorphism of gender identity from conception to maturity.* Baltimore: John Hopkins University Press.

NIMH (1983) Workshop on premenstrual syndrome, Rockville, Maryland, April 14–15 1983.

Nolen-Hoeksema, S. (1987) Sex differences in unipolar depression; evidence and theory. *Psychological Bulletin,* **101,** 259–82.

Nottelmann, E. D., Susman, E. J., Inoff-Germain, G., Cutler, G. B., Loriaux,

D. L. & Chrousos, G. P. (1987) Developmental processes in early adolescence. Relationships between adolescent problems and chronologic age, pubertal stage, and puberty related serum hormone levels. *Journal of Pediatrics* (St Louis), **110**, 473–80.

Nottelmann, E. D., Inoff-Germain, G., Susman, E. J. & Chrousos, G. P. (1990) Hormones and behavior at puberty. In Bancroft, J. & Reinisch, J. (eds.) *Adolescence & Puberty*. Third Kinsey Symposium. New York: Oxford University Press, pp. 88–123.

Nyborg, H. (1983) Spatial ability in men and women; review and new theory. *Advances in Behavioural Research and Therapy*, **5**, 89–140.

Olweus, D. (1975) Development of a multi-faceted aggression inventory for boys. University of Bergen, reports from the Institute of Psychology No. 6.

Olweus, D., Mattson, A., Schalling, D. & Low, H. (1980) Testosterone, aggression, physical and personality dimensions in normal adolescent males. *Psychosomatic Medicine*, **42**, 253–69.

Persky, H., Smith, K. D. & Basu, G. K. (1971) Relation of psychological measures of aggression and hostility to testosterone production in man. *Psychosomatic Medicine*, **33**, 265–77.

Pfeiffer, E., Verwoerdt, A. & Davis, G. C. (1972) Sexual behavior in middle life. *American Journal of Psychiatry*, **128**, 1262–7.

Porter, R., Bock, G. & Clark, S. (eds.) (1987) *Antidepressants and receptor function*. Ciba Foundation Symposium 123. Chichester: Wiley.

Rada, R. T., Laws, D. R. & Kellner, R. (1976) Plasma testosterone levels in the rapist. *Psychosomatic Medicine*, **38**, 257–66.

Rapkin, A. J., Edelmuth, E., Chang, L. C., Reading, A. E., McGuire, M. T. & Su, T.-P. (1987) Whole blood serotonin in premenstrual syndrome. *Obstetrics and Gynecology*, **70**, 533–7.

Regier, D. A., Boyd, J. H., Burke, J. D., Rae, D. S., Myers, J. K., Kramer, M., Robins, L., George, L. K., Karno, M. & Locke, B. T. (1988) One month prevalence of mental disorder in the United States. *Archives of General Psychiatry*, **45**, 977–86.

Reinisch, J. M. (1977) Prenatal exposure of human foetuses to synthetic progestin and oestrogen affects personality. *Nature*, (London), **266**, 561–2.

Reinisch, J. M. (1981) Prenatal exposure to synthetic progestins increases potential for aggression in humans. *Science*, **211**, 1171–3.

Reinisch, J. M. & Karow, W. G. (1977) Prenatal exposure to synthetic progestins and estrogens: effects on human development. *Archives of Sexual Behavior*, **6**, 257–88.

Reinisch, J. M. & Sanders, S. A. (1982) Early barbiturate exposure, the brain, sexually dimorphic behavior and learning. *Neuroscience and Biobehavioral Reviews*, **6**, 311–9.

Reinisch, J. M. & Sanders, S. A. (1987) Behavioral influences of prenatal hormones. In Nemeroff, C. B. & Loosen, P. T. (eds.) *Handbook of Clinical Psychoneuroendocrinology*. New York: Guilford, pp. 431–48.

Robins, L. N., Helzer, J. E., Weissman, M. M., Orvaschel, H., Gruenberg, E., Burke, J. D. & Regier, D. A. (1984) Lifetime prevalence of specific psychiatric disorders in three sites. *Archives of General Psychiatry*, **41**, 949–67.

Rosenthal, S. (1968) The involutional depressive syndrome. *American Journal of Psychiatry*, **124** (suppl), 21–35.

Rubin, R. T. (1990) Mood changes during adolescnece. In Bancroft, J. & Reinisch, J. (eds.) *Adolescence and Puberty.* Third Kinsey Symposium. New York: Oxford University Press, pp. 146–56.

Rubinow, D. R., Roy-Byrne, P., Hoban, M. C., Gold, P. W. & Post, R. M. (1984) Prospective assessment of menstrually related mood disorders. *American Journal of Psychiatry,* **141,** 684–6.

Rubinow, D. R., Roy-Byrne, P. P., Hoban, M. C., Grover, G. N., Stambler, N. & Post, R. M. (1986) Premenstrual mood change: characteristic patterns in women with and without premenstrual syndrome. *Journal of Affective Disorders,* **10,** 85–90.

Rutter, M. (1990) Changing patterns of psychiatric disorder over adolescence. In Bancroft, J. & Reinisch, J. (eds.) *Adolescence and Puberty.* Third Kinsey Symposium. New York; Oxford University Press, pp. 124–45.

Sachar, E. J. (1967) Corticosteroids in depressive illness. *Archives of General Psychiatry,* **17,** 544–67.

Sanders, D., Warner, P., Backstrom, T. & Bancroft, J. (1983) Mood, sexuality, hormones and the menstrual cycle. I. Changes in mood and physical state: description of subjects and method. *Psychosomatic Medicine,* **45,** 487–507.

Scaramella, T. J. & Brown, W. A. (1978) Serum testosterone and aggressiveness in hockey players. *Psychosomatic Medicine,* **40,** 262–5.

Schiavi, R. C. (1990) Sexuality and aging in men. *Annual Review of Sex Research,* **1,** 227–99.

Seligman, M. E. P. (1975) *Helplessness: on depression, development and death.* San Francisco: Freeman.

Sharma, V. & Saxena, M. (1981) Climacteric symptoms: a study in the Indian context. *Maturitas,* **3,** 11–20.

Sherwin, B. B. & Gelfand, M. M. (1987) The role of androgen in the maintenance of sexual functioning in oophorectomised women. *Psychosomatic Medicine,* **49,** 397–409.

Sherwin, B. B., Gelfand, M. M. & Brender, W. (1985) Androgen enhances sexual motivation in females; a prospective cross-over study of sex steroid administration in the surgical menopause. *Psychosomatic Medicine,* **47,** 339–51.

Shore, J. H., Tatum, E. L. & Vollmer, W. M. (1986) Psychiatric reactions to disaster: the mount St. Helens experience. *American Journal of Psychiatry,* **143,** 590–5.

Shuckit, M. A., Daly, V., Herrman, G. & Hineman, S. (1975) Premenstrual symptoms and depression in a university population. *Diseases of the Nervous System,* **36,** 516–7.

Steiner, M. & Haskett, R. F. (1987) The psychobiology of premenstrual syndrome: the Michigan Studies. In Ginsburg, B. E. & Carter, B. F. (eds.) *Premenstrual Syndrome: ethical & legal implications in a biomedical perspective.* New York: Plenum, pp. 369–85.

Stout, A. L. & Steege, J. F. (1985) Psychological assessment of women seeking treatment for premenstrual syndrome. *Journal of Psychosomatic Research,* **29,** 621–9.

Stout, A. L., Steege, J. F., Blazer, D. G. & George, L. K. (1986) Comparison of lifetime psychiatric diagnoses in premenstrual syndrome clinic and community samples. *Journal of Nervous and Mental Disease,* **174,** 517–22.

Surtees, P. G., Kiff, J. & Rennie, D. (1981) Adversity and mental health: an empirical investigation of their relationship. *Acta Psychiatrica Scandinavica*, **64,** 177–92.

Taylor, D. L., Mathew, R. J., Ho, B. T. & Weinman, M. L. (1984) Serotonin levels and platelet uptake during premenstrual tension. *Neuropsychobiology*, **12,** 16–8.

Thomson, B., Hart, S. & Durno, D. (1973) Menopausal age and symptomatology in general practice. *Journal of Biosocial Science*, **5,** 71–82.

Treloar, A. E. (1981) Menstrual cyclicity and the premenopause. *Maturitas*, **3,** 249–64.

Treloar, A. E., Boynton, R. E., Behn, D. G. & Brown, B. W. (1967) Variation of the human menstrual cycle through reproductive life. *International Journal of Fertility*, **12,** 77–126.

Udry, J. R., Billy, J. O. G., Morris, N. M., Groff, T. R. & Raj, M. H. (1985) Serum androgenic hormones motivate sexual behavior in adolescent boys. *Fertility and Sterility*, **43,** 90–4.

Udry, J. R., Talbert, L. M. & Morris, N. M. (1986) Biosocial foundations for adolescent female sexuality. *Demography*, **23,** 217–29.

Vollman, R. F. (1977) *The menstrual cycle.* Philadelphia: Saunders.

Warner, P. & Bancroft, J. (1990) Factors related to self-reporting of premenstrual syndrome. *British Journal of Psychiatry*, **157,** 249–60.

Warner, P., Bancroft, J., Dixson, A. & Hampson, M. (1991) The relationship between premenstrual mood change and depressive illness. *Journal of Affective Disorders*, in press.

Weissman, M. M. & Klerman, G. L. (1977) Sex differences and the epidemiology of depression. *Archives of General Psychiatry*, **34,** 98–111.

Weissman, M. M., Leaf, P. J., Holzer, C. E., Myers, J. K. & Tischler, G. L. (1984) The epidemiology of depression – an update on sex differences in rates. *Journal of Affective Disorders*, **7,** 179–88.

Weissman, M. M., Leaf, P. J., Tischler, G. L., Blazer, D. G., Karno, M., Livingston Bruce, M. & Florio, L. P. (1988) Affective disorders in five United States communities. *Psychological Medicine*, **18,** 141–53.

Wetzel, R. D., Reich, T., McClure, J. N. & Wald, J. A. (1975) Premenstrual affective syndrome and affective disorder. *British Journal of Psychiatry*, **127,** 219–21.

Winokur, G. (1973) Depression in the menopause. *American Journal of Psychiatry*, **130,** 92–3.

Yalom, I. D., Green, R. & Fisk, N. (1973) Prenatal exposure to female hormones: effects on psychosexual development in boys. *Archives of General Psychiatry*, **28,** 554–61.

11 Epilepsy and anticonvulsive drugs

H.-CH. STEINHAUSEN AND C. RAUSS-MASON

INTRODUCTION

Epilepsy is a relatively common neurological disorder with an average frequency of about 0.5–1% in the general population. A consensus has prevailed throughout history that closely associates epilepsy with psychopathology. Although the prejudice and social stigma regarding the epileptic continue, they have been modified with time.

Most studies support the notion that children with epilepsy have a significantly higher rate of psychiatric disorder than either healthy children or children suffering from other chronic diseases. There has been a concern to identify those variables that are specific to epilepsy and which predispose the person with epilepsy to cognitive impairment and to psychopathological disorder. In addition, the family is also at risk for psychosocial disturbances.

Clearly, methodological problems related to such factors as selection and methods of assessment continue to impede research; early studies of emotional and behavioural disorders among children with epilepsy are so seriously flawed that they are of historical interest only (Corbett & Trimble, 1983). The first studies employing an epidemiological approach began in 1960. It was not until the 1970s that the methodological flaws that limited most of the early epidemiological studies were overcome with the Isle of Wight study by Rutter and his colleagues (Rutter *et al.*, 1970) and shortly thereafter by Mellor and his colleagues (Mellor *et al.*, 1971: cf. Corbett & Trimble, 1983). Rutter *et al.* found that 29% of the children with uncomplicated epilepsy exhibited psychiatric disorders, compared with 7% in the general population sample.

Mellor *et al.* (1971) studied 308 children with epilepsy from schools in northeast Scotland and found the rate of psychiatric disorder in this group to be 27% compared with 15% in matched controls. These studies and others of children attending special schools for epilepsy confirm that the rates of emotional and behavioural disorders are higher in children with epilepsy than in the control groups, and even higher in children with complicated epilepsy, i.e. epilepsy 'with associated structural brain disorder' (Rutter *et al.*, 1970).

Research indicates that a number of variables are associated with this increased vulnerability. These will be dealt with later in this chapter. Before doing so, the behavioural and cognitive correlates of epilepsy will be discussed. Then, after addressing the issue of mechanisms involved in the relations between epilepsy and behaviour as well as cognition, issues pertaining to long-term outcome will be dealt with. Thereafter, the concept of so-called 'epileptic equivalents' will be presented. Furthermore, the side-effects of anticonvulsive drugs will be outlined, after which some conclusions will be drawn.

BEHAVIOURAL AND COGNITIVE CORRELATES

Psychiatric and personality features

There are a number of studies that have sought to determine the specific psychiatric disorders for which the epileptic child is at risk. The notion of an *epileptic personality* has been discredited (Tizard, 1962) and replaced by studies indicating that the nature of behaviour problems in epileptic children does not differ from that of other children, but rather that they suffer from such problems more frequently. Rutter *et al.* (1970) found that the majority of neuroepileptic children with psychiatric disorder suffered from neurotic or antisocial conditions. Bagley (1972) also found that the main types of psychiatric disorder observed in epileptic children fell into similar categories to those for non-epileptic children. He summarized the main types of disorder as follows: neurotic–anxious, depressed; aggressive–antisocial; over-active behaviour; mental handicap; and mixed. Forty-three per cent of the epileptic children were described as having psychiatric disturbances comparable in degree to children in a child guidance clinic.

Ounsted and his colleagues (Ounsted *et al.*, 1966) found 26 children with the hyperkinetic syndrome in its classical form in their series of 100 children suffering from temporal lobe epilepsy. The factors identified as being most important in potentiating the development of the hyperkinetic syndrome were male sex, the nature of the initiating insult, status epilepticus, and very early onset of epilepsy. In addition, the intellectual development of these children was significantly retarded. However, as the authors stated later, the classic hyperkinetic syndrome is now rare owing to certain changes in the clinical picture. In the more developed countries the number of children affected with severe brain damage due to infections and insults has decreased, as has the use of anticonvulsants such as phenobarbital and primidone, which are known to potentiate hyperkinetic behaviour (Ounsted & Lindsay, 1981).

In a more recent study, Epir *et al.* (1984) found that epileptic children in a low-income area of Turkey had significantly more behavioural problems of all types than either their siblings or the control group. These findings are based upon observation, maternal interviews and questionnaires, as well as a teacher rating scale. When compared with their peers, only problems related to fears and anxieties were significantly greater. When compared with their siblings, epileptics suffered more problems related to fears and anxieties as well as to conduct, disobedience and attentional problems. The non-epileptic children and the siblings did not differ significantly in any problem area.

Dependency

Increased dependency is a recurring issue in studies of psychological disorder among epileptics. The effects of parental attitudes on dependency, and the fact that many studies have indirectly assessed children through questionnaires answered by the parents, have certainly coloured the resulting picture. It has been suggested that over-protective attitudes of parents lead to strong dependency and that such attitudes are particularly prevalent in epileptic families. Verduyn (1980) noted that 'the effects of parental attitudes have been much commented upon and in fact little researched' (p. 180).

Stores (1978), using the Self-Administered Dependency Questionnaire (SADQ), investigated boys and girls with epilepsy. The scores of the epileptic children were compared with those of the population norms supplied by the SADQ. It was found that primary-school aged boys were more dependent in the areas of 'affection' and 'travel' whereas secondary-school aged boys scored higher in their needs for assistance in practical matters. Epileptic girls obtained scores that were not significantly different from those of the female population norms. Stores also found an increased need for physical and emotional contact with the mother in both boys and girls with a persistent left temporal spike discharge.

Hoare (1984b), also using the SADQ, compared four groups of children to determine whether epileptic children developed inappropriate dependency. The four groups studied were a newly diagnosed and a chronic group of epileptic children, as well as two comparable groups of diabetic children. Hoare's (1984b) results are generally comparable with those of Stores (1978), except that he found that girls with chronic epilepsy also exhibited increased dependency. He suggested that both the small number of subjects in his study as well as the confounding effects between inappropriate dependency and psychiatric disturbance may account for the differences between his study and Stores'. The findings strongly suggest that inappropriate dependency is dependent upon the nature of the illness rather than invariably belonging to chronic disease.

Using projective tests, interviews and self-esteem scales, Viberg *et al.* (1987) found that during interview sessions epileptic children and adolescents tended to emphasize their *independence* in relation to friends and parents. These researchers suggested that this tendency may be interpreted as a psychological defence mechanism employed in response to the actual dependence upon other people for medical treatment and over-protection at home.

Suicide

Suicide, too, has been reported as being more frequent among epileptics. A re-evaluation of older studies estimated the suicide rate to be about four times that of the general population (Brent, 1986). These studies, however, are not age-adjusted and therefore cannot be compared with the rate of suicide in the general population. When the suicide rates of epileptic children and non-epileptic children were compared, an increased rate for the epileptic children was found. Brent (1986) also noted that some authors observed a high incidence of the use of phenobarbital as the agent of drug overdose. There is, unfortunately, no explicit mention of the various anticonvulsant medications used by the subjects or of their types of seizure disorder. This seriously limits the interpretations of the findings, although the possibility that the therapeutic use of phenobarbital as an anticonvulsant could be associated with the suicidal behaviour was considered.

Brent (1986) tried to overcome some of these shortcomings in his own study. He evaluated, through a chart review, 131 consecutive suicide attempts made by 126 children and adolescents aged 7–17. This group included both epileptic subjects and non-epileptic controls. In this series 11 of the attempts were made by nine epileptics. With an estimate of 4.53/1000 prevalence rate of epilepsy in school age children, the frequency of attempts made by epileptics is 15.8 times greater than a probability prediction. Eight of the nine patients were diagnosed as having tonic–clonic seizures and four of the nine showed a temporal lobe focus on the EEG. Seven of the nine patients were on phenobarbital and an eighth was treated with a combination of phenobarbital and phenytoin. All patients treated with phenobarbital utilized this drug for their suicidal overdose. The ninth patient, who had a diagnosis of psychomotor epilepsy, was treated with carbamazepine.

None of the demographic factors – age, sex, race, parental occupation, one- vs. two-parent households – proved significant. The epileptic group tended to function better in school than the non-epileptic group.

Otherwise, there were no significant differences in the familial or social factors such as peer and family relationships, family discord, or the number of stressful life events experienced in the year prior to the suicide attempt. The proportion of major or minor affective disorder diagnosed among the epileptic attempters was greater than the non-epileptic group, though not significantly so. Continued suicidal intent after the attempt was more likely among the epileptic patients.

The ratings of certain variables characterizing the suicide attempt were significant in differentiating the epileptic group. The medical seriousness of the risk and the total suicide intent were greater in the epileptic group. This group also evidenced less desire for rescue and tended to spend more time preparing for the suicide attempt. These patients were twice as likely to use medicinal medications and much less likely to use over-the-counter preparations in their drug overdose.

This study supports three hypotheses concerning suicide risk factors and epilepsy: (a) epilepsy in childhood is related to a higher risk for suicidal behaviour; (b) the medical seriousness of the intent and the degree of suicidal intent are greater among epileptics; and (c) the use of phenobarbital as an anticonvulsant is implicated in suicidal behaviour among epileptics. This association between phenobarbital and suicidal behaviour needs to be further investigated in a larger sample and with additional controls regarding the type of anticonvulsant medication and the type of epilepsy involved (Brent, 1986).

Locus of control and self concept

Matthews *et al.* (1982) have described certain pervasive emotional concomitants that distinguish childhood epilepsy, and have formulated a number of congruous hypotheses that arise from these distinguishing attributes. Three such features are: (a) the unpredictability of the seizure with regards to time, place, and social circumstances; (b) the overt manifestation of a symptom that is often perceived by the child and by others as being frightening and grotesque; and (c) the loss of control that the convulsive seizure represents for the child and possibly for those around him.

The experience of *loss of control* might conceivably be generalized to other aspects of the child's life so that the child would be hindered in developing a belief in an internal *locus of control,* i.e. the perception that an event is contingent upon one's own behaviour or one's own relatively permanent characteristics rather than upon external sources – powerful others or unknown sources such as fate or chance.

When testing this theory experimentally with epileptic children and matched clinical (diabetic) and healthy controls, Matthews and her colleagues found that the children with epilepsy experienced the source of control over events in their lives to be external and often as having an unknown source. Although all of the groups tended to experience external sources as responsible for their failures, both chronically ill groups were more likely to perceive unknown sources – as opposed to powerful others – as being responsible for their failures. Epileptic children, however, tended to attribute even their own successes to unknown sources. Regarding competency domains, epileptic children, as compared with the healthy and diabetic children, were more likely to perceive their social competency as being externally controlled by either powerful others or by unknown sources.

Epileptic children also had lower self-concept scores and lower self-esteem. Anxiety was significantly greater among epileptic children as compared with the healthy children, but not significantly greater than the scores of the diabetic group. The epilepsy-significant variables revealed by the parental report are similar to those in other studies. The findings of this study are directly related to the 'learned helplessness' theory of Seligman and with the clinical implications connected with this theory (Seligman, 1975). Feelings of helplessness, lack of control, low self-esteem and anxiety have been described as cardinal symptoms of depression and as significant risk factors in suicide (Matthews *et al.*, 1982). It appeared that epileptic children may be at greater developmental risk for depression, which often goes undetected or is misdiagnosed in children (Birleson, 1981). Furthermore, there is evidence that styles of interaction in epileptic familes contribute to and help sustain the experience of helplessness and lack of control (Ritchie, 1981).

Cognitive deficits

Although most studies place children with uncomplicated epilepsy within the normal IQ range, it is noted that they often score at its lower end (Corbett & Trimble, 1983). The occurrence of seizure disorders increases in mental retardation and rises with the degree of retardation (Corbett *et al.*, 1985; Rutter *et al.*, 1970). Close analysis of the Wechsler Intelligence Scale for Children (WISC) verbal-performance discrepancies among uncomplicated epileptic children in the Isle of Wight Study suggested subtle cognitive disabilities even among these children. In addition, 18% of the children exhibited significant reading retardation (Rutter *et al.*, 1970).

Complicated epilepsy is also associated with lowered IQ scores (Corbett & Trimble, 1983; Corbett *et al.*, 1985; Bourgeois *et al.*, 1983). Bourgeois and his colleagues studied 72 newly diagnosed children. Children with complicated epilepsy scored less well – mean IQ 89 – than those with uncomplicated epilepsy – mean IQ 103 – but the initial scores of the non-epileptic siblings of 45 patients were not significantly different from those of their epileptic siblings, regardless of whether the epilepsy was complicated or uncomplicated.

Unfortunately, there is a paucity of studies of specific areas of cognitive and neuropsychological function among epileptics. In order to assess neuropsychological impairment in relation to cognitive deficits, Farwell *et al.* (1985) undertook a detailed neuropsychological investigation which included the WISC and the Halstead–Reitan battery. The epileptic group had significantly more impairment than the controls on all measures of brain function.

Epir *et al.* (1984) compared children with uncomplicated epilepsy and a matched control group. The performance of the epileptic children was poorer on most of the cognitive tests, although significantly poorer on only two. Receptive language skills were inferior to those of the healthy children. Only in the drawing tests, where the children reproduced geometric designs from memory, was there any indication of significantly inferior functioning in perceptuomotor skills. There was no difference between the two groups on design recognition. Children who did poorly on the drawing test tended to have more problematic behaviour. No such relationship was found between language skills and behaviour problems.

In contrast, Bolter (1986), in his review, concluded that no specific pattern of impairment has yet been identified as characteristic of children with epilepsy. While there is some support for a specific attentional deficit in these children, as a rule they manifest only mild and non-specific impairments, none of which are found in every case.

Performance

Performance and achievement are directly related to both psychosocial and cognitive development. It is not surprising, therefore that a lower level of school performance and academic achievement is found among epileptic children as compared with non-epileptic, chronically ill children or healthy children. There is also some indication that individuals with childhood epilepsy may have a poor long-term social prognosis (Addy, 1987; Farwell *et al.*, 1985).

Underachievement in reading has been widely reported, especially for boys with focal epilepsy. Boys are apparently also more inattentive in school than their non-epileptic peers (Stores, 1978). Seidenberg *et al.* (1986) examined relations between certain demographic and clinical seizure variables and academic achievement. On the whole, the epileptic children obtained academic achievement levels lower than expected for their IQ levels and age levels. Academic deficiencies were greatest for arithmetic and spelling, followed by reading comprehension and word recognition.

Of the demographic variables and clinical seizure variables investigated, those with significant predictive value were: the age of the child, age of seizure onset, and lifetime total seizure frequency. The predictive relations were strongest for spelling and arithmetic. Academic vulnerability in all four areas was greatest for older children as compared with younger children.

Seizure type correlated with poor achievement scores in arithmetic. Children with generalized seizures performed more poorly than those with partial seizures, and those with both absence and tonic–clonic seizures performed most poorly of all. Increased lifetime seizure total was found to be related to neuropsychological functioning of children with tonic–clonic seizures and was also related to lower achievement scores in arithmetic.

The higher levels of reading among female children was attributed by Seidenberg *et al.* (1986) to the fact that girls tend to acquire language earlier than boys do. A relationship between academic vulnerability and the site of EEG foci did not evolve as a significant predictor variable. And, unlike many previous studies, the number of anticonvulsive medications was not significantly correlated with academic functioning in this study.

Other studies from the United States, England and Italy (as summarized by Aird *et al.*, 1984b) indicated that epileptic children are more apt to receive special schooling than are their healthy peers. School failure, however, may be primarily related to complications related to epilepsy rather than to the occurrence of seizures *per se*.

MECHANISMS INVOLVED AND CLINICAL IMPLICATIONS

Prerequisites for the development of epilepsy clearly include heredity and/or brain-related factors. Evidence of genetic factors have been obtained from clinical examinations of epileptic patients and their relatives. When all individuals who have suffered at least one seizure are taken into account 30–40% of the unselected seizure patients have a positive family history, with up to 10% epilepsy cases arising in the offspring. This genetic trend is particularly evident in those instances in which epilepsy is one manifestation of an inherited single-gene disorder. The actual incidence is rare and, as a rule, epilepsy is only one part of a generalized disorder which can manifest itself in various other ways – e.g. as a physical malformation, mental retardation, or as a neurological defect (Aird *et al.*, 1984a).

When considering the spectrum of seizure types, there is a distinct genetic component in the generalized seizure disorder, tonic–clonic seizures, absence attacks, photosensitive epilepsy, and febrile convulsions. This trend has not been definitively shown to exist for partial and symptomatic seizures. In addition to the evidence in support of positive family history as an operant factor in the aetiology of certain seizure types, electroencephalographic data also support the view that genetic factors play an important role in the aetiology of epilepsy. Specific electroencephalographic patterns frequently associated with epilepsy, including generalized spike-and-wave discharges, the centrotemporal spike, and the photoconvulsive response appear with greater frequency among susceptible relatives.

Finally, the high concordance rate of epilepsy found in monozygotic twins (up to 90%) contrasts with the much lower rate in dizygotic twins (10–15%), indicating a strong genetic component – possibly polygenic in type (Newmark & Penry, 1980). However, this does not necessarily imply that genetic factors play a major role in the aetiology of psychiatric disorders of epileptic patients. Given the non-specific pattern of psychiatric symptoms in epileptic children and the variety of phenotypes of personality features due to both genetic and environmental variation in normal development, it is unlikely that genetic factors shape behaviour in epileptic children to a greater extent than in healthy children. Specific empirical evidence is lacking. Cognitive functioning, however, may be affected by heredity. In cases where epilepsy is a part of autosomal dominant, autosomal recessive, or *X*-linked genetic disorders, and where it is associated with organic and neurological defects, mental retardation is present. However, this accounts for only a small number of cases. In general, there are other factors that are of greater significance for understanding the mechanisms that determine the behavioural and cognitive sequelae of epilepsy.

Hermann & Whitman (1984) emphasized that accurate assessment of the psychopathological implications of a specific epileptic seizure type – such as temporal lobe epilepsy – requires consideration of other variables predictive of psychopathology in epilepsy. However, the relative aetiological importance of these variables is difficult to estimate due to varying degrees of intercorrelation and other such methodological and interpretive difficulties.

Furthermore, Hermann & Whitman proposed that the risk variables can be divided into three main categories: (a) *brain-related factors* – neurological, EEG, epilepsy and neuropsychological variables; (b) *non-brain-related factors* – chronic illness, epilepsy, developmental/epilepsy and demographic/subject variables; and (c) *treatment-related factors*. Following this conceptual model, the most frequently occurring risk variables as they appear in the literature are discussed below.

Brain-related variables

The brain-related factors that are most frequently discussed in psychological and psychiatric literature are those that belong to the subclass *epilepsy* variables. The *age of onset* and the duration – *chronicity* – of the seizure disorder are, of course, interrelated. Age of onset and chronicity were not correlated with behaviour disorders in those studies that specifically controlled for these two variables (Berg *et al.*, 1984; Hoare, 1984a,b). They do, however, appear to have aetiological significance for cognitive and emotional development. Verduyn (1980) referred to a survey by Pond & Bidwell (1960) that correlated early onset with psychological difficulties in childhood and with work difficulties and lower social class in adulthood. Other studies (Bourgeois *et al.*, 1983; Corbett & Trimble, 1983; O'Leary *et al.*, 1983; Seidenberg *et al.*, 1986) found strong correlations between early seizure onset and cognitive impairment. Some authors suggest that the inclusion of infantile epileptic syndromes that are associated with mental retardation – such as infantile spasms or Lennox–Gastaux syndrome – might be responsible for this correlation (Addy, 1987; Corbett & Trimble, 1983). Aicardi (1985) noted that epilepsy is most common in infancy and childhood. The age of onset is therefore also closely associated with the degree of neurological maturation at the time of the seizure onset.

Not only do the syndromes change according to the age of the child, but the neurological, psychological and sociological effects of seizures also vary with age. This applies as well to the causes of epilepsy, metabolism of anticonvulsive medication and to the prognosis.

Seizure frequency and *seizure control* are two further interrelated risk variables for behaviour and cognitive vulnerability. Hartlage *et al.* (1972) found a negative correlation between frequency of seizures and social maturity, and Verduyn (1980) reported that poor seizure control puts a child at increased risk for psychological difficulties. Similarly, in a more recent study, Hermann *et al.* (1989) found seizure control to emerge as the most significant predictor variable of behaviour problems. Berg *et al.* (1984), however, did not find this variable to be significantly correlated with behavioural vulnerability. Reviewing the literature, Corbett & Trimble (1983) noted that seizure frequency is often entangled with other factors, such as brain damage, which makes it difficult to interpret the data. Recent studies have shown a negative effect of seizure frequency and learning ability (Seidenberg *et al.*, 1986). No conclusive correlation was found between seizure frequency and cognitive development in the study by Niemann *et al.* (1985), which, however, used an atypical population. Farwell *et al.* (1985), though, did find a positive correlation between good seizure control and higher IQ.

A number of studies have compared *seizure type* to determine whether this variable has predictive value for behaviour or cognition. Various methods and criteria for determining seizure type have been used as the dependent measure for making the comparisons. Most comparison studies have compared temporal lobe epilepsy (TLE) with generalized epilepsies or primary generalized epilepsies to determine if sufferers from TLE were predisposed to psychopathology. A number of studies inconclusively suggest an increased risk of behavioural pathology (Hoare, 1984a). The studies of Stores (1978) and of Whitman *et al.* (1982) limit this vulnerability to boys. There does not appear, however, to be any evidence of a specific pathology or pattern of behaviour associated with seizure type (Corbett *et al.*, 1985).

The relationship between seizure type and intelligence also seems to be quite inconclusive, although there is evidence that patients who suffer from more than one type of seizure are more at risk for cognitive deficits (Addy, 1987; Corbett & Trimble, 1983). Stores (1978) found reading retardation and attention deficits in boys with TLE, and Farwell *et al.* (1985) reported differences in full-scale IQ measurements in children with different seizure types. Those children with minor motor or atypical absence seizures were most at risk. All other seizure types, except classic absence, were associated with a mean measured intelligence below that of the controls.

Hermann & Whitman (1984) discussed some of the methodological difficulties involved in studies of seizure type. In a number of studies either a diagnosis and classification of epilepsy on purely clinical grounds sufficed, or the presence of epileptiform EEG patterns alone was the determining factor in defining the seizure type. Some studies failed to define their selection criteria. There appears to be a very basic problem related to the definition of epilepsy *per se* and of the interictal state, not to mention the specification of seizure type (Aird *et al.*, 1989). These problems prevailed even in those studies where both EEG and clinical confirmation were required to meet selection criteria.

Even when the diagnosis was verified on both clinical grounds and with an EEG, difficulties still remain in determining the adequacy of the various EEG techniques. Certain procedures are more sensitive than others and may detect epileptiform activity that other approaches fail to uncover. For example, nasopharyngeal or sphenoidal electrode placements are believed to be more sensitive for detecting abnormal activity deep in the temporal lobe and the associated limbic structures. This technique has led to delineating subgroups of TLE patients found to be more vulnerable to psychiatric disorders (Hermann & Whitman, 1984).

The definition of the interictal period is an equally important consideration. Hermann & Whitman (1984) noted that researchers 'appear to implicitly consider the interictal period to be a somewhat fixed and homogeneous state during which clinical seizures do not occur. Electroencephalographically, however, the interictal period is anything but a quiescent state' (p. 481). They suggest that the interictal period be considered 'a fluid and dynamic state' (p. 481) and reason that abnormal epileptiform discharges during the interictal period have been found to affect cognitive functioning and may, therefore, affect the adequacy of behavioural functioning and emotion (see below).

The presence or absence of *brain damage* is a further brain-related variable that has generated inquiries concerning its role as a risk variable in epilepsy. Most studies have differentiated between uncomplicated or idiopathic epilepsies, and complicated epilepsy in which structural brain disorder is manifest. Corbett *et al.* (1985) surmised on the basis of various studies that:

> . . . it seems likely that children with epilepsy, associated with overt brain damage, are more vulnerable to environmental influences, including family, school, and societal adversity . . . The importance of brain damage and brain dysfunction as pervasive underlying factors, accounting for the high rates of psychiatric disorder and cognitive impairment seen in children with epilepsy, is supported by the finding of an early age of onset of seizures in . . . children with complicated epilepsy. (Corbett *et al.*, 1985, p. 22)

Rutter *et al.* (1970) have pointed out that brain abnormalities play an important – though not exclusive – role in the development of psychopathology in epileptic children. Additional factors that were strongly associated with psychiatric disorder are language retardation, low intelligence, and reading retardation. The authors considered that the effect of brain dysfunction was essentially to render the child more liable to react adversely to the stresses and strains that may impair the development of any child.

Hermann (1982) found that behavioural and social disorders as well as pathologic aggression in children and adults with epilepsy were more closely associated with 'clinical, radiologic, or EEG evidence of diffuse, bilateral, or deep cerebral pathology than with simple seizure type'. The poor neuropsychological functioning of these patients, as assessed with the age-appropriate Luria–Nebraska Battery, supported these findings. On the other hand, Niemann *et al.* (1985) reported no significant difference in the cognitive performance of epileptics with underlying brain damage. The results of his study, however, cannot be generalized to other epileptic populations for a number of reasons. The subjects were residents in an epileptic colony and were described as being either learning disabled or retarded. Twenty-seven of the subjects tested positive for brain damage with a CT scan and the other 10 subjects were found to be marginally-normal to normal. It is also possible that their measures were not adequately adjusted to this special population.

It is apparent that more research in this area is imperative and, considering the relatively recent advances in medical technology and in the disciplines of neuroscience, it is evident that this research will be of an increasingly interdisciplinary nature.

Non-brain-related variables

There are a number of *non-brain-related* variables and subclasses of these variables that need to be considered for their risk value in epilepsy. The need to discriminate between chronic-illness variables and those variables that are specific to epilepsy has been undertaken in several studies in which the target group was compared with another group of chronically ill children – usually children with diabetes or cystic fibrosis – and often a third control group of healthy children. These studies support the hypothesis that there are risk variables associated specifically with epilepsy (Ferrari *et al.*, 1983; Hartlage *et al.*, 1982; Hoare, 1984a,b; Matthews *et al.*, 1982).

Developmental epilepsy variables include: age of onset and variables involving the family as a unit and the parents as caretakers, family psychiatric history, peers and school, early experiences and developmental milestones, parental attitudes and expectations, personality, and environment. There has been little research done on these complex issues so far. Some findings indicate, however, that both parents, especially the mothers, as well as the siblings, show an increased rate of psychiatric disturbance in families with an epileptic child. Siblings in 'newly diagnosed families' have lower rates of disturbance than those in 'chronic families' where epilepsy has long been present (Hoare, 1984b). Rutter *et al.* (1970) concluded from their study that it is most likely the mental abnormalities in a parent that contribute to the child's emotional and behavioural difficulties. In part, the association may be mediated by the inheritance of abnormalities detected by EEG, but it is also clear that disorder in the child may often be due to the disturbed family relationship. Clearly, psychiatric disorder in epileptic children is multifactorially determined.

Demographic and subject variables which have been identified include socioeconomic status, age, sex, premorbid personality, and premorbid psychological status – including IQ and level of functioning in school. Socioeconomic status is an especially confounding variable because many of the studies have compiled their samples from patients attending large university epilepsy clinics, which serve a high proportion of disadvantaged populations. Such populations may also have a disproportionate rate and degree of psychopathology (Hermann & Whitman, 1984). In epidemiological studies by Rutter *et al.* (1970), epileptic children whose fathers had manual jobs were more likely to have psychiatric disorders than children of higher socioeconomic status, but this correlation may have arisen by chance. The same study revealed no sex differences with regard to psychiatric disturbances.

The third category associated with psychopathology as outlined by Hermann & Whitman (1984), namely *treatment-related factors*, will be discussed in the penultimate section on the behavioural and cognitive side effects of anticonvulsant drugs.

When considering the central question as to how these different factors operate and finally contribute to cognitive-behavioural functioning in the epileptic child, one would end with mere speculation. So far, research has tended to evaluate the vast majority of variables in relative isolation, without considering the potential interactive effects. While it is clear that epilepsy, as a neurobiological condition, constitutes a major risk for psychiatric disorders and that some brain-related factors have a strong impact on behaviour and cognition, much less is known about the relevance of developmental and psychosocial factors. The latter are among the most difficult variables to assess and interpret objectively. As Verduyn (1980) remarked:

> There is a problem of extricating the relevant factors and then it is often all too easy to attribute causality. For instance, it is not always clear whether difficult behaviour in a child causes a more negative parental attitude or is an effect of it, or both. It is clear that behaviour disturbance is a result of complex interactions between a number of variables . . . (Verduyn, 1980, pp. 181–182)

So far, these complex interactions have not been studied sufficiently. Hypothetically, the different groups of variables – i.e. brain dysfunction, developmental and psychosocial factors, and treatment related factors – might explain different proportions of variance for the various cognitive-behavioural functions.

In addition, little is known about the protective influences that enable some children to cope successfully with certain biological hazards. These protective and nurturing psychosocial factors need to be identified and analysed. Here, a closer look at family functioning and parenting might prove rewarding. There is some indication, for instance, that parental attitudes that foster social maturity and socialization skills and that encourage activity and self-initiated behaviour correlate with higher academic achievement in epileptic children (Hartlage & Green, 1972). Further evidence with regard to protective factors and resistance to psychiatric disorder in epileptic children is still to be discovered. Research in this area might benefit from what is known about resilience in the face of adversity in other fields of developmental psychopathology (Rutter, 1985).

LONG-TERM OUTCOME

As Rodin (1987) noted in his review, the general prognosis of epilepsy varies with the type of seizures. For instance, *neonatal seizures* are associated with a relatively low risk for epilepsy. *Infantile spasms* (hypsarrhythmia) mainly occur as a result of pre-existing brain damage and, therefore, carry a poor prognosis for cognitive development (Cavazuti *et al.*, 1984). Similarly, the prognosis for seizures beginning in the first year of life depends upon the presence of pre-existing or co-existing brain damage.

Febrile convulsions are the most common type of seizure in childhood, especially between the ages of 6 months to 3 years. The overall risk of developing epilepsy in this group is about five times that of the general population. In addition, these children have a higher than expected incidence of reading difficulties, although their mean intelligence is well within the normal range (Wallace, 1987). Children who have pre-existing central nervous system (CNS) damage and/or have suffered a complicated initial febrile seizure carry a higher risk of developing epilepsy than those who suffered a 'benign' febrile seizure; even in the latter group, the risk is twice that of the general population. On the whole, the prognosis for febrile convulsions is relatively benign compared to the prognosis of the epilepsies.

Petit mal absences tend to respond well to adequate anticonvulsive treatment. The prognosis is poorer for girls and when tonic–clonic seizures present as a second seizure type. As stated above with regard to temporal lobe epilepsy, *partial seizures* in childhood and adolescence have a better long-term prognosis than was once considered. The prognosis is better for simple partial seizures than for complex partial seizures, in which the persistence through adolescence into adulthood is associated with poor social outcome (Rodin, 1987).

Unfortunately, knowledge derived from longitudinal studies concerning the development and course of the *psychiatric sequelae* of epilepsy in childhood is very limited. Ounsted & Lindsay (1981) reported on the course of temporal lobe epilepsy in 100 children, 88% of whom also suffered from *grand mal* attacks. In their original report, 85% of these patients exhibited 'more or less grave disorders of personality' (Ounsted *et al.*, 1966). Thirteen years later an entirely different picture emerged. At this time, 70% of the adult survivors were reported as having no psychiatric disorder whatsoever when 5 patients with severe cognitive defects were excluded. Among 87 patients, 9 had developed overt schizophrenia, 12 exhibited antisocial disorders, and only 5 had, as adults, been treated for neurotic symptoms. Adult outcome, in terms of social and economic independence, was negatively affected by the following seven prognostic factors: low IQ, early onset of epilepsy, high frequency of temporal lobe seizures, a left-sided EEG focus, the hyperkinetic syndrome, catastrophic or so-called 'cataclysmic' rage, and a history of special schooling. Disordered homes in childhood bore no significant relationship to the likelihood of adult psychiatric problems. As with psychiatric follow-up studies, there is also a paucity of longitudinal data with regard to cognitive development. The topic has not received the attention it deserves. Rodin (1989) has stated, nevertheless, that the prognosis for intellectual function is good in uncomplicated epilepsies where there is only one seizure type which responds promptly to a simple anticonvulsant regimen. This especially applies for epilepsies in which onset begins in later childhood or adolescence. Because of the sparcity of longitudinal data, the prognosis for early-onset childhood epilepsies in which the seizures have remitted remains uncertain.

In addition to these limited findings coming from longitudinal studies of epileptic children and adolescents, the association of epilepsy and psychiatric disorders in adult life may shed some further light on the long-term outcome of these patients. *Interictal disorders* include both psychotic illnesses and neurotic disorders, which are predominantly affective in nature and characteristically of the depressive type. It has been suggested that depressive disorders are common among epileptics and that frequency increases when the epilepsy is of late onset. While some studies have reported associations between depression and temporal lobe epilepsy and complex partial seizures, other studies failed to verify any such relationship between seizure type and depression. As is the case with epileptic children and adolescents, suicide is much more common among adult epileptics than in the general population. Anxiety states, including fearfulness of attacks and phobias, are also not uncommon among epileptic patients (Fenwick, 1987).

As stated above, the global notion of the 'epileptic personality', which refers to alleged changes in the personalities of patients with epilepsy, has been discredited. Certain forms of personality change have, however, been related to specific types of epilepsy. These changes have been most strikingly observed in connection with seizures affecting the limbic system. Such seizures primarily involve patients with complex partial seizures. Damage to the limbic system frequently appears to occur when complex partial seizures repeatedly generalize into severe tonic–clonic convulsions. The limbic system is an essential structure involved in the storage and retrieval of memories and in the elaboration of the affective component of experience. It is also involved in certain aspects of sexual activity. Because of this, certain behavioural tendencies observed in epileptic patients have been attributed to altered limbic system functioning. These include emotionality, i.e. rapid fluctuation in mood; over-attention to detail; alteration in memory; and changes in sexuality. As Aird *et al.* (1984b) argued, owing to the failure to recognize the secondary involvement of the temporal lobe in long-standing generalized epilepsy, many studies failed to confirm that these changes are specific to TLE. More recent studies have confirmed that certain personality changes are more common among patients with TLE.

Finally, the interictal *psychoses* occurring in adult life deserve some consideration. These psychoses include hallucinatory or delusional episodes as well as brief episodes of manic or depressive mood swings. In some patients a persistent psychosis develops, taking the form of schizophreniform syndromes and, more rarely, manic-depressive illness (Aird *et al.*, 1984b; Fenwick, 1987). The prevalence of psychotic disorders among persons with epilepsy has been estimated at about 2–4%. This is a distinctly higher rate of prevalence than that found for the general population. While the acute confusional psychoses are commonly periictal and related to primary generalized epilepsy, the more chronic forms – especially the subacute and chronic paranoid and the hallucinatory episodes – are more closely related to the temporal lobe and the limbic system.

There are some additional features of interest concerning the paranoid/hallucinatory psychoses in adult epilepsy. Such psychoses most commonly begin in middle life, usually from 10 to 20 years after the onset of seizures. While the onset of the psychosis may be associated with a worsening of temporal lobe spikes, psychotic patients experience fewer psychomotor seizures. In approximately 30% of the patients, however, the onset coincides with cessation of seizures and improvement of the EEG (so-called forced normalization). The psychosis may be precipitated through control of seizures and alleviated by the recurrence of seizures. In the majority of cases the psychotic episodes are short-lived and periodic, however, in about 30% of the cases recurrent attacks lead to chronic psychosis.

THE CONCEPT OF SO-CALLED 'EPILEPTIC EQUIVALENTS'

Relations have been found to exist between paroxysmal EEG abnormalities and behaviour or cognition, even in the absence of overt clinical seizures. This connection between epileptiform activity in the EEG and behaviour or cognition has led some encephalographers to coin the terms *subclinical seizures* or *epileptic equivalents* (Martinius, 1990; Stores, 1987).

In general, the concept of behavioural disturbance due to electrophysiological dysfunction without clinical manifestation of seizures has not received much scientific investigation. In contrast, the association between cognition and EEG discharges without overt clinical seizures has received more attention. Both these aspects, however, have been addressed more often in studies with adults than in studies with children and adolescents.

Paroxysmal EEG abnormalities and behaviour

The association between specific types of behavioural problems and a given EEG abnormality has been repeatedly studied. Nuffield (1961) described a significant relationship between spike-and-wave abnormalities of the temporal lobe and aggressive behaviour as well as between 3 cycles per second spike-and-wave discharges and neurotic behaviour in epileptic children. Ritvo *et al.* (1970), however, observed no significant relationship between clinical diagnosis and the EEG in hospitalized patients. Similarly, Kaufman *et al.* (1980) were not able to replicate Nuffield's findings.

When analysing a large series of EEGs recorded over an extended period of time these authors detected only a very small number of patients who had abnormal EEG patterns that were consistent over time. They concluded that the previously reported neuropsychiatric correlations based upon 'pure' EEGs may have resulted from chance findings only.

Besides the clear association with organic brain syndromes, paroxysmal EEG abnormalities also occur both in non-organic mental states as well as in healthy people. Among a variety of electroencephalographic patterns described by Fenton (1986), only the positive spike phenomena has any significance for children and adolescents. Such anomalies are commonly observed in children and adolescents and reach a prevalence peak of 25% at the age of 13–15 years. Owing to the relatively high prevalence, these phenomena are regarded by most encephalographers as normal variants. Nevertheless, positive correlation has been noted to exist between certain paroxysmal EEG patterns and some behavioural and cognitive events – for example, stubbornness, attention deficit, hyperactivity, disturbed peer relationships, and school problems. The literature has also reported an association between this EEG pattern and dyslexia, behaviour disorders, and neurovegetative symptoms (Cavazutti *et al.*, 1980; Fenton, 1986).

Recently developed techniques may in the future clarify this controversy. Research units that carry out preoperative depth recording in epileptic patients have convincingly documented that subcortical seizure activity need not necessarily propagate to the cortex and that some of these subcortical discharges may be accompanied by changes in behaviour (Fenwick, 1988). Depth recordings performed on adult patients by Wieser (1988) and Wieser & Kausel (1987) have convincingly documented the presence of limbic seizure discharge producing aggressive behaviour without affecting cortical activities at all.

EEG discharges and cognition

The occurrence of so-called *transitory cognitive impairment* (TCI) during generalized subclinical EEG discharges has been repeatedly assessed in both patients who appeared to be seizure-free and in non-epileptic persons. According to Binnie (1988), intellectually demanding tasks, particularly those that demand high rates of information processing, are most likely to be affected by TCI. Simple reaction time as well as simple repetitive motor or mental tasks – such as tapping, counting, reciting, operation of a pursuit rotor – are relatively insensitive to the effects of subclinical discharges. TCI is demonstrated most often during prolonged, generalized, symmetrical, and regular 3 cycles per second spike-and-wave discharges.

The therapeutic implications of these subclinical EEG discharges are a matter of controversy for many clinicians, as Binnie (1988) has recently stated. Poor school performance in such a child might lead some clinicians to advocate a trial of anticonvulsants, while others would reserve this level of intervention for the suppression of overt seizures. This dispute, in fact, centres on the definition of epileptic seizure; an episodic impairment of cognition might conceivably be considered as a clinical manifestation of seizure activity and meet current definitions of epileptic seizure if it is accompanied by cerebral dysrhythmia.

In trying to circumvent this semantic debate, Binnie (1988) considered whether subclinical discharges affect the performance of everyday tasks and referred to recent studies where this effect has been observed, at least in the laboratory. A significant improvement of cognitive function and social adaptation has been demonstrated when subclinical discharges were suppressed by anticonvulsants. Considering, however, that the criteria for identifying those patients with subclinical discharges has not been established, the question remains open as to whether such treatment is indicated in a large portion of those people or rather in a smaller subgroup.

Stores (1987), on the other hand, advocated some kind of clinical intervention based on the duration of the subclinical seizure discharge: (a) *prolonged* – in excess of several minutes, extending in some cases to hours, days or even longer; (b) *brief* – more than three seconds and up to several minutes; and (c) *transient* – three seconds or less. In order to prevent impairment of intelligence and learning ability, and to avoid possible brain damage due to prolonged subclinical seizure disorder – as detected by long-term EEG monitoring – he advocated treatment with appropriate and continuous medication in an attempt to terminate the seizure discharge. While Stores (1987) described the clinical management of brief and of transient discharges as being less clear, he nevertheless concluded from some recent studies reviewed in his article that the suppression of subclinical EEG discharges might improve the performance of at least some of these patients as well.

BEHAVIOURAL AND COGNITIVE SIDE EFFECTS OF ANTICONVULSIVE MEDICATION

There are two sources of evidence that suggest that anticonvulsive drugs have effects on behaviour and cognition that extend beyond their therapeutic action. First, a number of recent reviews have reported on the clinical observations and controlled studies that deal with the side effects of anticonvulsive medication in epileptic patients (Parnas *et al.*, 1979, 1980; Tollefson, 1980; Rivinius, 1982; Corbett & Trimble, 1983; Mayer, 1988; Trimble & Cull, 1988). In addition, there is some further evidence concerning the behavioural and cognitive effects of anticonvulsive medication coming from a more recent approach in which the late sequelae of intrauterine exposure to these agents have been studied in the offspring of epileptic women.

Direct drug effects

The side effects of anticonvulsive medication in epileptic patients have been underestimated for quite a number of years. It was assumed that drugs played only a minor role among the other aetiological factors related to behavioural and cognitive disturbances. In recent years, however, clinicians and researchers have become increasingly aware that, besides the side effects due to overdose or to idiosyncratic responses in certain individuals, or even to potentiation caused by the interaction of different drugs, there are certain side effects that arise in the normal therapeutic range as well.

With regard to the most frequently prescribed anticonvulsive drugs used in clinical practice, non-specific behavioural problems – e.g. sedation, irritability, hyperactivity, aggression – occur most frequently with phenobarbital and clonazepam and appear least often with valproate and carbamazepine. The so-called psychotropic effects of certain drugs – e.g. carbamazepine and valproate – have been seriously questioned (Parnas *et al.*, 1979). Cognitive impairments occur with phenytoin, are less evident with valproate, and are minimal with carbamazepine (Trimble & Cull, 1988).

The combination of different drugs has been increasingly criticized for its failure to demonstrate therapeutic superiority over monotherapy. According to Bourgeois (1988), (a) numerous pharmacokinetic interactions are documented; (b) toxicity can be assumed to be at least partially cumulative; (c) interpretation of serum drug measurement is confused by drug combination, making the efficacy of any single drug more difficult to evaluate; and (d) idiosyncratic toxic interactions leading to dramatic clinical pictures – e.g. stuporous states – have been observed. In addition, behavioural and cognitive side effects may be underestimated. A number of studies have shown that reduction or removal of polytherapy led to improvement of certain neuropsychological parameters (Giordani *et al.*, 1982; Thompson & Trimble, 1982). Unfortunately, research findings so far have been overshadowed by a number of methodological shortcomings, which, according to Mayer (1988), may be grouped into the following major classes:

(1) *Samples.* With regard to the type of epilepsy, most samples are rather heterogeneous and clinical description is insufficient in a number of studies. Furthermore, the lack of a common system of classification of seizures has jeopardized comparability of findings. In addition, in many studies a number of important variables have not always been controlled for, including the patient's age at the onset of the disease, the duration of illness, and seizure frequency. Some studies have even neglected to control for the age of the patient, which has led to the naive assumption that side effects might be similar for all groups. Small sample sizes have imposed limitations on homogeneity and have contributed to a reduction of internal validity. Finally, the impact of higher intellectual levels which, in contrast with lower levels, might compensate drug effects, has not been considered so far. Taken together, these shortcomings have serious impact on the generalization of empirical findings.

(2) *Methods.* Similar to a number of sampling problems, there is a wide variety of methods which result in heterogeneity of empirical results. Further problems derive from the insufficient reliability and validity of methods and poor standardization. For cognitive assessment, standard intelligence tests have been the most frequently employed measures. Owing to the emphasis on reliability, however, these tests are quite insensitive for measuring the dimension of change. Neuropsychological variables, such as memory, attention, and visual perception have only rarely been studied.

(3) *Time of measurement.* The design of the studies varied considerably with regard to the assessment schedule, i.e. the number of measurements and the frequency or time span between these measurements. When the time span increases so does the likelihood that other variables besides the drug may be responsible for whatever change is observed or measured. While most studies have been restricted to simple *pre–post* designs, it is evident that *multiple measurements* are clearly warranted.

(4) *Theory.* Finally, research on drug effects in epileptic children has not been stimulated by any major theoretical concept which would serve to guide questions and research designs. The majority of researchers quite obviously believe in the lack of specificity of psychological side effects related to anticonvulsant drugs. Others have simply categorized side effects according to the variables of existing test batteries. This lack of conceptualization, combined with the problems involved in identifying and measuring the variables, may be responsible for the contradictory findings described above.

Among four existing concepts of behavioural toxicity, Novelly *et al.* (1986) have advocated *Luria's* theory, which emphasizes integration. According to this theory, side effects will be more apt to manifest themselves in functions of higher levels of integration. For instance, visuomotor functions are more likely to be affected than are highly trained gross-motor functions. The second theoretical concept hypothesizes a *selective vulnerability* in which the functions of the dominant hemisphere are believed to be less vulnerable than those of the non-dominant hemisphere. A third model – the so-called diathesis–stress model – proposes that specific behaviours already at risk or impaired by an epileptogenic lesion may be particularly vulnerable to drug effects. Finally, there has been a proposal to use *Cattell's* theory of crystallized and fluid intelligence to stimulate future research projects concerning the cognitive side effects of anticonvulsive medication. According to this model, the ability to acquire new or novel behaviour (fluid intelligence) may be more easily affected by antiepileptic drugs.

Teratogenic effects

In the recent past a number of studies have been started to control for the teratogenic effects of anticonvulsive medication during pregnancy. Children of epileptic mothers had been assessed with respect to drug effects on early motor and intellectual development. While some authors have observed an unusually high rate of mentally subnormal children in this sample, others have not confirmed these findings. For a review see Helge (1982).

These contradictions may be explained to a certain extent by the fact that the studies did not always indicate whether monotherapy or polytherapy was employed. There is, in fact, some evidence that polytherapy during pregnancy is more harmful to the developing child than monotherapy (Majewski *et al.*, 1980). In addition, further conditions may affect the mother's mode of treatment and the development of the child.

The issue of potential teratogenic effects on behaviour resulting from intrauterine exposure to antiepileptic drugs cannot be studied in isolation from genetic and environmental factors. In an attempt to disentangle the relative impact of these factors in our own research (Hättig & Steinhausen, 1987; Steinhausen *et al.*, 1982; Steinhausen *et al.*, 1984) we included three clinical groups, namely: (1) children born to epileptic mothers who were treated with anticonvulsant drugs during pregnancy, (2) children born to epileptic mothers who were not treated with anticonvulsant drugs during pregnancy, (3) children born to epileptic fathers. In addition, three control groups matched to the clinical groups for socioeconomic status, age of both parents, number of abortions, number of children, amount of smoking during pregnancy, and ethnic group were included in the study. The assessment procedures used were multidimensional and took account of aspects of infant and early childhood development including different developmental tests and a structural psychiatric examination.

Our data analysis, based on cross-sections, indicates that there are some drug effects due to intrauterine exposure. The level of functioning with regard to motor, regulation of state, and autonomic stability during the first week and second week of life – assessed with the *Brazelton Neonatal Behavioral Assessment Scale* (BNBAS) (Brazelton, 1973) – was poorer in infants who were exposed to anticonvulsive drugs than in the controls. Only with regard to autonomic stability was there a significant difference at the time of the third examination during the fourth week of life. Further analysis of the material indicated, however, that the data collected from the third examination were distorted due to certain assessment limitations inherent in the BNBAS. Neonatal behaviour as assessed by the BNBAS easily reaches the optimal end of the scale at the age of 4 weeks and leads to homogeneous behaviour in both the clinical groups and the control groups, thus reflecting a ceiling effect in the test.

Evidence of operating teratogenic factors was more clearly manifested when we compared the findings of a group of toddlers during their second year of life. Here it was clearly demonstrated that the behavioural and cognitive scores of those children with intrauterine exposure to anticonvulsant drugs were significantly lower than the other groups as assessed by the *Bayley Scales of Infant Development* (Bayley, 1969). Further corroboration of these findings came from a sample of preschool children. Again, those children with intrauterine exposure to anticonvulsant drugs scored significantly lower on measures of intelligence, psycholinguistic abilities, and visual perception.

In summary, the findings obtained from three different cross-sections of this longitudinal project serve to cross-validate the conclusion that intrauterine exposure to anticonvulsive drugs affects developmental outcome. In addition, there is further indication that these effects correlate with the mode of treatment. The incidence of developmental side effects is most pronounced in those children who were prenatally exposed to polytherapy. Our preliminary analyses, however, leave open the question as to whether or not further factors, (i.e. seizure type and frequency) contribute to this effect. It is evident that multivariate analysis is necessary in order to disclose the various factors contributing to the poor developmental outcome in some of the children affected by prenatal exposure to anticonvulsive medication.

CONCLUSIONS

There is overwhelming evidence that epilepsy in children constitutes a major risk for psychiatric disorder. This increased vulnerability does not imply any specific type of psychopathology. However, recent research has shown that certain problems arise more frequently. Owing to increased dependency, epileptic children – like children with other chronic medical conditions – tend to be impaired with regard to psychosocial functioning. Even graver implications arise from the studies that reveal that these children have a higher rate of suicidal behaviour, greater medical seriousness of the suicidal intent, and that anticonvulsants – namely phenobarbital – may play a major role in suicidal behaviour.

In addition, recent research on attitudinal style and self-concept has shown that epileptic children frequently have a rather poor self-concept and suffer from low self-esteem. These personality features may be linked to some extent to depression and suicidal behaviour and may derive, at least partly, from experiences related to chronic illness. There are two implications stemming from these recent findings. First, new approaches and theories that have been discussed extensively in the psychological literature in recent years – such as *locus of control* and *self-concept* – have turned out to be quite fruitful notions for revealing the impact of psychosocial and developmental variables on psychopathology in epileptic children. Research might benefit even further from the inclusion of the concept of *coping* in order to analyse the impact of protective factors. Secondly, some of these personality variables might serve as psychological markers to identify children at risk in order to consider more intensive psychiatric assessment and treatment.

Not only is behaviour negatively affected in a large number of epileptic children, but cognition and performance may be negatively affected as well. This is particularly true of children with complicated epilepsy. However, there is no specific neuropsychological pattern of impairment in these children. Because cognitive function is related to both chronicity of the disease and certain treatment factors, close clinical monitoring – including repeated psychological testing – is clearly indicated.

When considering the mechanisms involved in the relationship between epilepsy and psychiatric disorder, there is evidence that brain-related variables play a major role. Certain factors, such as age at onset or chronicity are clearly related to cognitive/behavioural functioning and to the course of the disease. Research findings are inconclusive, however, with regard to other factors, such as seizure frequency or type of seizure. It is evident that among the non-brain-related variables there are specific *epilepsy* risk factors – as opposed to general *chronic illness* factors – which are correlated with increased psychiatric vulnerability in children with epilepsy. The impact of developmental and psychosocial variables deserves further investigation since few studies have dealt with them so far. In general, owing to the isolated evaluation of variables little is known about the mechanisms that mediate in the relationship between epilepsy and psychiatric disorder. Thus far, the potential of multivariate analysis has not been sufficiently recognized. Analogously, there is a paucity of longitudinal studies that might shed some light on the process of development and psychosocial adaptation in these children.

The concept of behavioural disturbance due to so-called epilepsy equivalents or subclinical seizures has not been thoroughly investigated in children. There was very little evidence in the past of behavioural deficits due to electrophysiological dysfunction unaccompanied by overt seizures. More recently, however, depth recordings performed in adults have documented a connection between limbic seizure discharges and aggressive behaviour without abnormal cortical activity. Thus, the concept of subclinical seizures may be in need of theoretical revision which might then reactivate the clinical debate as to whether or not anticonvulsive treatment is indicated. The current discussion is founded primarily upon the phenomenon of transitory cognitive impairment during generalized subclinical EEG discharges, which has been investigated in several studies.

Finally, there is sufficient evidence that anticonvulsants have behavioural and cognitive side effects. The evidence comes from studies of both epileptic patients as well as the offspring of epileptic mothers who were treated with anticonvulsants during pregnancy. Although the research concerning the side effects of anticonvulsive medication in children is impaired by a number of methodological shortcomings, it is evident that polytherapy as well as specific drugs – i.e. phenobarbital – have quite remarkable side effects on behaviour and cognition and, therefore, should be restricted in clinical practice. Research involving single-case-study research design with time-series-analysis would make it possible to monitor the cognitive/behavioural side effects and, at the same time, contribute to the management of the individual patient. The documented correlation existing between intrauterine exposure to anticonvulsive drugs and developmental outcome not only verifies the impact that this sort of medication has but calls forth the need for preventive measures in order to protect the developing child.

REFERENCES

Addy, D. P. (1987) Cognitive function in children with epilepsy. *Developmental Medicine and Child Neurology*, **29**, 394–404.

Aicardi, J. (1985) Epileptic syndromes in childhood – overview and classification. In Ross, E. & Reynolds, E. (eds.) *Paediatric perspectives on epilepsy.* Chichester: John Wiley, pp. 65–70.

Aird, R. B., Masland, R. L. & Woodbury, D. M. (1984a) Genetic aspect of epilepsy. In Aird, R. B., Masland, R. L. & Woodbury, D. M. (eds.) *The epilepsies: a critical review.* New York: Raven Press, pp. 117–34.

Aird, R. B., Masland, R. L. & Woodbury, D. M. (1984b) Associated disorders. In Aird, R. B., Masland, R. L. & Woodbury, D. M. *The epilepsies: a critical review.* New York: Raven Press, pp. 158–80.

Aird, R. B., Masland, R. L., & Woodbury, D. M. (1989) Introduction to 'Hypothesis: the classification of epileptic seizures according to systems of the CNS', by Aird, R. B., Masland, R. L. & Woodbury, D. M. *Epilepsy Research*, **3**, 77–81.

Bagley, C. (1972) Social prejudice and the adjustment of people with epilepsy. *Epilepsia*, **13**, 33–45.

Bayley, N. (1969) *Bayley Scales of Infant Development.* New York: Psychosocial Corporation.

Berg, R. A., Bolter, J. F., Ch'ien, L. T. & Cummins, J. (1984) A standardized assessment of emotionality in children suffering from epilepsy. *The International Journal of Clinical Neuropsychology*, **4**, 247–8.

Binnie, C. D. (1988) Seizures, EEG discharges and cognition. In Trimble, M. R. & Reynolds, E. H. (eds.) *Epilepsy, behaviour and cognitive function.* Chichester: John Wiley, pp. 45–49.

Birleson, P. (1981) The validity of depressive disorder in childhood and the development of a self-rating scale: a research report. *Journal of Child Psychology and Psychiatry*, **22**, 73–88.

Bolter, J. F. (1986) Epilepsy in children. In Obrznt, J. E. & Wittynd, G. (eds.) *Child neuropsychology*, Vol. 2. Orlando: Academic Press, pp. 59–81.

Bourgeois, B. F. G. (1988) Problems of combination drug therapy in children. *Epilepsia*, **29** Suppl. 3, S20–S24.

Bourgeois, B. F. G., Prensky, A. L., Palkes, H. S., Talent, B. K. & Busch, S. G. (1983) Intelligence in epilepsy: a prospective study in children. *Annals of Neurology*, **14**, 438–44.

Brazelton, T. B. (1973) Brazelton Neonatal Behavioral Assessment Scale. Philadelphia: J. B. Lippincott.

Brent, D. A. (1986) Overrepresentation of epileptics in a consecutive series of suicide attempters seen at a children's hospital, 1978–1983. *Journal of the American Academy of Child Psychiatry*, **25**, 242–6.

Cavazutti, G. B., Cappella, L., & Nalin, A. (1980) Longitudinal study of epileptiform EEG patterns in normal children. *Epilepsia*, **21**, 43–55.

Cavazutti, G. B., Ferrari, P. & Lalla, M. (1984) Follow-up study of 482 cases with convulsive disorders in the first year of life. *Developmental Medicine and Child Neurology*, **26**, 425–37.

Corbett, J. A. & Trimble, M. R. (1983) Epilepsy and anticonvulsant medication. In Rutter, M. (ed.) *Developmental neuropsychiatry.* New York: Guilford Press; Edinburgh: Churchill Livingstone, pp. 112–29.

Corbett, J. A., Trimble, M. R. & Nichol, T. C. (1985) Behavioral and cognitive impairments in children with epilepsy: the long-term effects of anticonvulsant therapy. *Journal of the American Academy of Child Psychiatry*, **24**, 17–23.

Epir, S., Renda, Y. & Baser, N. (1984) Cognitive and behavioural characteristics of children with idiopathic epilepsy in a low-income area of Ankara, Turkey. *Developmental Medicine & Child Neurology*, **26**, 200–7.

Farwell, J. R., Dodrill, C. B. & Batzel, L. W. (1985) Neuropsychological abilities of children with epilepsy. *Epilepsia*, **26**, 395–400.

Fenton, G. F. (1986) The EEG, epilepsy and psychiatry. In Trimble, M. R. & Reynolds, E. H. (eds.) *What is epilepsy?: The clinical and scientific basis of epilepsy*. Edinburgh: Churchill Livingstone, pp. 139–60.

Fenwick, P. (1987) Epilepsy and psychiatric disorders. In Hopkins, A. (ed.) *Epilepsy*. London: Chapman and Hall, pp. 512–52.

Fenwick, P. B. C. (1988) Seizures, EEG discharges and behaviour. In Trimble, M. R. & Reynolds, E. H. (eds.) *Epilepsy, behaviour and cognitive function*. Chichester: John Wiley, pp. 51–66.

Ferrari, M., Matthews, W. S. & Barabas, G. (1983) The family and the child with epilepsy. *Family Process*, **22**, 53–9.

Giordani, J., Sackellares, C., Miller, S., Sutula, T. & Dreifuss, F. (1982) Changes in neuropsychological test performance following improved seizure control and elimination of barbiturate antiepileptic drugs. *Epilepsia*, **23**, 437.

Hartlage, L. C. & Green, J. B. (1972) The relation of parental attitudes to academic and social achievement in epileptic children. *Epilepsia*, **13**, 21–6.

Hartlage, L. C., Green, J. B. & Offutt, L. (1972) Dependency in epileptic children. *Epilepsia*, **13**, 27–30.

Hättig, H. & Steinhausen, H.-Ch. (1987) Children of epileptic parents: a prospective developmental study. In Rauh, H. & Steinhausen, H.-Ch. (eds.) *Psychobiology and early development*. Amsterdam: Elsevier Science Publishers B.V. (North-Holland), pp. 155–169.

Helge, H. (1982) Physical, mental, and social development, including diseases: review of the literature. In Janz, D., Dam, M., Richens, A., Bossi, L., Helge, H. & Schmidt, D. (eds.) *Epilepsy, pregnancy and the child*. New York: Raven Press, pp. 391–395.

Hermann, B. P. (1982) Neuropsychological functioning and psychopathology in children with epilepsy. *Epilepsia*, **23**, 545–54.

Hermann, B. P., & Whitman, S. (1984) Behavioral and personality correlates of epilepsy: a review, methodological critique, and conceptual model. *Psychological Bulletin*, **95**, 451–97.

Hermann, B. P., Whitman, S. & Dell, J. (1989) Correlates of behavior problems and social competence in children with epilepsy, aged 6–11. In, Hermann, B. P., Whitman, S. & Dell, J. (eds.) *Childhood epilepsies: neurological, psychosocial and intervention apsects*. New York: John Wiley, pp. 143–57.

Hoare, P. (1984a) The development of psychiatric disorder among schoolchildren with epilepsy. *Developmental Medicine and Child Neurology*, **26**, 3–12.

Hoare, P. (1984b) Does illness foster dependency? A study of epileptic and diabetic children. *Developmental Medicine and Child Neurology*, **26**, 20–4.

Kaufman, K. R., Harris, R. & Shaffer, D. (1980) Problems in the categorization of child and adolescent EEGs. *Journal of Child Psychology and Psychiatry*, **21**, 333–42.

Majewski, F., Raff, W., Fischer, P., Huenges, R. & Petruch, F. (1980) Zur terotogenität von antikonvulsiva. *Deutsche Medizinische Wochenzeitschrift*, **105**, 719–23.

Martinius, J. (1990) Cognitive correlates of abnormal EEG waveforms in children. In Rothenberger, A. (ed.) *Brain and behavior in child psychiatry*. Berlin: Springer, pp. 125–30.

Matthews, W. S., Barabas, G. & Ferrari, M. (1982) Emotional concomitants of childhood epilepsy. *Epilepsia*, **23**, 671–81.

Mayer, H. (1988) *Neuropsychologische nebenwirkungen antiepileptischer therapie*. University of Tübingen, unpublished dissertation.

Mellor, D. H., Lowit, I. & Hall, D. J. (1971) Are epileptic children different from other children? Paper presented at Annual Meeting of British Group of Paediatric Neurologists, Oxford, 1971.

Newmark, M. E. & Penry, J. K. (1980) *Genetics of epilepsy: a review*. New York: Raven Press, pp. 95–6.

Niemann, H., Boenick, H. E., Schmidt, R. C. & Ettlinger, G. (1985) Cognitive development in epilepsy. The relative influence of epileptic activity and of brain damage. *European Archives of Psychiatry and Neurological Science*, **234**, 399–403.

Novelly, R. A., Schwartz, M. M., Mattson, R. H. & Cramer, J. A. (1986) Behavioral toxicity associated with antiepileptic drugs: concepts and methods of assessment. *Epilepsia*, **27**, 331–40.

Nuffield, E. J. A. (1961) Neurophysiology and behaviour disorders in epileptic children. *Journal of Mental Science*, **107**, 438–58.

O'Leary, D. S., Lovell, M. R., Sackellares, J. C., Berent, S., Giordani, B., Seidenberg, M. & Boll, T. J. (1983) Effects of age of onset of partial and generalized seizures on neuropsychological performance in children. *Journal of Nervous and Mental Disease*, **171**, 624–9.

Ounsted, C., & Lindsay, J. (1981) The long-term outcome of temporal lobe epilepsy in childhood. In Reynolds, E. H. & Trimble, M. R. *Epilepsy and psychiatry*. Edinburgh: Churchill Livingstone, pp. 185–215.

Ounsted, C., Lindsay, J. & Norman, R. (1966) *Biological factors in temporal lobe epilepsy*. London: Heinemann.

Parnas, J., Flachs, H. & Gram, L. (1979) Psychotropic effects of antiepileptic drugs. *Acta Neurologica Scandinavica* **60**, 329–43.

Parnas, J., Gram, L. & Flachs, H. (1980) Psychopharmacological aspects of antiepileptic treatment. *Progress in Neurobiology*, **15**, 119–38.

Pond, D. & Bidwell, B. (1960) A survey of epilepsy in 14 general practices: II. social and psychological aspects. *Epilepsia*, **1**, 285–99.

Ritchie, K. (1981) Research note: interaction in the families of epileptic children. *Journal of Child Psychology and Psychiatry*, **22**, 65–71.

Ritvo, E., Ornitz, E. M., Walter, R. D. & Hanley, J. (1970) Correlations of psychiatric diagnoses and EEG findings: a double-blind study of 184 hospitalized children. *American Journal of Psychiatry*, **126**, 988–96.

Rivinius, T. M. (1982) Psychiatric effects of the anticonvulsant regimens. *Journal of Clinical Psychopharmacology*, **2/3**, 165–92.

Rodin, E. (1987) Factors which influence the prognosis of epilepsy. In Hopkins, A. (ed.) *Epilepsy*. London: Chapman and Hall, pp. 339–71.

Rodin, E. (1989) Prognosis of cognitive functions in children with epilepsy. In Hermann, B. P., Whitman, S. & Dell, J. (eds.) *Childhood epilepsies*:

neurological, psychosocial and intervention aspects. New York: John Wiley, pp. 133–50.

Rutter, M. (1985) Resilience in the face of adversity. *British Journal of Psychiatry*, **147**, 598–611.

Rutter, M., Graham, P. & Yule, W. (1970) *A neuropsychiatric study in childhood.* (Clinics in Developmental Medicine Nos. 35–36). London: Spastics International Medical Publications—Heinemann Medical Books.

Seidenberg, M., Beck, N., Geisser, M., Giordani, B., Sackellares, J. C., Berent, S., Dreifuss, F. E. & Boll, T. J. (1986) Academic achievement of children with epilepsy. *Epilepsia*, **27**, 753–9.

Seligman, M. E. (1975) *Helplessness: on depression, development, & death.* New York: W. H. Freeman.

Steinhausen, H. Ch., Huth, H. & Koch, S. (1984) The offspring of epileptic mothers: a high risk population? In Call, J. D., Galenson, E. & Tyson, R. L. (eds.) *Frontiers of infant psychiatry.* Vol. 2, New York: Basic Books, pp. 472–9.

Steinhausen, H. Ch., Nestler, V. & Huth, H. (1982) Psychopathology and mental functions in the offspring of alcoholic and epileptic mothers. *Journal of the American Academy of Child Psychiatry*, **21**, 268–73.

Stores, G. (1978) School-children with epilepsy at risk for learning and behaviour problems. *Developmental Medicine and Child Neurology*, **20**, 502–8.

Stores, G. (1987) Effects of learning of 'subclinical' seizure discharge. In Aldenkamp, A. P., Alpherts, W. C. J., Meinard, H. & Stores, G. (eds.) *Education and epilepsy.* Lisse, Amsterdam: Swets & Zeitlinger, B. V., pp. 14–20.

Thompson, P. J. & Trimble, M. R. (1982) Anticonvulsant drugs and cognitive functions. *Epilepsia*, **23**, 531–44.

Tizard, B. (1962) The personality of epileptics: a discussion of the evidence. *Psychological Bulletin*, **59**, 196–210.

Tollefson, G. (1980) Psychiatric implications of anticonvulsant drugs. *Journal of Clinical Psychiatry*, **41**, 295–301.

Trimble, M. R. & Cull, C. (1988) Children of school age: the influence of antiepileptic drugs on behavior and intellect. *Epilepsia*, **29**. Suppl. 3, S15–S19.

Verduyn, C. (1980) Social factors contributing to poor emotional adjustment in children with epilepsy. In Kulis, B. M. (ed.) *Epilepsy and behavior '79.* Lisse, Amsterdam: Swets & Zeitlinger, B. V., pp. 177–84.

Viberg, M., Blennow, G. & Polski, B. (1987) Epilepsy in adolescence: Implications for the development of personality. *Epilepsia*, **28**, 542–6.

Wallace, S. J. (1987) Febrile convulsions. In Hopkins, A. *Epilepsy.* London: Chapman and Hall, pp. 443–67.

Whitman, S., Hermann, B. P., Black, R. B. & Chhabria, S. (1982) Psychopathology and seizure type in children with epilepsy. *Psychological Medicine*, **12**, 843–53.

Wieser, H. G. (1988) Human limbic seizures: EEG studies, origin, and patterns of spread. In Meldrum, B. S., Ferendelli, J. & Wieser, H. G. (eds.) *Anatomy of epileptogenesis.* London: John Libby & Co,, pp. 127–37.

Wieser, H. G. & Kausel, W. (1987) Limbic seizures. In Wieser, H. G. & Elger, C. E. (eds.) *Presurgical evaluation of epileptics.* Berlin/Heidelberg: Springer-Verlag, pp. 227–47.

Index